Manual of
Perioperative Care

An Essential Guide

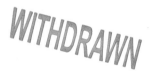

Manual of
Perioperative Care
An Essential Guide

Edited by

Kate Woodhead RGN DMS
Lesley Fudge MSc BA(Hons) RGN

WILEY-BLACKWELL

A John Wiley & Sons, Ltd., Publication

Library of Congress Cataloging-in-Publication Data

Manual of perioperative care : an essential guide / edited by Kate Woodhead, Lesley K. Fudge.
      p.   cm.
   Includes bibliographical references and index.
   ISBN 978-0-470-65918-2 (pbk. : alk. paper)
1. Therapeutics, Surgical–Handbooks, manuals, etc.   I. Woodhead, Kate.   II. Fudge, Lesley K.
   RD49.M264 2012
   617.9'1–dc23

                                       2012005849

A catalogue record for this book is available from the British Library.

Contents

About the Editors

Kate Woodhead RGN, DMS

Kate qualified as a nurse in London in late 1970s. After she had undertaken her specialist perioperative qualification, she travelled and worked in Australia for two years. She progressed into theatre leadership at The Radcliffe Infirmary Oxford in 1986. She left the National Health Service in 1998. Kate now runs her own healthcare consultancy business, specialising in the perioperative field.

She is a former President of the International Federation of Perioperative Nurses (2002–2006), and between 1998 and 2001 served as Chair of the National Association of Theatre Nurses (now the Association for Perioperative Practice).

She has recently been involved as a temporary advisor with WHO Patient Safety Global Challenge 'Safe Surgery Saves Lives'.

In her spare time, she is Chairman of Friends of African Nursing, which has been delivering perioperative workshops in Africa since 2001, in conjunction with Ministries of Health.

Lesley Fudge MSc, BA(Hons), RGN

The majority of Lesley's career has been spent in theatres, with a short spell in the community. Lesley was Theatre Manager at Frenchay Hospital in Bristol with a clinical background in plastic and reconstructive and neurosurgery. She then became one of the first procurement nurses in the UK and her final NHS post was as Head of Clinical Purchasing for three major Trusts.

Lesley became an independent consultant in 2003 and links with a large range of clients.

She is a past National Secretary of the Association for Perioperative Practitioners (AfPP) (formerly NATN) and is the Vice Chairman of the Latex Allergy Support Group. She was also a co-founder and past CEO of Friends of African Nursing and served as Treasurer of the International Federation of Perioperative Nurses. Lesley has a BA(Hons) degree in Philosophy and Art and a Master of Science degree in Biomedical Ethics and Healthcare Law.

Contributors

Sue Bacon RGN, SCM

Sue trained at St Thomas's Hospital in London 1972 followed by midwifery training at Queen Charlotte's Hospital in 1976. She holds a Diploma in Health Studies from York University 2010 and was a specialist nurse in thrombosis in Scarborough from 2005 to 2009, when she moved to North Bristol NHS as a specialist nurse in 2009, her current role. Sue is a member of the steering group of the UK Thromboprophylaxis Forum and is a previous member of the VERITY steering group on thromboembolism.

Libby Campbell OBE, MPhil, MSc, RN, RM

After specialising in operating theatre nursing, Libby pursued a career in NHS management and leadership, holding various operational and strategic posts, most recently, as Director of Nursing for Acute Services in Lothian based at the Royal Infirmary of Edinburgh. Previously National Chairman of NATN (now the Association for Perioperative Practitioners), she has been a motivational speaker, has published work on leadership, communication and legal issues and completed a Master of Philosophy in Medical Law and Ethics in 2007. Libby has now retired from full-time NHS practice and is working on a consultancy basis on legal and health-related projects.

Helen Carter RSCN/RGN

Helen trained at Great Ormond Street Hospital, London and the Royal Berkshire Hospital, Reading and has over 20 years of paediatric theatre experience. For the past five years she has worked as a paediatric surgical care practitioner at the Leeds Teaching Hospitals following training at Manchester University.

Russell Chilton SODP, BA(Hons), Dip Ed, Plast Tech, NEBSM, CGLI 752

Clinical Tutor, Royal Devon & Exeter NHS Foundation Trust. Russell is a retired Royal Navy medic, consultant and unit author for the Open University Foundation Degree in Operating Department Practice (2010) as well as AfPP South West Regional Team Lead and multi-agency child protection trainer. He is passionate about developing the very best for the health community, at all levels.

Felicia Cox MSc, RN

Felicia is the lead Pain Management Nurse Specialist at Royal Brompton & Harefield NHS Foundation Trust. She is regularly invited to write and speak on pain and is the Editor of the *British Journal of Pain* for the British Pain Society and has a seat on the RCN Pain and Palliative Care Steering Group.

Joanne Dickson BSc, RN

Lead Nurse – eMedicines, Leeds Teaching Hospitals NHS Trust. Jo has had a varied career in adult nursing, including working in general and neurosurgery, and as a pain management nurse specialist. She now works as a medicines management nurse, leading on electronic prescribing and medicines administration, as well as continuing to support non-medical prescribers in a large acute teaching hospital trust.

Chris Earl RGN, ENB176 and 998, ENB N77 & D10 (SCP qualification), MSc (Cardiff) Advanced Surgical Practice, BA(Hons) Humanities and Classical Studies

Chris trained in 1987 and worked in theatres until training as a surgical care practitioner in 2001, working mainly in trauma and emergency theatres. He worked as a surgical care practitioner in the renal transplant unit at Manchester Royal Infirmary 2002–2012 and recently emigrated to Queensland, Australia to work as a clinical nurse in theatres at Mt Isa Hospital. Chris served as a Nursing Officer (Major) in the TA medical services, having been commissioned since 1992.

Diane Gilmour RN, PGCEA, BN, DANS, Diploma in Infection Control Nursing, ENB 176

Diane was President of AfPP 2009–2010 and has had an extensive portfolio of roles within the perioperative environment over 25 years, including those in practice development, education, managerial as well as having led key projects in this area. Diane has published and presented nationally and internationally and is now involved in commissioning services for patients in the community and primary care.

Rita Hehir RN, RM, BA(Hons) Health and Nursing studies. MA. Sociology and Social Policy

Programme Leader Operating Department, Edge Hill University, Ormskirk. Rita has a special interest in social policy, social inclusion and discrimination in healthcare settings. She is currently researching the transition in the gender make-up of operating department practitioners, which is perceived as a 'male' role to the present recruitment trends which indicate a bias towards females.

Kevin Henshaw BSc(Hons), PGCHETL, Cert Ed RODP

Kevin has been a senior lecturer in operating department practitioner (ODP) education at the Faculty of Health and Social Care at Edge Hill University for five years and previously worked as an ODP at the Walton Centre for Neurology and Neurosurgery (WCNN) Liverpool for 12 years. He spent two years working as an anaesthetic technician at the Rhyiad al Kharj (RKH) Military Hospital in Saudi Arabia and was actively involved in brainstem testing at RKH and taking part in many organ donations at the WCNN. These experiences helped to raise his awareness of some of the differences in cultural attitudes when dealing with perioperative deaths.

Johnathan Hewis BSc(Hons), Diag Rad, Pg Dip Med Imag, Pg Cert LTA HE, Pg Cert Barium Enema, FHEA

Senior Lecturer/Associate Professor in Medical Imaging at Central Queensland University. Johnathan qualified as a diagnostic radiographer in 1998 and has a broad range of clinical experience including specialising in MRI and radiographer reporting. He has been teaching radiography at both undergraduate and postgraduate level for the last seven years and previously worked as a senior lecturer at Sheffield Hallam University. He is currently completing a doctorate in his own time researching anxiety in clinical MRI.

Saheba Iaciofano RGN, MBA, Oncology Cert

Saheba has extensive knowledge and experience as a clinical lead in operating theatres, endoscopy and ambulatory care, where she has project managed new builds and development of new services. As the Surgical Services and Decontamination Lead for 13 years at the Princess Grace Hospital, which is part of HCA International, she was involved in developing and managing bariatric surgery within the independent sector, covering all aspects of care pathways. Her role at HCA International – London included being the designated Lead for Human Tissue Authority and Decontamination for which she has ISO 13485 Leaders' training. Saheba also has expertise and interest in change management and lean processes. She has held various posts overseas in Belgium and Vancouver, Canada and is a member of the Comparative Health Knowledge System survey team.

Jane Jackson SRN, MPhil, MCGI

Immediate Past Chair Preoperative Association and Consultant Nurse Preoperative Assessment, West Hertfordshire NHS Trust. Jane qualified in 1980 from SRN training at University College Hospital, London and has since worked in the field of surgery – both within acute and elective ward areas as well as intensive care. Jane is passionate about patient preparation as being an essential element in safe admission for elective surgery, creating this as a service in 1993, working with the inter-professional team to create a service that provides patient preparation, including health education, for every patient prior to admission. Jane works with the Department of Health operational board on Patient Reported Outcome Measures and the Enhanced Recovery programme.

Joanne Johnson EN, RN, Dip ENB 176, BA(Hons), PG Cert Ed

Leeds Institute for Skills Training and Assessment, Leeds Teaching Hospitals NHS Trust. Joanne has worked in the perioperative environment since qualifying in 1985. In 1991 she moved to the Leeds Teaching Hospital NHS Trust, where she specialised in upper gastrointestinal and colorectal surgery (laparoscopic and open). She currently manages LISTA, the Leeds Institute for Skills Training and Assessment.

Martin Kiernan MPH, RN, ONC Dip N (Lond.)

Martin is Nurse Consultant, Infection Prevention at Southport and Ormskirk NHS Trust. He has worked in the field of infection prevention and control for 22 years in a variety of settings. Martin is a member of the Department of Health Expert Advisory Committee on Antimicrobial Resistance and Healthcare-associated Infection and is a past President of the Infection Prevention Society.

Liz McArthur RSCN, Dip Paediatric Pain Management, BSc Advanced Nursing, MSc Pain Management, Extended and supplementary Prescribing, Paediatric clinical examination

Liz trained in Edinburgh and initially worked in burns and plastic surgery, which awakened her interest in pain management. This led to her most recent post from which she has now retired as a clinical nurse in pain and sedation at the Royal Liverpool Children's NHS Trust. For many years running alongside this work was a project looking at how to gain the views and experiences of children and young people in the healthcare setting. This work has been facilitated with experts such as the Children's Society and Investing in Children.

Rosanne Macqueen RGN, BN Pg Cert THE

Rosie has recently taken up a post at NHS Greater Glasgow and Clyde as Patient Safety Programme Coordinator. This position is linked to emergency care and medical services as well as regional services. Her role is designed to help deliver the Scottish Patient Safety Programme. She holds Chairmanship of the Royal College of Nursing Perioperative Forum and within AfPP holds positions on the governance committee, education and research group and is Educational Lead for the regional team in East of Scotland. Rosie is a reviewer for the *Journal of Perioperative Practice* and for the RCN's *Nursing Standard*. She has 12 years of perioperative experience.

Fiona Martin MB CHB, BSc(Hons), FCARCSI, Dip (Clin) Ed, Cert Mgmt

Fiona is a locum consultant anaesthetist at the Royal Devon and Exeter Hospital.

Adrienne Montgomery RGN, RM, RCNT, Dip N., MN

Adrienne is Director of Masters programmes at the National University of Ireland. She has responsibility for the specialist modules in the Postgraduate Diploma in Nursing (Perioperative Nursing) and is link lecturer to all the operating departments in the region.

Zena Moore PhD, MSc, PG Dip, FFNMRCSI, Dip First Line Management, RGN

Zena is a registered nurse from Dublin, Ireland, and has worked as a lecturer in wound healing and tissue repair and research methodologies at the Royal College of Surgeons in Ireland since 2002. She has undertaken a number of systematic reviews with the Cochrane wounds group and the Cochrane renal group and has also published over 70 articles and book chapters. She has over 20 years of clinical experience in the field of tissue viability, where her research focus is specifically on pressure ulcer prevention and management.

Sarah Naylor DCR, MSc, PgC

Sarah is a senior lecturer at Sheffield Hallam University. She has been a diagnostic radiographer for over 25 years, working in various teaching, management and advanced practice roles. Sarah currently teaches on a variety of undergraduate and post graduate modules. Her previous teaching experience at post graduate level was at the Nottingham International Breast Education Centre and at National Vocational Qualification level for assistant practitioners at Nottingham City Hospital. Advanced practice interests have been in breast cancer diagnosis and bladder pressure studies.

Ross Palmer RGN, BSc(Hons) in Nursing Studies

Modern Matron for Trauma and Orthopaedics, UHCW NHS Trust. Ross is currently studying for an MSc in Advancing Healthcare Practice. He has 16 years' experience working in vascular, colorectal, general surgery and trauma and orthopaedics.

Hazel Parkinson RGN, BSc(Hons), MSc

Hazel trained at the Queen Elizabeth Hospital in Birmingham and has over 20 years' experience of the perioperative environment. For the past 10 years she has been Professional Development Practitioner for Operating Theatres across the Leeds Teaching Hospitals NHS Trust, responsible for the education and training of all perioperative staff.

Susan Pirie RGN, MA in Healthcare Ethics and Law

Susan is an experienced nurse with over 20 years' experience in perioperative practice in many specialities, in both the private sector and the NHS. She is a published author on the importance of safe patient positioning in relation to the safety of the patient and staff, and currently developing a bespoke manual handling course for theatre staff. She is currently a Practice Educator at Surrey and Sussex Healthcare NHS Trust.

Natalie Quine DipHE, RN, BSc(Hons) Peri-Operative Award

Natalie has worked in the post-anaesthetic care environment since 2001. She is currently employed as PACU Sister at Spire Gatwick Park Hospital and prior to this at the Queen Victoria Hospital NHS Foundation Trust. She is the Chairman of the British Anaesthetic and Recovery Nurses Association (BARNA) and has been involved with the development of clinical competencies for the PACU area.

Professor Mark Radford BSc(Hons), RGN, PGDip (ANP), MA(Med ed), FHEA

Mark is currently the Deputy Director of Nursing at University Hospitals Coventry & Warwickshire NHS Trust and Visiting Professor of Nursing at Birmingham City University. Mark has worked in perioperative and surgical care as a practitioner through to consultant nurse.

Paul Rawling MSc, BA(Hons), RODP, Cert Ed

Paul has 25 years of perioperative clinical experience and 6 years' experience in higher education, working as a Senior Lecturer in Pre and Post Registration Education. He has special interests in perioperative care and research.

Melissa Rochon BSc(Hons) Nursing

Melissa has worked for many years as a clinical nurse specialist in surveillance for the Royal Brompton and Harefield NHS Foundation Trust. Current projects include developing surveillance for wound infections in implant devices (pacemakers, internal cardiac defibrillators and loop systems) and maintaining surgical site infection reporting as a quality indicator for the Trust.

Eileen Scott RGN, BA(Hons), M.Litt, PhD

Patient Safety Coordinator, Surgical Directorate, North Tees & Hartlepool NHS Foundation Trust. Since qualifying as a nurse in 1989, Eileen has always specialised in anaesthetics and recovery and was a member (and Chair) of the Royal College of Nursing's Perioperative Nursing Forum for some years. Her research interests (PhD obtained in 2000) centre on tissue viability and temperature management in the perioperative environment. Eileen was closely involved in the NICE Clinical Guideline relating to the management of perioperative hypothermia, and has published widely on these subjects and has also contributed to many national and international conferences. She also has experience of research and development in the NHS and the academic sector (Durham University). Her current work on clinical governance in an NHS Foundation Trust is concerned with ensuring that systems are in place to ensure risk management and patient safety is maintained.

Pat Smedley MSc Nursing, BA(Hons), RGN, RN, PGCE

Pat is an independent consultant in post-anaesthetic care, with many years of practical experience in this speciality. Until recently Pat was Senior Lecturer in Perioperative Care at Kingston University. Currently she is President of the British Anaesthetic and Recovery Nurses Association and has worked to raise the profile and knowledge base of post-anaesthetic care nursing in the UK for over 20 years.

Jane Smith RGN, SCM, Dip in Health Studies

Jane is currently employed as Matron for Outpatients and Medical Imaging at Barnsley Hospital NHS Foundation Trust. Prior to this she was Matron for Women and Children's Services, GUM, OPD and Medical Imaging for two years. Jane has 30 years of perioperative experience in a variety of roles, her last being Lead Nurse for Orthopaedics, Trauma and Emergency Surgery. She continues to be an active member of AfPP in a number of guises. For the past three years she has been part of a UK perioperative team who conduct complex orthopaedic surgery on children in India.

Wayne Spencer Ieng, MIHEEM AE(D)

Wayne is an independent decontamination consultant based in the UK. He is also an Authorising Engineer (Decontamination), a UK-specific role for independent review of decontamination validation processes. Wayne worked for the Department of Health as a technical advisor until 2005 and chaired the department's decontamination investment process that delivered £90 million to the NHS.

Ross Thompson Dip HE, ODP, Cert Ed

Resuscitation Officer, Royal Devon & Exeter NHS Foundation Trust. Ross has worked in the NHS for over 17 years, across community services and critical care. Has has spent six years within NHS education and training, with a paper published in *CODP Journal*

'The Technic'. Ross believes in expanding the career options for all health practitioners and developing transferable skills.

Louise Wall RGN

Louise is an independent nurse practitioner in upper and lower endoscopy and is facilitator for the Gastrointestinal Endoscopy for Nurses (GIN) programme for North Bristol NHS Trust. Having worked in theatres and endoscopy from 1985 to 1998, she then moved to endoscopy full time as a clinical nurse manager. She completed upper and lower nurse endoscopist training in 2001.

Foreword 1

Perioperative practice unifies the many disciplines that work toward the assurance of good clinical outcomes and patient safety in operating rooms of inpatient and ambulatory services, providing elective, urgent and emergency surgery. Surgical suites are unquestionably exciting, energy charged and stimulating environments and highlight on a daily basis the priorities of accountability, advocacy and ethical care, the challenges of complexity and human error that can so easily be compounded by complacency or disregard for patient and staff safety, the aggressive march of technology and innovation that tests us all, the contribution of effective teamwork and communication and the vital importance of compassion and professional commitment to safeguard patients, when they are at their most vulnerable.

Throughout my career first as a student enjoying placement, a 'newbie' staff nurse, post-qualifying green hat or 'course nurse' (a title reserved those fortunate to pursue a JBCNS or ENB programme in the 1980s), Sister, Manager, Commissioner, Educator and National Advisor, I have been engaged in and associated with the perioperative arena. I could not imagine working in a speciality more rewarding, stimulating and exciting and I consider myself privileged to have enjoyed the career path that I have and to have worked with so many exceptional perioperative staff and leaders, willing to take the risks that they have to benefit patients, to ask the difficult question to safeguard safety and who have championed change, to realise service improvements at scale.

Although my current portfolio means I am engaged in research and Board Assurance, and less frequently involved in direct patient care (regular bank shifts still keep me current and clinically credible), I am acutely aware that the central tenets of perioperative practice (clinical quality, patient safety, governance, controls assurance and clinical effectiveness) are enduring and focused themes of my work, as relevant to my practice today as they were when I first set foot in an operating theatre. I also know in my heart that my passion for our discipline is as strong today as it was when I started out 30 years ago and that the many opportunities and challenges I have encountered working in this environment have shaped who I am, how I think, how I care, how I lead and the career choices I have made over the years.

Would I have done anything differently? Not a bit of it. Might another speciality have given me and tested me as much? No way. As all the students I have encouraged to take up this discipline will testify, this environment, our practice, is like no other and gets under your skin. While surgery is not without stress, and delivering patient care in the circumstances and conditions that we do can be uniquely challenging, it is none the less an incredible privilege that encourages us to give of our best every day.

Sound knowledge and honed skills are key to us giving of our best and underpin our individual clinical competence and team effectiveness. This manual outlines the background knowledge required of staff who wish to ensure they deliver good safe and effective perioperative care, and have ambitions on advancing their career through the specialty.

It is practical in focus, addressing principles rather than procedures and logically structured around the patient's journey, the five discrete sections providing further structure to guide the reader. Each chapter, prepared by respected leaders and academics of the field, contains useful guidance and the theoretical underpinning of the core subjects pertaining to perioperative practice; as an 'essential guide' it provides nurses and operating department practitioners (ODPs) with answers and rationales to many of the questions that arise in the day-to-day delivery of care. Although aimed principally at nurses and ODPs, the quality and depth of the information is so extensive it will prove an excellent reference resource for those (medical and nursing students, surgical trainees and industry partners) seeking to understand the dimensions and diversity of the discipline.

At a time when the rising popularity of handheld electronic devices raises questions regarding the long-term future of hard copy, I think we can be confident that however we avail ourselves of the information we need, the greater priority will always concern the quality and validity of what we access rather than how. The principles and foundations of each chapter, once understood, internalised and practised will facilitate the delivery of high-quality, evidence-based, patient-focused perioperative care and I commend them to you.

Jane H. Reid, RN, DPNS Enb 176, BSc(Hons), PGCEA, MSc

President International Federation of Perioperative Nursing

Visiting Professor Bournemouth University

Fellow NHS III Safer Care and Improvement Faculty

Foreword 2

Teamwork in the perioperative environment is a fundamental aspect of professionals working together to deliver the best care possible for patients undergoing surgery. One of the key aspects of good surgical practice, from all team members is situation awareness; the ability to 'see' or hear the clues in the environment, analyse the situation with sufficient knowledge to apply it to what is occurring and be able to make judgements about their relevance to the patient, at that moment. As a practising surgeon, it goes without saying that reducing risks to patients and awareness of patient safety is implicit in each practitioner's practice in the perioperative environment.

There has been a renewed emphasis on the importance of patient safety within the surgical environment since the work undertaken by the World Health Organization's second Global Challenge 'Safe Surgery Saves Lives'. The National Patient Safety Agency's publication of the surgical checklist and the subsequent acceptance of this in operating theatres throughout the UK and beyond has without doubt helped teams to focus on what is important in the minutes before surgery starts. This has ensured that everyone in the team concentrates on the patient not only at that point in the surgery but as the operation proceeds.

Organisations need to be flexible in order to demonstrate that they understand the requirement to continuously improve the quality of care to patients. Clinicians should focus on the evidence and being knowledgeable practitioners so that they have the ideas and energy to innovate. Many of the actions which denote quality care and an improved patient experience can be shown to come from ideas generated in clinical practice, such as the redesign of care pathways and the changing roles and responsibilities of staff delivering the care. Innovation may come from inspired leadership or quite simply from a group of staff asking the question 'how can we do this differently?'

For the individuals and team members, answers to that question may come from ideas gleaned from any number of sources. The expertise of the authors in this book, the *Manual of Perioperative Care – An Essential Guide*, should help to generate solutions and be the inspiration for innovation.

Patient safety is a key theme running through almost every chapter of this book. The book is helpfully divided into sections, so that the key subjects are highlighted. All the customary chapters that you would expect to find in a perioperative text book are included and in addition a section on different patient care groups which further defines how perioperative practice can be delivered with particular focus on the patient's age or specific physiological considerations. A final section on the new approaches to traditional surgical approaches highlights the dynamic and ever changing face of surgery.

The purpose of new textbooks especially when a fundamentally practical approach is taken to the topics in hand is to add to the body of knowledge which is practised every day and for every patient. All practitioners in the team are expected to maintain and improve their knowledge in order to provide evidence-based care, focused on each individual patient. Lifelong learning is a concept which is well rehearsed within healthcare in the twenty-first century and applies to each member of the team.

Professor Lord Ara Darzi PC, KBE
Paul Hamlyn Chair of Surgery, Imperial College London

Section 1

Foundation for Safe Perioperative Care

CHAPTER 1

The Context of Perioperative Care

Kate Woodhead and Lesley Fudge

What is Perioperative Practice?

The word 'perioperative' is a fairly recently devised term. The Association for Perioperative Practice (AfPP 2005) describes the perioperative environment as the area utilised immediately before, during and after the performance of a clinical intervention or clinically invasive procedure.

Previously, the care of the patient undergoing a surgical procedure was separated into distinct and separate areas of care. In the case of elective surgery the majority of patient journeys began with a visit to the GP, followed by a wait, hopefully appropriate to the urgency of their disease needs, for a referral to a specialist surgeon to come to fruition and then again, subject to urgency, another wait for an admission date to a hospital for surgery possibly after a series of investigations. Once admitted, the patient started on another journey in less familiar surroundings which, dependent on age, ethnicity and language, competence and understanding may have caused anxiety and fear which the healthcare professionals responsible for the care of the patient must make every effort to resolve as part of their service to the people who need their help and support.

It was then at this point that the perioperative care in anaesthesia, surgery and postanaesthetic recovery took place as suggested by the AfPP.

More recently, the patient has been considered holistically and the term 'perioperative' now much better describes the care of the patient from initial referral and diagnosis to full recovery, or as full as that recovery might be for their physical condition. That final outcome may inevitably be death and it is not necessary to deem that conclusion as a failure.

The word 'peri' derives from the Latin 'around', so perioperative means around the operation or intervention. Therefore perioperative care should start with good-quality information-giving and sharing with the patient from the first time they interact with a healthcare professional in the doctor's surgery or possibly in the emergency department of a hospital. Today's elective patients are likely to have investigated their own symptoms, often using unregulated internet sites and may arrive for their first healthcare consultation believing that they have already discovered their own diagnosis. The patient's first interaction and continuing care may be as part of the caseload of a surgical

Manual of Perioperative Care: An Essential Guide, First Edition. Edited by Kate Woodhead and Lesley Fudge.
© 2012 John Wiley & Sons, Ltd. Published 2012 by John Wiley & Sons, Ltd.

nurse consultant or advanced surgical care practitioner, who may care for the patient throughout their surgical journey and should be considered as perioperative.

All patients should be treated as individuals and not as a diagnosis or surgical operation. Sometimes, in this busy pressurised world, there may a tendency to forget that the patient does not experience the surgical environment every day as do the specialised healthcare professionals. Even the least complex procedure in the perioperative environment may be a major event for the patient.

Where Does it Take Place?

Historically, perioperative care was undertaken in an operating theatre or suite of theatres in an acute hospital, but more recently the settings for surgery have expanded after recognition that as long as the allocated area meets standards required for asepsis and infection management, conventional environments are not necessarily the only available option. These various settings can include doctors' surgeries and treatment centres for routine and more minor cases, keeping the acute or tertiary setting for the most complex and urgent surgeries. Patients can therefore access their surgical care closer to home and with less personal inconvenience and, it is hoped, with reduced waiting times. Healthcare is unfortunately enmeshed with the political system, but one of the better outcomes for patients over the last decade is that they usually have to wait less time than previously to see a specialist and receive appropriate treatment for non-urgent surgery.

In addition, in the current climate of global unrest, life-saving surgery is undertaken in conflict zones across the world and standards expected in more settled places may not be able to be fully met, the first priority being the saving of life. For example, surgery takes place in mobile operating rooms, in vehicles and ships, tents and other settings which will be completely alien to the practitioner who works in a standard hospital operating room. Working in the armed forces, for non-governmental organisations, charities and the like can broaden the practitioner's experience at the same time as engendering appreciation of their own high-quality operating suites within a recognised standard situation. Many advances in care and treatment have been innovated and initiated in times of conflict because of the needs of the patient with multiple trauma injuries.

Perioperative practice caregiving is delivered by a range of professionals who work collaboratively towards the best-quality outcome for the patient. There is a confusing range of these roles; names may differ across organisations and countries, but despite the differing titles their functions are similar. Boundaries have been crossed in recent times, with role expansion and development for many perioperative practitioners.

Many practitioner roles now have their own patient caseload and perform tasks within the surgical field that were previously only performed by medical staff. Through training and supervision, continuing assessment and quality outcome measurements, it has been shown that practitioners other than medical staff can perform many surgical procedures competently. The medical staff are then freed to perform more complex procedures. These less difficult cases are being performed competently and the stability or care delivery has been shown to have better outcomes for patients and the practitioners undertaking these advanced roles often become the instructors for junior medical staff, given their expertise and the stability of their role.

The Patient's Perspective – Consent and Competence

At all times it must be remembered that the patient must be at the centre of individualised care and unless their capacity to make decisions is compromised, their autonomy to make decisions for themselves must be respected. From an ethical perspective, each competent adult is an autonomous person and their own decisions about 'self' must be respected and followed.

Coercion to undergo treatment is unacceptable but difficult to avoid in a healthcare setting. With admission on the day of surgery becoming common practice, if consent has not been taken preadmission, then the patient has had insufficient time to ask further questions should they wish to gain the necessary information on which to base a decision. Decision-making on the morning of surgery or when the patient has already changed into a theatre gown is not appropriate or good practice.

As Martin Hind, senior lecturer in critical care, states 'it may be difficult to prevent some degree of coercion in securing consent from a patient, but misrepresentation of the facts or overt manipulation of the patient should be avoided' (Woodhead and Wicker 2005). What healthcare professionals must also always accept is that refusal to consent is as valid as agreement to consent to treatment, even if that decision is contrary to what they would advise.

Consent should be taken recognising the following conditions; these are not exclusive but examples of what may block fully informed consent being made by the patient:

- *Language*: Does the patient understand the person taking consent? Is the patient, deaf, blind, lacking understanding of the language being used or might they require support from a translator or signer? Does the consent taker, speak the patient's language sufficiently well? In a multi-ethnic system real comprehension of information given and received can be difficult.
- *Understanding*: Has the healthcare professional used medical terminology that can be understood by the patient? Without understanding of what the treatment entails, including any likely complications, the patient is not sufficiently able to make a fully informed decision. With good planning, the patient can be given language- and age-specific information about their disease, treatment, outcomes and complications along with frequently asked questions. Written information along with a verbal interaction between the patient and a competent information-giver, while sounding like utopia, is best practice and should be a clinical aspiration.
- *Capacity*: Is the patient a child or do they suffer from learning difficulties or another impairment such as unconsciousness or brain injury? Consent for minors under the age of 16 in the UK is taken from parents, legal guardians and legal caregivers. In cases where there are difficulties best interest principles must be used or the intervention of the legal system to ensure that the patient is at all times at the centre of the process and outcomes.
- *Best interest principles*: These have to be taken into account in a range of situations where the patient does not have the capacity to make a decision for themselves. The UK Mental Capacity Act 2005 identifies a single test for assessing whether a person lacks capacity to take a particular decision at a particular time.

So, for example a patient may be admitted unconscious and unidentifiable to an emergency department. Following examination, only emergency surgery will give the person a chance to survive. In other circumstances, this person may be competent and able to make decisions for themselves but in this situation and at this time the patient cannot, therefore others must make that decision for them and consent to surgical intervention will be foregone and surgery performed. As in any clinical situation, contemporaneous documentation must be made and the rationale for the decision recorded and signed by more than one clinician.

As in so many healthcare situations, unless decisions, actions and possibly rational omissions are contemporaneously documented, if the care records become part of a legal process at sometime in the future, the responsible carer will not be able to prove what they did or did not do for the patient.

The Nursing and Midwifery Council (2008) published principles of good record-keeping for nurses and midwives that is relevant for all healthcare professionals. They state that good record-keeping, whether at an individual, team or organisational level, has many important functions. These include a range of clinical, administrative and educational uses such as:

- helping to improve accountability
- showing how decisions related to patient care were made
- supporting the delivery of services
- supporting effective clinical judgements and decisions
- supporting patient care and communications
- making continuity of care easier
- providing documentary evidence of services delivered
- promoting better communication and sharing of information between members of the multi-professional healthcare team
- helping to identify risks, and enabling early detection of complications
- supporting clinical audit, research, allocation of resources and performance planning
- helping to address complaints or legal processes.

Evidence-Based Practice and Clinical Effectiveness

All care delivery should be based on evidence of its effectiveness by all healthcare professionals in the many multi-professional spheres. Where the evidence is derived from and how broad and deep the research has been behind the evidence should determine the practice delivered. Cochrane Reviews gather global information and create a matrix of the strength of the evidence based on the number of clinical papers that reach a similar outcome with comparable levels or breadth and depth and putting them into a scoring system to suggest efficacy (www.cochrane.org/cochrane-reviews).

Even with evidence, not all practitioners observe best practice principles. To cite a specific scientifically proven best practice perioperative principle – that shaving of body hair prior to surgery should be undertaken as close to the time of surgery as viable but not in the operating room – this is flouted on a daily basis across the world, while at the same time the antibiotics needed to protect the patient from postoperative infection possibly caused by bacteria introduced through shaving continue to outwit the scientists (Tanner *et al.* 2006).

Being fixed to the idea that all practice must be derived from clinical evidence and published science may, however, slow innovation in the clinical field and this, along with global and specific financial pressures in healthcare, carries a risk of a lack of progress. McKenna *et al.* (2000) make some valid points about considerations that should be taken into account in their paper on demolishing myths around evidence-based care and practice.

Staffing and skill mix

Staffing levels in nursing have always been a bone of contention. Nurses frequently, especially when asked, say that they have insufficient numbers to provide the quality of care that they would like to provide. Staff numbers on wards and in operating theatres have never been mandated in the UK, although in Victoria, Australia, unions and governments have agreed minimum levels of staff patient ratios which hospitals have to adhere to. In the UK we have an NHS Constitution which is enshrined in law, which states that patients have a right to be cared for by appropriately qualified and experienced staff in safe environments. The National Health Service Act 1999 ensures that the Board of any hospital is responsible for the quality of care delivered. In addition, regulatory bodies, such as the Nursing and Midwifery Council, stipulate nurses' responsibilities for safe staffing levels. In England, being able to demonstrate safe levels of staffing is one of the essential standards which all healthcare providers must meet to comply with the Care Quality Commission Regulations (Care Quality Commission 2010).

In operating theatres, recommendations from the AfPP make available online a formula for managers to use to ensure safe staffing levels (AfPP 2008). These include:

- one qualified anaesthetic assistant practitioner for each session involving an anaesthetic
- two qualified scrub practitioners as a basic requirement for each session, unless there is only once planned case on the operating list
- one trained circulating practitioner for each session
- one qualified post anaesthetic recovery practitioner for the immediate postoperative period. There may be occasions where two qualified staff are required if there is a quick throughput of patients requiring minor procedures, such as in a surgical day unit (AfPP 2011).

Skill mix

The term 'skill mix' is often used to describe the mix of posts, grades or occupations in an organisation or for a specific care group (e.g. within a department such as an operating suite or in a speciality ward).

Skill mix needs to be examined on a regular basis, so that managers and practitioners account for changing patient demographics, the skills of the practitioners available and acuity in the patient population. It is difficult, therefore, to give specific guidance on an ideal skill mix for a given situation. Reviewing the evidence, Buchan and Dal Poz (2002) identified that increased use of less-qualified staff would not be effective in all situations. Evidence on the nurse/doctor overlap suggests that there is unrealised scope in many systems for extending the use of nursing staff. In addition, they cite that many of the studies regarding skill mix are poorly designed and are often biased towards the qualified/unqualified argument focused on cost containment (Buchan and Dal Poz 2002).

Training and education

It is vital that, in order to provide the appropriate level of quality care, all staff have the necessary capability, skills, knowledge and competence to perform the role which they are employed to undertake. In order to reach, maintain and develop the appropriate level of skill and knowledge there needs to be a system in place that provides access to continuing professional development. This may include a level of mandatory education, on-the-job skills training and a continuing mechanism to ensure that competence is regularly assessed. Six main areas for consideration have been outlined by the AfPP (2011):

- educational support
- orientation and induction
- resources
- assessment

- professional development
- pre-registration learners.

Accountability and responsibility

The duty of care which nurses and other registered professionals owe to their patients can be found iterated within Codes of Conduct. The Nursing and Midwifery Council Code states 'As a professional, you are personally accountable for actions and omissions in your practice and must always be able to justify your decisions' and 'You must always act lawfully, whether those laws relate to your professional practice or personal life' (Nursing and Midwifery Council 2008).

If a nurse or midwife is asked to deliver care they consider unsafe or harmful to a person in their care, they should carefully consider their actions and raise their concerns to the appropriate person. Nurses and midwives must act in the best interest of the person in their care at all times (Nursing and Midwifery Council 2008).

The Health Professions Council, which regulates operating department practitioners, Code of Proficiency states that registrant operating department practitioners must:

- be able to practise within the legal and ethical boundaries of their profession
- understand the need to act in the best interests of service users at all times
- understand the need to respect, and as far as possible uphold the rights, dignity, values and autonomy of every service user including their role in the diagnostic and therapeutic process and in maintaining health and wellbeing (Health Professions Council 2008).

Accountability is integral to professional practice. Judgements have to be made in a wide variety of circumstances, bringing professional knowledge and skill to bear in order to make a decision based on evidence for best practice and the patient's best interest. Professionals should always be able to justify the decisions that they have made.

New roles

During the last 20 years many new roles have emerged to meet identified needs within the patient population as well as perceived needs for professionals to remain in clinical practice. The roles are many and varied. Roles change as professionals expand existing roles; many of the new roles fit within existing scope of professional practice, or they may be completely new and need specific developments and education. Whichever of the approaches an organisation decides is appropriate, a structured means of development is essential. The Career Framework sets out to standardise and describe roles at different levels of responsibility, supervision and knowledge and to illustrate career progression routes (Skills for Health 2006). Further detail has been identified into the Knowledge and Skills Framework, which is now the basis of job descriptions and competence assessment.

Nurses and others who develop their roles to include tasks or roles currently undertaken by other healthcare professionals must be aware of their legal boundaries. 'The rule of law' requires professionals to act within the law and 'the rule of negligence' requires the task or role to be delivered to the same standard as undertaken by another. Sufficient education and training are required to ensure the health professional is competent to perform the role to the required standard. In perioperative care, various roles are likely to be encountered. These include the following.

Surgical care practitioner

The role of the surgical care practitioner (SCP) is as a non-medical practitioner, working as part of the extended surgical team, under the supervision of a consultant surgeon. The SCP must be previously registered as a healthcare professional with either the Nursing and Midwifery Council or the Health Professions Council.

SCPs perform a range of duties, including examination, clerking and requesting investigation. They can assist and perform delegated duties in theatres, manage patients postoperatively, adjust treatment plans, discharge and follow-up (Association of Cardiothoracic Surgical Assistants 2011).

Advanced scrub practitioner

The Perioperative Care Collaborative provides the following definition of an advanced scrub practitioner (ASP). The ASP role can be defined as the role undertaken by a registered perioperative practitioner providing competent and skilled assistance under the direct supervision of the operating surgeon while not performing any form of surgical intervention (Perioperative Care Collaborative 2007).

Assistant theatre practitioner

The assistant theatre practitioner (ATP) carries out all the tasks of a senior theatre support worker but is also trained and competent to perform the scrub role for a limited range of cases. In addition, some ATPs work within the post-anaesthetic care unit, taking delegated care from registered practitioners (NHS National Practitioner Programme 2006).

Advancing practice

In recent years there has been a proliferation in the number of innovative advanced roles such as clinical nurse specialists, nurse practitioners and the broader role of consultant nurse. Role diversity is valuable if it improves health and well-being for patients and workers. The purpose of the consultant role is to improve practice and patient outcomes, strengthen leadership in the professions and help retain nurses by establishing a new clinical career opportunity. Some overlap occurs with specialist nursing posts in that half the consultant's time is spent in expert practice, but where the specialist works principally with patients in a clearly defined area of clinical practice, the consultant role is expected to be more strategic and broad based, to improve the practice of others and occupy a leadership position in nursing similar to that held by medical consultants (National Nursing Research Unit 2007). Examples of all the specialist roles can be found within perioperative care across the UK.

Professional development

There are a variety of definitions of continuing professional development (CPD) across the professions but it is usually taken to mean learning activities that update existing skills. CPD requirements should be identified on the basis of the needs of individuals, within the context of the needs of the organisation and patients.

In the NHS, CPD is determined through appraisal with a personal development plan agreed between the individual professional and his or her manager with the commitment of the necessary time and resources. A key development in ensuring that health professionals maintain their competence is the move among the regulatory bodies to develop CPD strategies for the revalidation/recertification of their members (Department of Health England 2007).

In perioperative practice, CPD is required by the regulators to ensure that competence is maintained. For this purpose, resources and support should be made available within the work environment. Development needs are usually identified during the annual individual performance review and are recorded by the individual practitioner within his or her personal development plan. Registrants are also required to record continuing development in their portfolios, which may be requested by the regulator at regular re-registration to prove the practitioner's education and training on an ongoing basis.

References

AfPP (Association for Perioperative Practice) (2005) NATN definition of a perioperative environment. www.afpp.org.uk/filegrab/periopdef.pdf?ref=54 (accessed March 2012).

AfPP (2008) *Staffing for Patients in the Perioperative Setting*. Harrogate: AfPP.

AfPP (2011) *Standards and Recommendations for Safe Perioperative Practice*, 3rd edn. Harrogate: AfPP.

Association of Cardiothoracic Surgical Assistants (2011) Definition. http://acsa-web.co.uk/about-surgical-care-practitioners/ (accessed 4 December 2011).

Buchan J and Dal Poz M (2002) Skill mix in the healthcare workforce: reviewing the evidence. *Bulletin of the World Health Organization* 80(7): 575–580.

Care Quality Commission (2010) *Guidance about Compliance: Essential standards of safety and quality*. London: CQC.

Department of Health England (2007) http://webarchive.nationalarchives.gov.uk/+/www.dh.gov.uk/en/Managingyourorganisation/Workforce/EducationTrainingandDevelopment/PostRegistration/DH_4052507 (accessed 4 December 2011).

Health Professions Council (2008) *Standards of Proficiency for Operating Department Practitioners*. http://www.hpc-uk.org/assets/documents/10000514Standards_of_Proficiency_ODP.pdf (accessed March 2012).

McKenna H, Cutliffe J and McKenna P (2000) Evidence based practice: demolishing some myths. *Nursing Standard*: 14(16): 39–42.

National Nursing Research Unit (2007) Advanced nursing roles: survival of the fittest? *Policy*+issue 6. http://www.kcl.ac.uk/content/1/c6/03/25/81/PolicyIssue6.pdf (accessed March 2012).

NHS National Practitioner Programme (2006) *Introducing Assistant Theatre Practitioners: A best practice guide*. Assistant Theatre Practitioner Project, NHS East of England.

Nursing and Midwifery Council (2008) *The Code: Standards of conduct, performance and ethics for nurses and midwives*. www.nmc-uk.org/publications/standards (accessed March 2012).

Perioperative Care Collaborative (2007) *The Roles and Responsibilities of the Advanced Scrub Practitioner*. http://www.afpp.org.uk/careers/Standards-Guidance/position-statements (accessed March 2012).

Skills for Health (2006) *Key Elements of the Career Framework*. http://www.skillsforhealth.org.uk/images/stories/Resource-Library/PDF/Career_framework_key_elements.pdf (accessed March 2012).

Tanner J, Woodings D and Moncaster K (2006) Preoperative hair removal to reduce surgical site infection. *Cochrane Database of Systematic Reviews* 3: CD004122.

Woodhead K and Wicker P (2005) *A Textbook of Perioperative Care*. Oxford: Elsevier.

Further Readings

Association for Perioperative Practice (2011) *Standards and Recommendations for Safe Perioperative Practice*, 3rd edn. Harrogate: AfPP.

Gordon S, Buchanan J and Bretherton T (2008) *Safety in Numbers: Nurse to patient ratios and the future of healthcare*. New York: Cornell University Press.

Hood PA, Tarling M and Turner S (2011) *AfPP in your Pocket: Perioperative Practice*. Harrogate: AfPP

Hughes S and Mardell A (2009) *Oxford Handbook of Perioperative Practice*. Oxford: Oxford University Press

Professional Education in Practice (2009) *Advanced Surgical Care Practitioners*. http://pepractice.co.uk/course_advanced_scrub_practitioner.html (accessed March 2012).

Wicker P and O'Neill J (2010) *Caring for the Perioperative Patient*, 2nd edn. Wiley-Blackwell.

Woodhead K and Wicker P (2005) *A Textbook of Perioperative Care*. Oxford: Elsevier.

CHAPTER 2

Preoperative Assessment

Jane Jackson

So, the first principle must be 'do no harm.' When it goes wrong in the NHS, patients suffer and patients die. Safety for patients is at the heart of quality care and if the professional responsibility of nurses and doctors. So there is no trade off between safety and efficiency.

(Rt Hon Andrew Lansley, June 2010)

Patient Preparation for Anaesthetic and Surgery

No anaesthetic or surgical procedure is without its risks, in addition to the risks associated with patient co-morbidity. The role of patient preparation is to identify the patient's current health status, to weigh up the risks and to put a process into place to optimise the patient prior to admission and thereby minimise the risk of complications. There will be occasions when the risks of anaesthesia or surgery outweigh the risks of deteriorating health associated with the disease. In these cases informed consent will provide the patient with the understanding of why surgery is not the best option.

Patient preparation – or preoperative assessment (POA) – should be undertaken for all patients who are referred for surgery. The form that the patient preparation takes may differ for the type of procedure, anaesthetic or patient's fitness, but in essence, the patient should be prepared for the surgical admission (National Patient Safety Agency 2011).

This chapter will address the principles and application of patient preparation.

Definition of Patient Preparation

Accurate patient preparation will identify a patient's fitness and willingness to proceed with surgery and anaesthetic and ensure appropriate action is taken when the patient is not fit or willing to proceed.

Patient preparation is a process by which a patient's known co-morbidities are made known to the relevant healthcare professionals who will interpret the information, decide on additional investigations or examinations and then determine the risk factors associated with the patient's health and the anticipated anaesthetic and surgical intervention.

The patient must be informed of the risk and benefits of surgery and anaesthetic, and be provided with sufficient information to ensure an informed choice. It may be, at the end of the patient preparation stage that the patient decides not to proceed with surgery. Admission and discharge planning will be addressed during patient preparation. Integral to patient preparation is anticipation of potential outcomes, length of hospitalisation, ability to complete activities of daily living and discharge planning. The process will involve the patient and their carers and all healthcare professionals appropriate to the individual patient, in primary and secondary care.

Aims and Objectives of Patient Preparation

The overall aim is to ensure that the care for each patient is well planned and appropriate to the patient's needs. The objectives should be considered from both the healthcare and the patient's view.

The exchange of information both from the patient – giving the healthcare provider a full understanding of their health, social and medication requirements – and from the healthcare provider – providing the patient with information (verbal, written or visual format) – is essential to ensure a full awareness and understanding of each patient's health needs, and to allow the healthcare professional to identify any specific patient requirements. This exchange of information about health to date, and proposed treatment/investigation – together with risks and benefits – will assist the patient in forming a decision as to the surgery or anaesthetic. This is informed consent (NHS Brand Guidelines 2010).

The patient should be provided with the opportunity to negotiate their admission date, and be informed on the expected duration of their hospital stay so that discharge planning is arranged prior to admission. For the healthcare professional, having a detailed medical and social history will help in identifying potential risks during the perioperative period. Mechanisms can then be put into place to reduce those risks and to optimise the patient's health prior to the admission. This will form the basis of trust between patient and healthcare provider.

Inter-professional Teamwork

The process of patient preparation is one of inter-professional teamwork, involving primary and secondary care. The general practitioner (GP) will first see the patient and determine from their presentation if investigation or referral is required. The GP will consider the patient's health prior to referral and perform initial checks, such as haemoglobin levels, correcting any anaemia; regularity of pulse to identify atrial fibrillation; body mass index, referring the patient to weight management if necessary; factors such as smoking, referring them to smoking cessation; or social issues requiring attention prior to referral. In addition, radiology or pathology input may be required prior to referral to secondary care. The patient should be offered delayed referral until the known health concerns are optimised.

The patient is seen in the outpatient department for the expert opinion of the consultant surgeon and/or their team. If surgery is recommended, then patient preparation for admission begins. Patient preparation is commonly led by a consultant anaesthetist and/or lead nurse, with a team of specialist appropriately trained registered general nurses (RGNs) and/or foundation year one house officers (FY1s) and healthcare assistants (HCAs). Within the team in some patient preparation services are pharmacy prescribers who provide a valuable input regarding the medication/allergies and advice on omitting drugs prior to admission.

Clear protocols for patient preparation and patient surgical care pathways are applied by the team, who should be trained to complete accurate assessment. Conducting patient interviews and recording an accurate medical, surgical, anaesthetic, medication and allergy history are essential skills for the assessor. Patient examination and ordering of appropriate investigations will add to the information from which the assessor will need to judge the patients fitness to proceed with the procedure or their need to address specific ill-health. The anaesthetist will provide their expertise in determining the support required for those patients due to undergo complex major surgery or who have complex ill-health. Additional specialist support will be provided as required, for example the cardiology team for those patients who present with cardiac history and who require echocardiogram or cardiac consultation.

Enhanced Recovery

Enhanced recovery (ER) is an approach to surgical care that should be applied for every patient admitted to secondary care (Figure 2.1). Patients' quality of care is provided by minimising patient stress, both physical and psychological prior to admission, and maintaining normal activities during the perioperative phase. The role of patient preparation is to manage patient safety and expectations. It also ensures that the patient has had appropriate optimisation of co-morbidities prior to admission and has received education on their health and the procedure and discharge planning implemented.

Collating the Patient Information

The patient's medical record contains information that is confidential. All information should be accurate and non-judgemental. All records should be written/typed with clarity to enable others to read what has been written without supposition. The patient's medical record is a legal document and may be used in court.

It is important at patient preparation to gather in full all the relevant information to ensure that a considered opinion can be made as to the patient's co-morbidities. This will then guide the assessor as to what investigations/interventions are required prior to weighing the risks of surgery and/or anaesthesia with the potential outcome if surgery is not undertaken.

The reference points for gathering the patient information will come from multiple sources. It is important to read all available information prior to the patient interview so that concentration can be given to the direct patient contact. Potential sources of information will include the following.

- *Patient personal history* either directly from the patient or via an interpreter. Written or verbal communication may be challenging because of a language barrier where English is not the first language or where the patient is unable to communicate because they lack mental capacity, for instance. In these cases a carer will usually accompany the patient and it should be recorded that the history has been obtained via a carer and not directly from the patient.
- *A GP referral letter*. This should contain a summary of past medical history, medical and allergies as well as the reason for the referral.

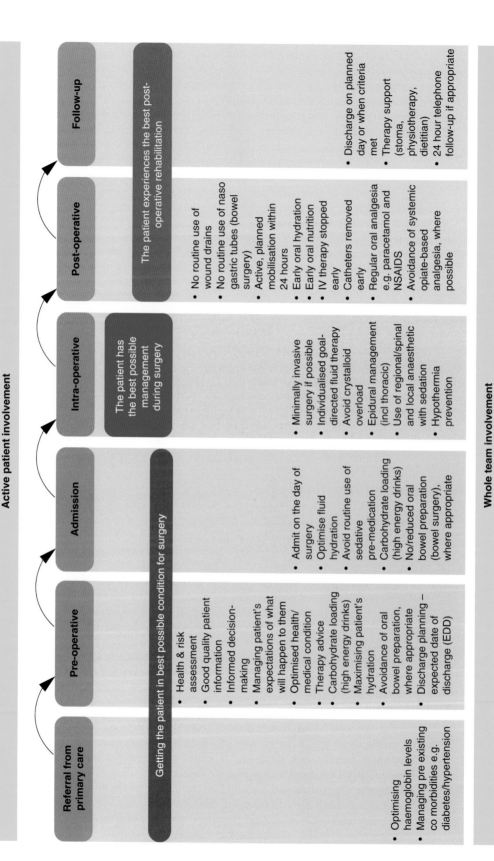

Figure 2.1 Enhanced patient recovery: Reproduced with permission from the Department of Health, UK.

- *A consultant clinic letter*. This should contain a summary of the patient symptoms, examination results and recommended course of action/treatment.
- *Hospital notes*, including copies of clinic outcomes/investigations performed elsewhere. This will often be the prime source of information and is particularly useful when the patient has seen multiple specialties such as cardiac, endocrinology as well as surgery.
- *Investigation results*. These provide a record of trends as well as the latest analysis. An abnormal reading may be an improvement on the patient's past results and will provide the assessor with the knowledge that the patient's health is responding to treatment.
- *The waiting list card*. This should provide full patient identification, their consultant, procedure planned and any special requirements, which may include special instruments or patient requirements.
- *The patient's prescription* and/or evidence of over-the-counter bottles/containers. This will provide the pharmacist and/or assessor with vital information about the patient's health.

There may be occasions when a patient-completed questionnaire will suffice in providing enough information about the patient's health to determine that no further assessment is required before clearing the patient to be added to the waiting list. Such questionnaires can be completed in the outpatient department or the assessment clinic by the patient and handed in to a member of the nursing team, or patients may be asked the questions as part of a telephone assessment. These tend to be used for patients booked for minor procedures, or as a prescreening questionnaire to determine if/when a full assessment is required and with whom.

For patients due to undergo inpatient surgery, or who have very complex co-morbidities and are for day surgery admission, attendance at an assessment clinic for a face-to-face assessment may be appropriate.

Anticipation of equipment and documentary requirements for each patient should allow for a prepared area that allows the assessment to take place in privacy, giving respect to patient dignity and confidentiality. Interruptions should be kept to a minimum.

The patient may be asked to provide a urine sample to investigate for urinary tract infection, haematuria or glucosuria. If the department uses electronic assessment, then the patient will complete demographic information with the HCA or RGN. Observations will then be taken including regularity of pulse, blood pressure, respiratory rate and oxygen saturation levels. The height, weight and body mass index will be measured and documented. Swabs will be taken from nose, groin, catheter sites and any wound area to test for MRSA (methicillin-resistant *Staphylococcus aureus*) status (see External factors required at time of patient preparation point 1). For patients with respiratory disease, a peak flow measurement will be made and recorded. For those patients with a cardiovascular history or due for major surgery, an ECG may be required (NICE 2003).

With the above documentation, the RGN/FY1 will then have a range of information ready for his or her intervention.

History Taking

The RGN or FY1 will interview the patient in a private room, ensuring privacy and dignity. They should read through all available information provided, gaining clarity on specific issues before progressing to the discussion on the procedure itself.

Accurate history taking and recording is important and can be broken down into the following stages.

Accurate record of past medical, surgical, anaesthetic and social history

Attention to detail is important to enable a full understanding of a patient's health or ill-health, co-morbidities, smoking or alcohol history. This will enable the assessor to gain insight into the past experiences of the patient, and to anticipate any potential areas that will require clarification or investigation. All records must at minimum be signed and dated and, if handwritten, be clear so as to avoid misinterpretation. Should a patient experience a clinical event (e.g. chest pain), it is important to record the time of the chest pain and its duration.

Complications from past medical, surgical or anaesthetic history

Unexpected outcomes and complications do occur and in order to minimise the chance of recurrence, it is important that the health professional has a clear understanding of what occurred, when and if possible why. This information allows the RGN/FYI to appropriately investigate potential causes/previously unknown health conditions, and thus optimise the condition prior to progressing with surgery. Investigations and resulting expert consultation with consultant and potential optimisation of the condition may delay the admission of the patient. The timing of the assessment should therefore be as early as possible in the surgical pathway.

Current symptoms/history

Having an understanding of the patient's current symptoms will assist the health professionals to tailor the intervention appropriately. Information provided by the patient should be recorded in the clinical notes accurately and with clarity, ensuring date and time are entered, particularly when symptoms are changing. This information will be used by other health professionals and, in conjunction with the procedure and past medical history, form the base from which any improvements or deterioration of symptoms can be judged.

For patients due to have a general anaesthetic, questions should be asked relating to orthopnoea. This is because it is important to judge the patient's ability to lay relatively flat for the length of the surgery without respiratory or cardiac distress. Questions could include the number of pillows a patient uses to sleep and if they sleep in a chair or bed and whether they suffer shortness of breath on exertion while climbing a flight of stairs or at night or at rest.

It is also useful to ascertain how far the patient can walk, and the reason why they stop, for example because of joint pain, dyspnoea, leg pains, chest pain, balance or fatigue. The response will lead the assessor to further questions and investigations.

Family history

Of particular note is immediate family incidence of reaction with anaesthetic, such as suxemethonium allergy or venous thromboembolism. These familial conditions are just two examples where the patient may have a predisposition and a full history and/or further testing may be required to reduce the risk of an untoward event.

Observations

Observations should be recorded during patient preparation and will form the baseline for changes in the observations during the perioperative period. The recorded results should be checked and any abnormal readings noted. It is good practice to repeat a raised blood pressure reading after 15–20 minutes.

Examination

The purpose of patient examination is to provide observation to accompany the history. Results will guide the assessor as to which investigations are required, if any, prior to reaching a decision as to the patient's fitness to proceed with the surgery and/or anaesthetic.

Any pallor of the patient's skin and signs of cyanosis, jaundice and anaemia should be observed, then checks made for oedema of the legs and sacrum, varicose veins, ulceration or pressure sores.

Checks on the patient's neck flexion and extension should be carried out, and Mallampati Score checking used (Figure 2.2) for any restrictions which could cause difficulty with laryngoscopy or intubation (Mallampati *et al.* 1985, Nuckton *et al.* 2006).

Modified Mallampati Scoring is as follows:

- Class 1: Full visibility of tonsils, uvula and soft palate
- Class 2: Visibility of hard and soft palate, upper portion of tonsils and uvula
- Class 3: Soft and hard palate and base of the uvula are visible
- Class 4: Only hard palate visible.

The chest may also be examined. The trained professional should observe the position of the trachea, checking for any obstructions, the shape of the thorax noting any abnormalities that may indicate long-term respiratory disease. The patient should be asked about any cough or sputum, including the colour of any phlegm such as yellow or green indicating infection, or if the sputum is frothy, or blood streaked indicating haemoptysis. The chest is then palpated, checking for air entry to right and left side of the chest, before auscultation. Auscultation will provide the trained assessor with evidence of respiratory flow or restrictions – and is usually followed by cardiac auscultation, checking the heart valves for signs of regurgitation.

The venous thromboembolism risk assessment may be completed by the FY1 or RGN while the patient is in attendance for preparation. If completed at this stage then the form would need to be countersigned on admission (NICE 2010, Department of Health 2009).

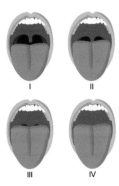

Figure 2.2 Modified Mallampati Scoring is as follows: Class I: Full visibility of tonsils, uvula and soft palate. Class II: Visibility of hard and soft palate, upper portion of tonsils and uvula. Class III: Soft and hard palate and base of the uvula are visible. Class IV: Only hard palate visible. Reproduced from Wikimedia Commons – freely licensed media file. http://en.wikipedia.org/wiki/Mallampati.

Investigations

Routine investigations may be required for certain procedures according to local policy. History and examination will also prompt the assessor to request investigations to provide additional information prior to reaching a decision as to a patient's fitness to proceed with the surgery and, if appropriate, anaesthetic. It is the responsibility of the assessor to check results of all investigations ordered and to take appropriate action on the findings.

Medication and Allergies

The pharmacist is key in patient preparation and several assessment clinics have pharmacist involvement. Where a pharmacist is not present then this role is undertaken by the RGN or FY1.

Many patients attending patient preparation are already prescribed medication in the form of tablets, injections, inhalers, ointments, drops and so on. The majority of the patients will arrive with their prescription or their medication. If the medication is not in its appropriate containers then the assessor should use the opportunity to stress the importance of keeping medication in its clearly labelled container.

The pharmacist is key to providing advice to the patient on their medication, its effects and side-effects as well as advice on what should be omitted prior to admission, and on drug interactions. Often the pharmacist will raise concerns with the patient's GP or seek clarity on duration of drug therapy.

The qualified prescriber will commence the medication chart including, if appropriate, any prophylactic treatment as this will reduce the chance of medication omissions.

Many patients take over-the-counter medication that has not been prescribed and that may adversely affect the action of their prescribed medication, for instance reducing the affect of antihypertensive agents. Patients should be advised of this and encouraged to advise their GP of any over-the-counter medication taken.

Education

During the course of the patient preparation assessment, a rapport is built between patient and assessor(s). It is essential that the procedure is discussed, what is involved, the likely outcome and the effect that this may have for the individual patient. Risks and benefits should be included as well as the expected length of hospital stay. Every effort should be made to provide the patient with written information (Bunker 1983, Audit Commission 1993).

Patient preparation is also the ideal opportunity to discuss health promotion, for example on reducing alcohol or drug dependency, and to give particular emphasis to the benefits of smoking cessation (Smokefree 2012). The patient should be encouraged to cease smoking permanently as early as possible, quitting eight weeks before surgery for maximum benefit (Warner 2005).

Obesity is also a growing problem! The latest Health Survey for England data shows us that nearly 1 in 4 adults, and over 1 in 10 children aged 2–10, are obese (Bourn 2001). Obesity has life-long effects for the patient and their care, giving rise to an increase in diabetes, cardiovascular disease, respiratory and musculoskeletal conditions. The patient should be helped to understand the ramifications of their weight on their health and encouraged to seek the support of their GP to discuss their weight and consider weight reduction.

Discharge Planning

The patient's admission, hospital stay and appropriate discharge should all be addressed during patient preparation. For elective surgery the approximate length of stay in secondary care can be anticipated and the patient and/or relatives advised. For many patients additional support following surgery is minimal, but for a few patients, it will be necessary to make arrangements for help with catering or housework until the patient is able to return to their level of independence prior to admission. Care should be planned prior to admission to ensure that discharge is not delayed once the patient is fit to return to primary care.

Determining the Outcome from Patient Preparation

The trained assessor will be alert to the risks of anaesthesia and surgical intervention, and will consider any risks to the patient as soon as she or he identifies the patient's medical history. Detailed questioning of the patient will determine the past and present status for each co-morbidity and will provide evidence on the stability of the condition(s). The assessor will pay particular attention to cardiovascular and respiratory disease, diabetes and thyroid and renal conditions as these have the greatest bearing upon a patient's fitness for anaesthesia/surgery. Appropriate investigations will identify evidence of the condition at the time of investigation, and together with the physical examination of the patient will alert the assessor to potential areas of concern.

Many patients will be declared fit for admission at the time of assessment, but a few will require review. There should be clear protocols within the patient preparation department which allow the competent assessor to make a judgement on the patient's suitability for admission, or will guide the assessor to refer the patient to the consultant anaesthetist or consultant cardiologist for their opinion.

Anaesthetic Consultation/Referral

The consultant anaesthetist has a key role in the preparation of patients prior to admission (Association of Anaesthetics of Great Britain and Ireland 2010). The role is one of education for the assessors, monitoring the latest evidence-based research and where appropriate applying these within the department. The anaesthetist will be the person the assessor approaches for advice if the patient has multiple, often unstable, co-morbidities.

The anaesthetist will review the result from the assessment and will be able to advise further investigation such as echocardiogram, lung function test, cardiopulmonary testing or, in the case of patient with multiple unstable co-morbidities, a meeting with the patient and/or relatives to discuss the risks and benefits of the surgery/anaesthetic. This shared decision-making is particularly important for those patients who have particularly high risk from anaesthesia where the risk of death from the disease is less than that of recovery from the anaesthetic and surgery. Increasingly the consultant anaesthetist needs to share these conversations and communicate the decision back to the consultant surgeons, pharmacist and to the patient's GP.

Where a pharmacist is not present at patient preparation, they may, however, be the professional who prescribes venous thromboembolism prophylaxis and provide guidance on medication cessation such as aspirin/clopidogrel, or hypoglycaemic agents prior to admission.

Recording the Findings

Records may be kept via paper or electronic format. All records should be fully documented, clearly and accurately ensuring inclusion of date, time, signature and name in capitals (Nursing and Midwifery Council 2009).

Investigation results should be contained within the notes, detailing abnormalities and action taken to address them. There will be occasions when the results are abnormal yet the patient is at optimal fitness within the confines of their condition(s), or perhaps the patient has a latex allergy. It is particularly important for these cases that the anaesthetist, surgeon and support teams are informed that this patient may require additional support during the perioperative period.

External Factors Required at Time of Patient Preparation

Within the busy environment of patient preparation there are several factors that need to be included, yet whose requirement is outside of the patient preparation area or Trust control. These requirements ensure adherence with government directives, for example NICE clinical guidelines and Department of Health policies. The patient preparation team will need to ensure compliance with the following mandatory requirements.

- *MRSA screening*: Patients due for elective or emergency admission should be screened to ascertain their MRSA status. There are certain exception groups (Department of Health 2010).
- Identification of patients at risk of *variant Creutzfeldt–Jakob disease (vCJD)* (Department of Health 2011a): An assessment should be carried out before surgery and/or endoscopy to identify patients with, or at risk of, CJD or vCJD. All patients due for surgery should be asked the question 'Have you ever been notified that you are at increased risk of CJD or vCJD for public health purposes?' This should be a routine question asked during patient preparation for surgery. If the patient replies that they have been so informed, then guidance is available on transmissible spongiform encephalopathy (TSE) from the Department of Health (2011b).
- *Venous thromboembolism (VTE)* risk assessment (NICE 2010): The VTE risk assessment must be undertaken for all adult admissions, and should be completed on admission. The form (Department of Health 2011c) can be initiated at time of patient preparation but must be reconfirmed for any changes on admission.

In addition to the above three clinical requirements, there is a clinical governance mandatory requirement that all NHS Trusts in England comply with patient reported outcome measures (PROMS):

- *PROMS* began as a questionnaire issued to patients undergoing hip replacement, knee replacement, groin hernia or varicose vein procedures. The purpose is to gain the patient's perspective of their health or health-related quality of life and independence prior to and following surgery (Department of Health 2008). The questionnaire should be completed prior to surgery, and this is followed up by a second questionnaire sent to the patient three months post surgery following hernia or varicose vein procedures or six months following hip or knee surgery. The results are analysed and available on line by commissioners, Trusts and public (NHS 2011).

Legal Issues Related to Patient Preparation

There is particular emphasis for the nurse working in autonomy in this field. The care undertaken by a nurse working in patient preparation must be to the same standard of care as that attained by the health professional who would have undertaken the role before the nurse.

Liability would be found against the nurse if he or she is found to be negligent, or caused harm as a consequence of being negligent. It is therefore essential that nurses working in the field of patient preparation – a specialism – identify any lack of competency or skills and undertake appropriate steps to attain the knowledge to allow them to perform their duties with responsibility.

Nursing staff working in patient preparation should comply with the Nursing and Midwifery Council Code (2008). These are standards set of conduct, performance and ethics set by the Nursing Midwifery Council designed to ensure a 'high standard of practice and care at all times'.

The nurse will be 'personally accountable for actions and omissions in your practice and must always be able to justify your decisions', and must 'have the knowledge and skills for safe and effective practice'.

The Code requires the nurse to 'maintain their professional knowledge and competencies' and continues that a nurse must ensure that she or he keeps updated with the knowledge and skills required for her or his practice (Dimond 2009).

Patient preparation or POA is a specialty in its own right. Before working in this field, registered nurses need to recognise their capabilities and seek appropriate training and competencies for the patient group they are expected to assess. Competency to complete assessments should be regularly undertaken – at least annually – to ensure best practice that complies with the latest protocols and provides patients with a high standard of care.

Summary

Preparation of a patient prior to potential surgery and/or anaesthetic is an inter-professional process. Starting in primary care, the patient has their known co-morbidities optimised prior to referral through to secondary care. Within secondary care, patient preparation provides the opportunity to identify a patient's fitness, willingness and ability to proceed with surgery and/or an anaesthetic. The patient should be fully informed of all risks and benefits of the anaesthetic and surgery so that she or he is able to provide an informed consent. All aspects of the patient's health and social needs should be considered so that the time spent in secondary care can be kept to a minimum to allow for discharge to the primary care environment as soon as medically fit. Patients who are not fit for surgery need to receive appropriate information to enable a full understanding of the issues and alternative treatment options.

Patient preparation is key to the surgical admission process, being the link between primary care referral and booking the patient onto the waiting list for surgery. It has been shown to be central to the development of essential advances to delivering quality patient care through Department of Health ER pathway (NHS Institute for Innovation and Improvement 2008).

References

Association of Anaesthetists of Great Britain and Ireland (2010) *Safety guideline 2. Pre-operative Assessment and Patient Preparation.* http://www.aagbi.org/ (accessed 6 December 2011).

Audit Commission (1993) *What Seems to be the Matter: Communication between Hospital and Patients.* London: HMSO.

Bourn J (2001) *Tackling Obesity in England*, HC 220, Session 2000–2001, 15 February. London: National Audit Office.

Bunker TD (1983) An information leaflet for surgical patients. *Annuals of the Royal College of Surgeons of England* 65: 242–243.

Department of Health (2008) PROMS. http://www.dh.gov.uk/prod_consum_dh/groups/dh_digitalassets/@dh/@en/documents/digitalasset/dh_092625.pdf (accessed 7 December 2011).

Department of Health (2009) *Venous Thromboembolism Prevention. A patient safety priority.* http://www.dh.gov.uk/en/Publicationsandstatistics/Publications/PublicationsPolicyAndGuidance/DH_101398 (accessed March 2012).

Department of Health (2010) *Screening for MRSA.* http://webarchive.nationalarchives.gov.uk/+/www.dh.gov.uk/en/Publichealth/Healthprotection/Healthcareassociatedinfection/DH_094120 (accessed 7 December 2011).

Department of Health (2011a) Assessment to be carried out before surgery and/or endoscopy to identify patients with, or at increased risk of, CJD or vCJD (Annex J). http://www.dh.gov.uk/dr_consum_dh/groups/dh_digitalassets/@dh/@ab/documents/digitalasset/dh_123586.pdf (accessed 7 December 2011).

Department of Health (2011b) Guidance for transmissible spongiform encephalopathy. www.dh.gov.uk/ab/ACDP/TSEguidance/DH_098253 (accessed 7 December 2011).

Department of Health (2011c) Risk assessment for VTE. http://www.dh.gov.uk/dr_consum_dh/groups/dh_digitalassets/@dh/@en/@ps/documents/digitalasset/dh_113355.pdf (accessed 7 December 2011).

Dimond B (2009) *Legal Aspects of Nursing*, 5th edn. London: Pearson, pp. 548 and 553.

Mallampati S, Gatt S, Gugino L, Desai S, Waraksa B, Freiberger D and Liu P (1985) A clinical sign to predict difficult tracheal intubation: a prospective study. *Canadian Anaesthesiologists' Society Journal* 32(4): 429–434.

National Patient Safety Agency (2011) National Research Ethics Service. Informed consent. http://www.nres.npsa.nhs.uk/applications/guidance/consent-guidance-and-forms/ (accessed 6 December 2011).

NHS (2011) Patient reported outcomes measures (PROMs). http://www.ic.nhs.uk/proms (accessed 7 December 2011).

NHS Brand Guidelines (2010) Patient information introduction. http://www.nhsidentity.nhs.uk/tools-and-resources/patient-information (accessed March 2012).

NHS Institute for Innovation and Improvement (2008) *Enhanced Recovery Programme.* http://www.institute.nhs.uk/quality_and_service_improvement_tools/quality_and_service_improvement_tools/enhanced_recovery_programme.html (accessed 7 December 2011).

NICE (National Institute for Health and Clinical Excellence) (2003) *Clinical Guidelines Number 3: Preoperative Tests: The use of routine preoperative tests for elective surgery.* http://publications.nice.org.uk/preoperative-tests-cg3 (accessed March 2012).

NICE (2010) *Clinical Guidelines Number 92: Venous Thromboembolism.* http://www.nice.org.uk/guidance/CG92 (accessed 7 December 2011).

Nuckton TJ, Glidden DV, Browner WS and Claman DM (2006) Physical examination: Mallampati score as an independent predictor of obstructive sleep apnea. *Sleep* 29(7): 903–908.

Nursing and Midwifery Council (2008) *The Code: Standards of conduct, performance and ethics for nurses and midwives.* London: NMC.

Nursing and Midwifery Council (2009) *Record Keeping: Guidance for nurses and midwives.* http://www.nmc-uk.org/Documents/Guidance/nmcGuidanceRecordKeepingGuidanceforNursesandMidwives.pdf (accessed March 2012).

Smokefree (2012) Smoking cessation. www.smokefree.nhs.uk (accessed March 2012).

Warner DO (2005) Helping surgical patients quit smoking: why, when, and how. *Medical Intelligence* 101: 481.

CHAPTER 3

Communication

Libby Campbell

Introduction

This chapter explores the issues around consent, confidentiality and documentation which are based on legal and ethical principles and the issues surrounding communication related to aspects of teamwork within the operating theatre.

Consent

When I first started working in operating theatres the attitude towards consent for surgery was, at best, haphazard. The forms were often completed by someone other than the surgeon who was planning to operate, often someone very junior, the explanation about what might be likely to happen was general in nature, rare but grave potential complications were not discussed in an attempt to allay anxiety and permission was frequently couched in terms that would enable further intervention if that was found to be required. This paternalistic approach to consent pertained until the move towards patient autonomy and human rights enabled the individual to become an equal partner in treatment rather than a passive recipient in what was regarded as 'their best interests'.

As a result of the desire for increased patient protection and, indeed, staff protection, along with the lessons learnt as a result of poor practice and findings in court cases, the need for valid consent to surgical intervention is fundamental to patient care in the operating theatre. Rather than just another form to be completed, it should be regarded as the reflection of a fundamental right of the individual to determine what should and should not happen to him or her.

Principles

The principles underpinning consent to treatment are based on the moral conviction of the right of self-determination about what happens to one's own body and in common law which recognises that every individual has the right to have his or her body protected against invasion by others (Mason and Laurie 2011). Except in a few narrowly defined

Manual of Perioperative Care: An Essential Guide, First Edition. Edited by Kate Woodhead and Lesley Fudge.
© 2012 John Wiley & Sons, Ltd. Published 2012 by John Wiley & Sons, Ltd.

circumstances, non-consensual touching by another may give rise to a civil action for damages or may even constitute a criminal assault. Thus, even when that 'touching' is designed to help an individual who needs treatment, every touch of a patient by way of medical treatment is potentially a battery or assault in law (Mason and Laurie 2011).

> Every human being of adult years and sound mind has a right to determine what shall be done with his own body, and a surgeon who performs an operation without the patient's consent commits an assault. (Cardoza 1914)

There are some limited exceptions to the need for consent, such as where the patient is in a state of impaired consciousness, particularly when life-saving treatment is required. In these circumstances it might be assumed that treatment is what the patient would wish if they were in a position to give consent. Even then, treatment is permissible only until the point at which the patient is able to give consent and only to the extent that is immediately required.

Even when consent has been given, it doesn't mean that the surgeon may do as they wish. In one case (*Murray* v. *McMurchy* 1949) the doctor had discovered during a caesarean section that the condition of the patient's uterus would make it hazardous for her to go through another pregnancy and he tied the fallopian tubes. The court took the view that it would not have been unreasonable to postpone the sterilisation until after consent had been obtained, in spite of the convenience of doing it at the time. By contrast, however, there are some instances where the courts have found that it would have been unreasonable to postpone. In one case (*Marshall* v. *Curry* 1933) a surgeon removed a testicle which he found to be diseased during an operation for repair of hernia. The surgeon stated that removal was essential or the health and life of the patient would have been imperilled had he not done so and the court agreed. The distinction between necessity and convenience therefore is finely balanced, especially in the light of some consent forms which can be rather vague.

Consent may be implied or expressed. Implied consent is reasonably indicated for example when a patient attends for treatment or acquiesces to the treatment routine. The weakness of implied consent, however, is that it is not always clear that the patient is agreeing to what the person treating them intends to do. A classic example is where an individual rolls up his or her sleeve to have a blood pressure reading taken but is given an injection instead.

There is no specific threshold for requiring an expressed consent in law, which relies on comparison with the practice of a reasonable doctor (*Bolam* v. *Friern Hospital Management Committee* 1957), but when it comes to surgical intervention it is essential to obtain expressed consent and to do so in writing so that it is clear to all involved, including the courts if necessary.

Furthermore, the consent must be valid in that it must be given voluntarily by a competent person without duress who is as fully informed about the potential risks as possible so that they can make up their own mind in the light of all the relevant circumstances.

It is not possible to explore here the interesting discussion about whether a patient can ever be fully informed, what constitutes significant risks or 'therapeutic privilege' that apparently justifies withholding of information that might cause undue anxiety. Suffice it to say that if a patient is not told of the potential risks, in their specific circumstances, consent will not be deemed to be valid.

Capacity

An adult, or a mature minor, will be deemed competent to consent unless it is proved that they lack the mental capacity to do so. Determining incapacity has also been considered in the courts and in one case (*Re MB* 1997) it was found that a person lacks the capacity 'if some impairment, or disturbance of mental functioning, renders the person unable to make a decision whether to consent to or to refuse treatment'. The case in question concerned a pregnant woman who suffered from a needle phobia, as a result of which she was unable to agree to have an injection that would precede a caesarian section. The High Court judge held that her needle phobia rendered her mentally incapacitated to take the decision but emphasised that had she been competent she could have refused the operation.

Provided the patient has the mental capacity in relation to the decision to be made, he or she can refuse to give consent for a good reason, a bad reason or no reason at all.

> The patient is entitled to reject (the) advice for reasons which are rational, or irrational, or for no reason. (Templeman 1985)

Neither does the presence of a mental disorder automatically mean that a person is incapable of making a decision in relation to the treatment being considered. In one case (*Re C* 1994) a 68-year-old man who was suffering from paranoid schizophrenia developed gangrene in his foot and doctors believed an amputation to be a life-saving necessity. He refused consent and sought an injunction restraining the hospital from carrying out surgery without his express written consent. He succeeded on the grounds that the evidence failed to establish that he lacked the understanding of the nature, purpose and effects of the proposed treatment. Instead the evidence showed that he had understood and retained the relevant information, he believed it and he had arrived at a clear choice. By contrast, in another case (*NHS Trust* v. *Ms T* 2004) a patient refused a blood transfusion which was required because she self-harmed. She described blood as being evil and it was held that this was evidence of mental disorder which made her incapable of using and weighing the relevant information.

Children

Parents have a legal duty to care for their children and act in their best interests until the age of majority, which is 18 years in England, Wales and Northern Ireland and 16 years in Scotland. This means that they would normally give, or withhold, consent for treatment, including surgery. That said, under Section 8 of the Family Reform Act (1969), a child of 16 or 17 years can give a valid consent to treatment and this presumption is now contained in the Mental Capacity Act (2005) (Section 1(2)) which states that a person must be assumed to have capacity unless it is established that he or she lacks capacity.

However, parents must give, or withhold, consent 'reasonably' and a third party, such as his or her healthcare professional, may be justified in ignoring an unreasonable giving or withholding of consent. Many of the issues of conflict associated with consent of minors have emerged from cases concerning continuing or withholding treatment, often life-saving treatment, rather than consent for surgical intervention, although the legal principles from those cases pertain generally (*Re J* 1992).

There is, however, a growing recognition of the need to involve children in decision-making regarding their own treatment as far as they are able to understand the implications. The Children's Act 1989 Section 1(3) (a) requires the courts to consider: 'the ascertainable wishes and feelings of the child concerned considered in the light of their age and understanding.'

The landmark case in relation to the maturity and understanding of a child to give valid consent was that of *Gillick* v. *West Norfolk and Wisbech Area Health Authority and the DHSS* (1985) and has led to the phrase 'Gillick-competent' being used in relation to children. Not only must legislation be acknowledged but professional guidance is available to safeguard children and must be followed (Royal College of Nursing 2003).

Religious cultures

There are a variety of religious cultures that impinge on medical practice but the most common is that of Jehovah's Witnesses and the need for blood transfusion, often in emergency situations. If a Jehovah's Witness is a competent adult, they are free to refuse blood transfusion as long as their refusal is valid. In a Canadian case (*Malette* v. *Shulman* 1991), an unconscious patient was given a life-saving blood transfusion despite the fact that she was carrying a card refusing such treatment. She was awarded damages because the doctor had ignored her written request not to give blood and this constituted a trespass on her person.

There is, however, more discussion about parents refusing blood transfusion as part of treatment on behalf of their children. In another case (*Re E* 1993) a youth aged 15 years 9 months required blood transfusion as part of his treatment for leukaemia. Both he and his parents were Jehovah's Witnesses and refused to give consent so the Health Authority applied for him to be made a ward of court and a declaration made that the treatment could proceed. The judge gave leave for the blood transfusion to be given and the consent of the patient and his parents dispensed with. As a judge in Canada observed, albeit in a peripheral context: 'Parents may be free to become martyrs themselves. But it does not follow that they are free in identical circumstances to make martyrs of their children' (*B* v. *Children's Aid Society of Metropolitan Toronto* 1995).

It is almost impossible to find a case in UK common law where a court has upheld a parental claim to authority to refuse recommended life-saving treatment on behalf of their child purely on their own religious convictions (Mason and Laurie 2011). The appropriate benchmark remains the best interests of the patient although emphasis may shift depending on the specifics of the case.

Research

Research and experimentation are commonly used interchangeably but there is a distinction. Research implies a predetermined protocol with a clearly defined end-point whereas experimentation involves a more speculative approach to an individual subject (Mason and Laurie 2011).

Following a notorious history, research is now governed by rules which set out principles, requirements and standards for acceptable research including the ethical dimension (Mason and Laurie 2011). Strict protocols need to be followed and explained fully to patients or their advocates who then have the choice of taking part or not. Choosing not to take part must not detract from treatment.

The status of the experimental doctor has always been uncertain since 1797 when a doctor was criticised in court for introducing what still remains the standard treatment for fractures of limbs (*Slater* v. *Baker and Stapleton* 1797). The difficulty is that there will not be 'a responsible body of medical opinion' against which the treatment can be measured, required under the 'Bolam test' (*Bolam* v. *Friern Hospital Management Committee* 1957). Without experimentation, however, 'it would be disastrous . . . for all inducement to progress in medical science would then be destroyed' (*Hunter* v. *Hanley* 1955).

Consent from the individual patient is paramount, in all aspects, but the balance between progress and patient interests is a fine one (Mason and Laurie 2011).

Prisoners in the perioperative environment

Prisoners do not forfeit their human rights by virtue of their deprivation of liberty but it is accepted that 'the manner and extent to which they may enjoy those other rights will inevitably be influenced by the context' (*Shelley* v. *United Kingdom* 2008).

Prisoners have the right to the same standard of care as is available to the rest of society (British Medical Association Medical Ethics Committee 1996) and to the same 'duty of care' embodied in the values of professional healthcare codes of practice (General Medical Council 2001).

However, the prison service has a duty to maintain prisoners in custody with effective security procedures, whatever the environment, and this includes the healthcare environment. Whatever the offence committed, prison staff are responsible for the security of the prisoner on behalf of the general public and society and when they are within the theatre environment they still retain that duty of care (Fyfe 2004).

Individual healthcare staff will have their anxieties, as indeed will the prisoner, therefore the risks need to be assessed in the light of specific circumstances. Prison officers and the healthcare team need to assess the risks jointly, especially since some prisoners present a danger of flight or violence to the public or healthcare staff. This assessment will include the level of restraint required, attendance of prison officers during anaesthetic, during surgery and in the recovery areas and any precautions required as a result of potential HIV status, known to be higher in the prison population.

Consent in practice

All of the information relating to consent merely serves to illustrate that the circumstances surrounding consent are not always quite as simple as we wish they were. In the vast majority of cases there will be no issue but if there is any doubt, it is always wise to seek guidance on the subject. And, indeed, guidance is available in abundance. There is, of course, legal guidance but there will be local policy and procedures which will reflect legal requirements, professional requirements and employer requirements. Professional requirements and local policy is often referred to as 'quasi-law' but practitioners must make themselves aware of it if they are considering deviating from the norm and must be able to provide evidence that they have done so for good reason that has been tested among their peers.

Confidentiality

Whether it is a carelessly constructed phone-call, or permitting photos to be taken without permission, or carrying patient identifiable information out of the hospital, or discussing an interesting case in the lift with colleagues, all of us at one time or another will have let down a patient by sharing information without their permission.

Others go further; a Sydney-based neurosurgeon was criticised for offering a visit to watch him work, including operating, as a prize for a charity auction (Robotham and Doherty 2011) and there are frequent requests for visits to the operating theatre in inappropriate circumstances.

Clearly there is information that must be shared in order to implement our collective duty of care but the occasional cavalier attitude towards personal information and the increasing applications that modern technology enables means that we have to develop better practice in relation to protection of what is very personal information.

Data protection

The legislation set out in the European Directive on Data Protection implemented in the UK by the Data Protection Act 1998 establishes a set of principles with which users of personal information must comply. The Human Rights Act 1998 (Article 8) also recognises an individual's right to private and family life manifest in several court injunctions to grant individuals life-time anonymity (Dimond 2008).

In addition to the statutory duties, the duty of confidentiality arises from the duty of care, the implied duties under the contract of employment, the duty to keep information that has been passed on in confidence, confidential and requirements set out as part of codes of professional conduct. Many of these duties are described in terms of the professional individual but employers also have duties to maintain data securely and to ensure that staff are trained accordingly. Any breach of confidentiality will be taken seriously and may result in dismissal.

However, there are exceptions to the duty of confidentiality and these include when the patient consents, if it is in the interests of the patient and when the police or the courts order disclosure. In addition, non-anonymised data may need to be made available to managers and others not bound by professional codes of conduct, such as occurs when adverse events or complaints are being investigated. Again, there needs to be a balance between maintaining confidentiality and enabling other agencies to meet their statutory requirements and memorandums of agreement are often set in place to deal with those situations sensibly.

There is excellent guidance available (Department of Health 2003) and there are individuals within NHS organisations, such as a data manager and Caldicott Guardian, who will give advice.

Documentation

When all goes well, the need for documentation is sometimes regarded as an arduous task that 'takes time away from patient care' (Pirie 2011), but when things go wrong, good communication can be the distinguishing factor between evidence of a professional approach to a legal duty of care and indication of a haphazard approach to practice.

> The quality of a registrant's record-keeping is a reflection of the standard of their professional practice. (Tune 2009)

Any document may be requested by the courts and therefore will constitute a 'legal' document and, in terms of omission, if a care procedure had not been documented, then in law it has not occurred (Wood 2010).

Practitioners must be aware of the documents that are required to be retained, whether manually or electronically, and they must be aware of common errors such as legibility, avoidance of abbreviations and signing and dating entries. There will be local policy that must be followed and there are national guidelines available (Nursing and Midwifery Council 2009).

Handover of care

Handover or transfer of care occurs at several points in the operating theatre and is recognised as a process that carries risks. Studies (Patterson *et al.* 2004, Catchpole *et al.* 2010) have confirmed that these are vulnerable points in care and investigations of adverse events frequently identify transfer shortcomings. Risks identified include misunderstanding and the lack of opportunity to ask questions, incomplete information and the lack of written documentation and diversions or interruptions during transfer.

It is, therefore, good practice to use standardised forms or checklists to ensure that information is not omitted or assumed and that these are reviewed regularly in the light of experience. Transfer should take place face-to-face in order to confirm understanding and identify priorities for care.

Communication

Communication is frequently mentioned as an integral part of successful teamwork in the operating theatre and the lack of it an indication of problems. There is no one model of teamwork to follow as teams need to form and reform according to the job required but we cannot assume that familiarity, worklists and procedure books will ensure adequate communication. Neither is there one model of communication to follow.

The first useful model for communication was designed to illustrate radio and telephone technologies and was described as having a sender, a communication channel and a receiver. It included the potential for 'noise' interfering with transmission of the message but was otherwise a simple but very basic concept (Shannon and Weaver 1949). Models have been developed over the years to elaborate on every part of the process, particularly the barriers to effective communication and the importance of transmission of meaning and factors that affect transmission (Pluckhan 1978). Further work recognised the elements of verbal and non-verbal aspects of communication (Argyle 1972) and these have been applied to work in the operating theatre (Campbell 1984, McGarvey *et al.* 1999). Increasingly, studies have concentrated on describing communication in practice, including operating theatre practice (Tanner and Timmons 2000) and on human factors that affect successful communication between team members (Lingard *et al.* 2004, Leonard *et al.* 2004).

Failures

Frequently, communication is not successfully achieved. One study highlighted that communication failures were at the root of over 60% of adverse events and found that approximately 30% of procedurally relevant exchanges among team members in the operating theatre failed; exchanges were too late to be effective, communication was not complete or accurate, key individuals were excluded or issues were left unresolved until the point of urgency (Lingard *et al.* 2004).

From various studies, the factors contributing to failure of communication in the operating theatre indicate three main aspects: cultural, individual and system.

- *Cultural aspects* include the difference in the way that doctors and nurses are trained, doctors being concise and nurses broad and narrative in their communications. In addition, doctors approach practice as an individual process rather than the collaborative process favoured by nurses, and professional hierarchies are seen as inhibiting people from speaking up.
- *Individual aspects* include human factors such as limitations to memory, effect of stress and fatigue, risks associated with distractions and interruptions and limited ability to multitask but also include process factors such as indistinct speech, lack of listening, background noise and difficulties with language (Nestel and Kidd 2006). In addition, personal and professional characteristics are also implicated (Firth-Cozens 2004) with lack of respect or discourteousness being mentioned (Nestel and Kidd 2006).

- *System aspects* that militate against effective communication include lack of training and supervision (Lingard *et al.* 2004), lack of feedback and styles of management.

In order to address some of those issues, safety checklists and briefings have been introduced and the effect has been remarkable.

Safety checklists and briefings

In June 2008, the World Health Organization (WHO) launched a challenge to reduce the number of deaths across the world by strengthening the commitment of clinical staff to addressing safety issues within the surgical setting. This included the WHO Surgical Safety checklist which has been adapted for use throughout the NHS and is a core set of safety checks, identified for improving performance at safety critical time points within the patient's intraoperative care pathway.

Team briefings are a simple way for the team to share information about potential safety issues and concerns about patients and are designed to foster an environment in which the team can share information and check assumptions openly. It is intended that they should be brief, taking only a few minutes and are normally led by the surgeon prior to surgery.

Included in the briefing is basic information such as the patient's name, intended procedure and equipment requirements but also anticipated critical events reviewed individually by the surgeon, the anaesthetist and the nurse. The nurse, for example will discuss with the team all specific patient concerns, equipment, implants, supplies, staffing and any other issues affecting patient safety. Importantly, all members of the team introduce themselves.

The briefings are designed to encourage discussion and to ensure that all team members have the same expectations. Observational studies have identified that using the team briefing methodology has reduced the number of communication failures and promoted collaborative team communication (Lingard *et al.* 2004) and although there has been scepticism from some surgeons there has been a positive impact on team cohesion.

Teamwork and Communication in Practice

- A common goal or purpose for the team needs to be identified or reiterated. It needs to reflect organisational goals and outcomes as well as acknowledging individual team goals and it need to be expressed in a way that outlines principles and behaviours acceptable to the whole team, highlighting respect for patients and colleagues.
- There needs to be a greater understanding of the roles that each member holds and how they contribute to the purpose of the team within their professional practice. Even agreeing a 'common goal or purpose' will enable a greater understanding of the different roles within the team.
- Inevitably, different individuals will bring different skills to the team, either as a result of their education, experience or personality. Assessment of skills, both technical and non-technical, is required along with multi-professional education and training to address the skills gaps.
- Leadership skills need to be identified and developed to enable learning, to understand the influences that affect teamwork and to minimise the negative effects of external issues.
- Communication issues need to be addressed on an ongoing basis and one of the most effective ways to do that is to introduce briefing before procedures and debriefing after procedures.

- Learning from successes and from adverse events is essential and, as well as reviewing relevant data on an ongoing basis, that needs to include human factors as well as procedural issues.
- Outcomes need to be measured, perhaps using some form of departmental 'scorecard', which will not only enable trends to be established and successful strategies identified but will also provide data for organisational purposes.
- An open and honest atmosphere is required that fosters trust and respect for individuals within the team rather than an informal approach to teamwork that fosters undue deference to hierarchy and individuals in an attempt to preserve the status quo.
- Concerns about time and work pressures to achieve all of this will need to be addressed but in order to minimise errors and to maintain an effective team, there is evidence that this is no longer an option.

References

Argyle M (1972) Non-verbal communication in human social interaction. In Hinde RA (ed.) *Non-Verbal Communication*. Cambridge: Cambridge University Press, pp. 243–269.

B v. Children's Aid Society of Metropolitan Toronto [1995] 1 SCR 315 at 433.

Bolam v. Friern Hospital Management Committee [1957] 2 All ER 118.

British Medical Association Medical Ethics Committee (1996) *Guidance for Doctors Providing Medical Care and Treatment to Those Detained in Prison*. London: BMA.

Campbell E (1984) A study of the socialisation of the student nurse into the operating theatre (unpublished). University of Edinburgh.

Cardoza J (1914) in *Schloendorff v. Society of New York Hospital* 105 NE 92 (1914).

Catchpole K, Sellers R, Goldman A, McCulloch P and Hignett S (2010) Patient handovers within the hospital: translating knowledge from motor racing to healthcare. *Quality and Safety in Health Care* 19: 318–322.

Department of Health (2003) *Confidentiality: NHS Code of Conduct*. London: Department of Health.

Dimond B (2008) *Legal Aspects of Nursing*, 5th edn. Harlow: Pearson Education.

Firth-Cozens J (2004) Why communication fails in the operating room. *Quality and Safety in Health Care* 13: 327.

Fyfe A (2004) Managing prisoners in theatre. *British Journal of Perioperative Nursing* 14: 559–562.

General Medical Council (2001) *Good Medical Practice*. London: GMC.

Hunter v. Hanley [1955] SC 200.

Leonard M, Graham S and Bonacum D (2004) The human factor: the critical importance of effective teamwork and communication in providing safe care. *Quality and Safety in Health Care* 13(suppl 1): i18–i19.

Lingard L, Espin S, WhyteS, *et al.* (2004) Communication failures in the operating room: an observational classification of recurrent types and effects. *Quality and Safety in Health Care* 13: 330–334.

Malette v. Shulman [1991] 2 Med LR 162.

Marshall v. Curry [1933] 3 DLR 260.

Mason JK and Laurie G (2011) *Law and Medical Ethics*, 8th edn. Oxford: Oxford University Press.

McGarvey HE, Chambers MGA and Boore JRP (1999) Exploratory study of nursing in the operating department: preliminary findings on the role of the nurse. *Intensive and Critical Care Nursing* 15: 346–356.

Murray v. McMurchy [1949] 2 DCR 442.

Nestel D and Kidd J (2006) Nurses' perceptions and experiences of communication in the operating theatre: a focus group intervention. *BMC Nursing* 5: 1.

NHS Trust v. Ms T [2004] EWHC 1279.

Nursing and Midwifery Council (2004) *Code of Professional Conduct: standards for conduct, performance and ethics*. London: NMC.

Nursing and Midwifery Council (2009) *Record-keeping: guidance for nurses and midwives*. London: NMC.

Patterson E, Roth E, Woods D, Chow R and Orlando J (2004) Handoff strategies in settings with high consequences for failure: lessons for health care operations. *International Journal for Quality in Health Care* 16(2): 125–132.

Pirie, S. (2011) Documentation and record-keeping. *Journal of Perioperative Practice* 21(1): 22–27.

Pluckhan ML (1978) *Human Communication: the matrix of nursing*. New York: McGraw-Hill.

Re C (an adult: refusal of medical treatment) [1994] 1 All ER 819.

Re E (a minor)(wardship: medical treatment) [1993]1 FLR 386 FD.

Re J (a minor)(wardship: medical treatment) [1992] 2 FLR 165.

Re MB (adult: medical treatment) [1997] 2 FCR 541.

Robotham J and Doherty P (2011) Surgery with spectators a good money-raiser, says Cancer Council. *The Sydney Morning Herald* 29 January.

Royal College of Nursing (2003) *Safeguarding Children and Young People – every nurse's responsibility.* London: Royal College of Nursing.

Shannon CE and Weaver W (1949) *The Mathematical Theory of Communication.* Chicago, IL: University of Illinois Press.

Shelley v. *United Kingdom* [2008] 46 EHRR SE16.

Slater v. *Baker and Stapleton* (1797) 95 ER 860.

Tanner J and Timmons S (2000) Backstage in theatre. *Journal of Advanced Nursing* 32(4): 975–980.

Templeman L in *Sidaway v Board of Governors of Bethlem Royal Hospital* [1985] 1 AC 171.

Tune M (2009) Interview. *Nursing and Midwifery Council News* 29.

Wood S (2010) Effective record-keeping. *Practice Nurse* 39(3): 20–23.

CHAPTER 4

The Perioperative Environment

Hazel Parkinson

Surgery takes place in patient care environments specifically designed for such purpose and can be in a wide variety of settings:

- inpatient operating theatres
- patient treatment centres
- day surgery facilities
- diagnostic imaging and interventional radiology departments
- outpatient departments
- endoscopy units
- community or GP settings
- mobile operating theatres (NHS Estates 2005).

Whatever the design or layout of these departments they should all meet current national and professional guidelines to ensure standards of patient care are met. This chapter aims to give an overview of these design issues and current guidance.

Division of the Operating Theatre Environment

Surgical intervention and treatment has evolved considerably over time and continues to develop and expand. The building or refurbishment of surgical care facilities should consider these developments (NHS Estates 2005) and be able to accommodate the use of new equipment, for example digitally based image enhancement, ultrasound equipment, plus innovations in anaesthetic and surgical equipment such as robotic laparoscopic surgery. Current guidelines advocate the need for increased space, and to ensure that facilities are flexible in use and cost effective. The speed of developments in technology will have significant implications for future design and layout of surgical facilities (NHS Estates 2005).

Throughout the design process the needs and experiences of the patient must be addressed (Association for Perioperative Practice, AfPP 2007). The needs of children should be considered in creating paediatric specific facilities designed not only for the child but also for accompanying parents or guardians (Department of Health 2003).

Manual of Perioperative Care: An Essential Guide, First Edition. Edited by Kate Woodhead and Lesley Fudge.
© 2012 John Wiley & Sons, Ltd. Published 2012 by John Wiley & Sons, Ltd.

BOX 4.1

Recommended areas in the operating department

Inpatient facilities (NHS Estates 2005)
- Reception
- Admission area
- Anaesthetic room
- Operating theatre
- Scrub room/area
- Preparation room
- Recovery (PACU)
- Disposal
- Storage facilities
- Staff facilities
- Anaesthetic department
- Education and training facilities
- Administration area

Day surgery facilities (NHS Estates 2007)
- Reception and waiting area
- Preassessment (optional)
- Admission with changing rooms
- Sub waiting area
- Anaesthetic room
- Operating theatre
- Scrub room/area
- Preparation room
- Recovery (PACU)
- Second-stage recovery
- Discharge lounge
- Disposal
- Interview room
- Storage facilities
- Staff facilities
- Education and training facilities
- Administration area

The needs of staff who work in surgical facilities should also be addressed at an early stage, to ensure their wellbeing and ability to deliver high-quality care.

Current recommended areas within an operating theatre department are listed in Box 4.1.

Ideally the main inpatient theatre department in an acute hospital should be central and in one location (NHS Estates 2005). This helps to maximise the flexibility of facilities and provides efficiency of staffing, equipment and supplies. Many hospitals have a number of surgical facilities, but however many areas there are, they should all be covered by the same policies and procedures to ensure a high standard of care and good clinical governance.

Other considerations that need to be taken into account in designing surgical facilities include:

- infection prevention strategies – infection prevention teams should be involved from the start and a key principle of perioperative care is patient safety with a duty of care to minimise the risks of postoperative infection
- protecting patients' privacy and dignity throughout their journey, including single sex accommodation (NHS Estates 2005)

- cultural considerations of patients and staff
- access for disabled people
- moving and handling of patients and equipment
- storage facilities
- wayfinding and signage.

Core Functions of Each Area

The reception area should be welcoming and staffed while the department is in use, acting as a point of entry and exit for patients and visitors.

The admission area is where formal identification of patients is made as they enter the department against the appropriate documentation to ensure the correct patient is received and their preparation for surgery is complete. In day surgery departments changing rooms are provided and patients then proceed to a sub-waiting area.

Anaesthetic rooms should provide a calm and undisturbed environment for the induction of anaesthesia (NHS Estates 2007). If used they need to be equipped with the same standard of monitoring as the operating theatre. Wall-mounted medical gas services – air, nitrous oxide, oxygen, vacuum and gas scavenging – are standard requirements. An adjustable ceiling-mounted examination lamp will be required for any clinical procedures (NHS Estates 2007). All anaesthetic rooms within a department should have the same layout for ease of use by staff and to decrease risks. Locked storage should be provided for drugs.

Operating theatres where the surgical procedures take place can be either conventionally ventilated or ultraclean ventilated.

Scrub rooms or areas designed for the scrubbing, gowning and gloving of surgical personnel should be large enough to accommodate several staff at any one time without the risk of contamination of sterile surfaces (NHS Estates 2007).

Preparation rooms are attached to the operating theatre and are used to lay up surgical instrumentation. They are good storage areas for essential supplies needed throughout surgical procedures, including a cabinet for warming fluids used in surgery. Ideally each theatre should have its own preparation room to avoid any potential risk of cross-infection (NHS Estates 2007). These rooms should also have a similar layout within departments for ease of use and minimising risk.

Patients are transferred post procedure to recovery rooms or post-anaesthetic care units (PACU) where they are cared for before discharge from the department. PACUs should be able to accommodate level 2 (and possibly level 3) patients for a period of time while they await transfer to a critical care bed. Each bay should have wall-mounted medical gases, vacuum and standard monitoring facilities. There should be an isolation bay for those patients with active infections. If children are cared for in adult areas, paediatric specific facilities and staffing must be considered to ensure the needs of both the children and their parents or guardians are met. The needs of the dying patient and their relatives should also be taken into consideration. PACU is often a central area in departments and is therefore used to store emergency and cardiac arrest trolleys and defibrillators (NHS Estates 2007).

Second-stage recovery in day surgery is used when patients have regained consciousness. They remain here until able to get dressed and transfer to the discharge lounge, where they continue to be monitored until allowed home (NHS Estates 2007). All patient care areas within the department should have an emergency call system that is linked to PACU and staff rest areas to be able to summon help (NHS Estates 2007).

Disposal areas are used for the immediate dismantling of used sterile trolleys, sorting equipment for reprocessing, disposal of sharps, body fluids and the processing of waste.

Cleaning equipment for the theatre between patients and at the beginning and end of operating sessions is stored here. Central disposal areas can be used to store equipment for reprocessing or waste for collection from sources external to the department.

Storage facilities are important and need to be replenished on a regular basis. They include: areas for storing supplies such as sterile instrument trays, sutures, swabs implants, etc.; areas to store equipment such as operating tables, mechanical vacuum, diathermy and image intensifiers; a clean linen store; a pharmacy store supplied from the main hospital pharmacy that has a lockable door and used to supply the anaesthetic rooms, theatres and PACU with drugs, lotions and fluids, etc.

There should be a rest room so that personnel can take breaks in a relaxed area, with facilities to make drinks and food. Secure staff changing facilities with lockers should be provided so that staff can change into appropriate theatre attire, with facilities for storage and cleaning of theatre footwear.

The anaesthetic department should ideally be located in close proximity to the theatre department, providing office space and administration support. Admin areas within the theatre department are needed for management of the department and staff.

Education and training is important for competence and ongoing development, therefore a seminar room is a useful addition as it enables easy access to training.

Additional facilities might include a laboratory area for blood gas analysis and blood glucose monitoring, plus the provision of a blood refrigerator.

Building Notes – Areas to Consider

Within the operating theatre the ventilation system has four main functions:

- control of temperature and humidity
- to dilute airborne bacterial contamination
- to control air movement to minimise the transfer of airborne bacteria from less clean to cleaner areas
- to assist with the removal of and dilution of waste gases (NHS Estates 1994).

A conventional ventilation system is designed to change the air within an operating theatre approximately 20 times per hour, forcing filtered air from the ceiling down and out through exhaust vents near the floor, thus creating a positive air pressure at all times (Hospital Infection Society 2005). To maintain the positive pressure and effectiveness of the ventilation doors should remain closed as much as possible, especially when surgery is taking place. Staff must consider their route through theatre to avoid having more than one door open at a time to ensure airflow is in one direction only (NHS Estates 1994, Williams 2008).

Ventilation systems are not normally turned off completely, to avoid the potential backflow of contaminated air, but can be turned to set back. There should be a visual indicator on the theatre control panel of the ventilation status plus an override facility if the system is on a timed cycle (Hospital Infection Society 2005).

Some clinical specialities, such as orthopaedics, where the risks and consequences of infection for patients are greater, need a higher specification of ventilation (Gilmour 2005). In ultraclean ventilation systems, filtered air descends in a unilateral flow over the patient thus creating a clean zone. The high flow of air is achieved by recirculating theatre air and passing it through HEPA (high-efficiency particulate air) filters. There are up to 300 air changes per hour in ultraclean systems (Hospital Infection Society 2004).

Piped medical gases supplied to the operating theatre, anaesthetic room and PACU include: oxygen, nitrous oxide, medical air, vacuum and anaesthetic gas scavenging.

While these supplies are wall mounted in anaesthetic rooms and PACU, in theatre they should be ceiling mounted. For greater flexibility a pendant should be placed at each end of the operating table, allowing the configuration of the theatre to be changed dependent on patient needs (NHS Estates 2005). All systems must be checked before each operating session to ensure competent supply. Back-up cylinders of oxygen and nitrous oxide should be attached to anaesthetic machines in case of pipeline failure, and a mechanical vacuum facility should be available in case of line failure.

Within the general department a source of natural light has an important role on the sense of wellbeing of patients and staff (NHS Estates 2005, 2007) and where possible the operating theatre, PACU and staff areas should have natural light.

Within the operating theatre there must be an even distribution of light, which is individually and collectively controlled for brightness. Operating table lights must meet the needs of the clinical speciality being undertaken and are designed to be easily cleaned and maintained, and staff should be competent to operate and position them to maximise the view of the surgical team (Hughes and Mardell 2009, p. 272). During laparoscopic procedures the main theatre lighting is reduced to allow visualisation of display screens. Staff need to make arrangements to spot illuminate anaesthetic monitors and instrument trolleys to ensure monitoring is maintained and to reduce the risk of contamination of sterile fields. Staff should be aware of the potential for slips and trips in darkened theatres.

The finish on walls must be durable and robust enough to withstand the impact of moving equipment and trolleys. Vulnerable areas such as doorways, corners and storage should be reinforced to avoid damage. Walls should have a hygienic finish that is impervious and able to withstand repeated cleaning and be painted a light, attractive colour that does not interfere with monitoring changes in patients' skin tone or colour (NHS Estates 2005). Damage should be repaired to avoid microbial contamination. Walls within operating theatres should be constructed to provide radiation protection (NHS Estates 2005). Ceilings within the operating theatre itself should be sealed to maintain microbiological standards (NHS Estates 2007) while other areas may have modular fittings to allow access for maintenance of estate.

Flooring must be able to withstand the movement of trolleys, operating tables and heavy equipment. It should be continuous and smooth between the floor and walls and have sealed or welded joints to avoid microbial contamination. Breaks or lifting of the surface should be repaired to avoid microbial contamination and the risk of slips, trips and falls (NHS Estates 2005). Floors need to be robust enough to withstand spillages and mopping, regular cleaning and be slip resistant (NHS Estates 2007). Floor markings are useful to denote the area covered by ultraclean ventilation hoods (NHS Estates 2005) and to denote the position of equipment for specific procedures for example robotic surgery.

Doors should close fully, usually with automatic closures, to aid the effectiveness of the ventilation system. Glass panels will reduce the risk of accidents, but should incorporate obscure glass for the privacy and dignity of patients. Doors should be lead-lined for radiation protection, and the glass should be laser proof (NHS Estates 2007).

While natural light is desirable if windows are present, they must be completely sealed and at least double-glazed (NHS Estates 2007), aiding noise reduction and energy conservation as well as ensuring positive air pressure (Weaving *et al.* 2008). To provide adequate blackout needed for certain procedures there should be electronically controlled blinds within the sealed units (NHS Estates 2007).

Storage facilities should avoid surfaces where dust can accumulate (i.e. horizontal) but be easy to reach, clean and use. Storage areas should be included on deep clean programmes and any damage to surfaces or fittings repaired promptly.

Each theatre should have a control panel that houses relevant controls for ventilation, lights, blinds, X-ray screening, clock and alarm systems. This should be accessible for maintenance from the theatre corridor.

IT facilities are needed within the operating theatres with enough stations provided for effective working. Touch screen monitors, flat wipeable keyboards or plastic covers for conventional keyboards should be utilised.

Telephones within patient care areas should be volume controllable or silent with a light indicator so that they do not disturb the surgical or anaesthetic teams during patient care (NHS Estates 2007).

For security, entry and exit points should have electronically controlled access to reduce the risk of unauthorised access, with CCTV monitoring in use at all times.

If laser is to be used within theatres, doors should lock from inside, and there must be warning lights at all entrances and exits to warn staff that laser is in use.

Electrical supply to departments should be continuous and monitored. If there is electrical failure it is important critical equipment is supplied by an uninterrupted power source (UPS) for example, anaesthetic monitoring and operating lights. Staff should be aware of the location of UPS sockets and use them for critical equipment only.

Handwashing facilities should be available throughout departments in easily accessible prominent positions to reinforce the importance of hand hygiene to staff (NHS Estates 2005). Hand basins should be wall mounted with curved sides, no plugs or overflows and with non-touch mixer taps, with ample space for soap and towel dispensers (NHS Estates 2007).

Patient Flow

Perioperative practice aims to achieve an absence of infection by controlling the movement within and entry to the environment to reduce airborne contamination (Hospital Infection Society 2004, Gilmour 2005). Sources of postoperative infection are either endogenous to the patient or exogenous – which includes airborne contaminants such as skin cells shed by staff movement and which may contain bacterial colonies (Gilmour 2005). Staff working in surgical care facilities must be educated and trained regarding the rules of movement and divisions within the department, to minimise traffic and keep air turbulence to a minimum (Hospital Infection Society 2005). Departments can be divided into areas where access is unrestricted, semi-restricted and restricted dependent on the function and the need to consider the cleanliness of the air (Hospital Infection Society 2005).

Unrestricted areas include the reception area for visitors, admission areas for patients and changing rooms. Some administration areas and training facilities are unrestricted dependent on layout of the department.

Semi-restricted areas include sterile storage areas, anaesthetic rooms, PACU and discharge areas. Movement of staff, patient and equipment is controlled to minimise flow and allow only that which is necessary.

Restricted areas include the theatres, preparation rooms and scrub rooms, and numbers of staff are kept to a minimum for patient safety while reducing the risk of contamination by air turbulence.

The flow of patients, staff and equipment throughout the departments should be agreed and adhered to. Traffic flows, deliveries, waste disposal and storage are separated from patient care areas so that there are clean and dirty zones designed to reduce cross-contamination (Williams 2008).

Movement of staff and equipment during procedures should be kept to a minimum, discouraging entry or exit directly from the theatre to avoid air turbulence, loss of positive air pressure and potential breach of patient dignity.

Within semi-restricted and restricted areas staff are required to wear theatre attire, appropriate footwear and hair covering. While there is little evidence that wearing hats reduces infection (Hospital Infection Society 2005), Weaving *et al.* (2008) argue it can act as a reminder of the vulnerability of patients.

In restricted areas staff must be aware of which areas and items are considered sterile and keep movement around these to a minimum, and a distance of 30 cm from a sterile field to avoid the risk of contamination. Constant vigilance of the sterile field is needed to ensure they remain so.

Waste

The management of waste is regulated by legislation and surgical care facilities need robust policies and procedures to ensure waste is disposed of correctly and in a timely manner (AfPP 2008). Such policies should comply with regulations governing health and safety, environment and waste and transport and reflect the most up-to-date recommendations, which lead to a unified approach across practice (Department of Health 2011).

Current European and UK legislation recommends adopting:

- a methodology for identifying and classifying infectious and medicinal waste
- a revised colour-coded best practice waste segregation and packaging system
- use of the European Waste Catalogue codes
- an offensive/hygiene waste stream to describe waste that is non-infectious (Department of Health 2011).

All staff involved in waste management have a duty of care to ensure it is dealt with correctly from the point of production to the point of disposal (Department of Health 2011).

Types of waste within theatres include:

- domestic – general household waste that is suitable for disposal by landfill
- clinical waste – produced from healthcare activities such as human tissue, blood or body fluids, excretions, swabs and dressings, syringes, needles or other sharp instruments that if not rendered safe may prove hazardous and could cause infection to anyone coming into contact with it (Department of Health 2011)
- medicinal waste that includes any expired, unused or contaminated pharmaceutical products, drugs and vaccines (Cytotoxic and cytostatic waste is treated separately as not all waste facilities are able to process these.)
- sharps – items that can cause cuts or puncture wounds and include suture needles, syringes with needles attached, scalpels and blades, glass ampoules and the sharps from infusion sets (Department of Health 2011).

It is important staff have training and education to deal with waste appropriately to avoid injury or contamination. Training should include:

- risks associated with waste
- segregation and handling of waste
- use of personal protective equipment (PPE) and personal hygiene
- storage and collection protocols
- day-to-day procedures
- procedures for spillages, accidents and emergencies.

> **BOX 4.2**
>
> **Key principles in waste management**
>
> - Access to equipment to include colour coded receptacles
> - Location of waste receptacles close to the point of waste production
> - Replacing receptacles when three-quarters full
> - Securely sealing receptacles using a swan neck and a plastic tie
> - Labelling receptacles to indicate their origin
> - Ensuring collection occurs on a frequent basis
> - Transport of waste in sealed containers that are washable and disinfection
> - Use of gels to solidify liquids before disposal
> - Correct use of PPE when dealing with all aspects of waste
> - Secure storage of waste ready for collection.

References

AfPP (Association for Perioperative Practice) (2007) *Standards and Recommendations*. Harrogate: AfPP.

AfPP (2008) *Standards and Recommendations for Surgery in Primary Care*. Harrogate: AfPP.

Department of Health (2003) *Getting the Right Start: National Service Framework for Children, Young People and Maternity Services. Standard for Hospital Services*. London: Department of Health.

Department of Health (2011) *Health Technical Memorandum 07-01: Safe Management of Healthcare Waste*. http://www.dh.gov.uk/en/Publicationsandstatistics/Publications/PublicationsPolicyAndGuidance/DH_126345 (accessed March 2012).

Gilmour D (2005) Infection control principles. In: Woodhead K and Wicker P (eds) *A Textbook of Perioperative Care*. Edinburgh: Elsevier.

Hospital Infection Society (2004) *Behaviours and Rituals in the Operating Theatre*. www.his.org.uk/resource_library/operating_theatres.cfm (accessed 4 December 2011).

Hospital Infection Society (2005) *Microbiological Commissioning and Monitoring of Operating Theatre Suites*. www.his.org.uk/resource_library/operating _theatres.cfm (accessed 4 December 2011).

Hughes SJ and Mardell A (eds) (2009) *Oxford Handbook of Perioperative Practice*. Oxford: Oxford University Press.

NHS Estates (1994) *Health Technical Memorandum 2025: Ventilation in Healthcare Premises, Design Considerations*. London: The Stationery Office.

NHS Estates (2005) *Health Building Note 26: Facilities for Surgical Procedures*, Vol. 1. London: Stationery Office.

NHS Estates (2007) *Health Building Note 10-02: Surgery. Day Surgery Facilities*. London: Department of Health Estates and Facilities Division.

Weaving P, Cox F and Milton S (2008) Infection prevention and control in the operating theatre. *Journal of Perioperative Practice* 18(5): 199–204.

Williams M. (2008). Infection prevention in perioperative practice. *Journal of Perioperative Practice* 18(7): 274–278.

Section 2

Infection Prevention in Perioperative Care

CHAPTER 5

Infection Prevention

Martin Kiernan

The prevention of transmission of microorganisms is of paramount importance in the perioperative setting. Although it is easy to think that infection prevention measures are primarily focused on minimising the risk of surgical site infections, these procedures and actions will additionally protect staff working in the perioperative environment. In addition to infection prevention being fundamental to patient safety, the occupational risks of the potential exposure to blood and body fluids must be considered. Standard precautions should be applied consistently in all settings and for all patients to ensure that all parties are protected from the transmission of potential pathogens.

Control of Substances Hazardous to Health

In the UK, potential risks of infection transmission are embodied in legislation centring on health and safety. The Control of Substances Hazardous to Health (commonly known as COSHH) Regulations (Statutory Instruments 2002), which are further supported by a code of practice (Health and Safety Executive 2005) covers agents likely to cause infection if transmitted. Further advice is available from a publication from the Advisory Committee on Dangerous Pathogens (2005). The legislation recommends risk assessment when there is the likelihood of contact with potential pathogens and states that such assessments must be 'suitable and sufficient'.

Risk Assessment in the Perioperative Environment

The Advisory Committee on Dangerous Pathogens (2005) recommends that any risk assessment should:

- reflect the nature of the work activity being assessed: the more hazardous a scenario, the more in-depth the assessment required
- draw on specialist advice as required (e.g. from the infection control department, health and safety advisors)

Manual of Perioperative Care: An Essential Guide, First Edition. Edited by Kate Woodhead and Lesley Fudge.
© 2012 John Wiley & Sons, Ltd. Published 2012 by John Wiley & Sons, Ltd.

- consider all those who may be affected by the work
- anticipate foreseeable risks
- be appropriate to the nature of the work and identify how long the assessment is likely to remain valid.

Control of risks normally falls into one of three categories:

1. The risk should be eliminated where possible (not possible in many theatre scenarios), generally applies to the laboratory setting.
2. The risk should be controlled at source, for example by using safety devices to prevent sharps injuries.
3. The risk should be controlled by the implementation of safe systems of working, for example by the implementation of hand hygiene policies or the use of personal protective equipment (PPE) to minimise the risk. Note that the legislation states that this should be the last resort if elimination or control at source is not possible.

Standard Precautions

In order to maintain practice that is safe for all who enter the perioperative environment, a standard set of precautions is advised for all situations. Standard precautions are a minimum set of protective measures that protect both the patient and the member of staff from the transmission of pathogens, reducing the risk of cross-infection. Microorganisms can be found both on intact skin and in body fluids and the strict adherence to standard precautions for all patients during all procedures will mitigate the risk of transmission of pathogens in either direction. Standard precautions apply to all actual and potential contacts with blood and other body fluids, including excretions and secretions and regardless of whether blood is evident. They also apply to contact with mucous membranes and non-intact skin.

Personal Protective Equipment

In addition to the use of scrupulous hand hygiene, standard precautions comprise the use of appropriate personal protective equipment, also known as PPE. Hand hygiene is important, especially following the removal of any items of PPE. The most commonly used items of PPE are gloves, which should be robust, the correct size and appropriate for the specific purpose. Other items of PPE that may be used will depend on a risk assessment of the potential pathogens that could be encountered and the procedure to be undertaken, where likely exposures can be considered. Plastic aprons and/or impervious gowns will protect from contamination with body fluids and if there is a risk of splashing onto facial mucous membranes a mask and eye protection should be used. The eye protection may take the form of goggles, a face shield or a combined mask and face shield. On rare occasions, leg and shoe covering may be necessary and these should be available.

All employers have a duty of care to undertake risk assessments of potential hazards that may present to staff members and to take steps to mitigate these risks. No staff member should be expected to work without access to the appropriate level of protective equipment.

The physical perioperative environment

The maintenance of a comfortable theatre environment is important to both patients and staff members. The factors that control this are temperature, humidity and the movement of air (Humphreys 1993). The room temperature should be maintained in the region of 19–23 °C (Department of Health 2007), which is comfortable for staff, reduces the risk of patients becoming excessively cooled and inhibiting for bacterial growth. In the USA it has been suggested that the relative humidity should be maintained at between 30% and 60%, as a lower humidity dries the air, resulting in excess dust and a higher humidity may result a moisture-rich environment that can promote fungal growth (American Institute of Architects 2006). In the UK it has been recommended that this humidity be maintained in the similar region of 30–65% (Department of Health 2007).

Ventilation

Specialised ventilation has been used in operating theatres for over 50 years. Positive pressure ventilation, where air flows from clean areas outward to less critical zones, has been in use since the 1940s. Some theatres are designated as ultra-clean air theatres, however there is no evidence that supports the raising of the standard of plenum (or conventional) ventilation in surgery that does not involve the placement of an implant (Humphreys and Taylor 2002).

The purpose of theatre ventilation is to reduce the opportunity for contamination of the wound, operative field and instruments from bacteria that may be present in the air. An effective ventilation system achieves this in two ways: by preventing contaminated air from entering the theatre through the use of positive pressure and by achieving the recommended amount of air changes so that the contamination arising from the particles of human skin generated within the room is diluted (Hoffman *et al.* 2002). Although older theatres often achieve 20 air changes (a volume of air that is equivalent to 20 times the volume of the room should be provided by the system per hour), modern theatres (and those undergoing major refurbishment) should achieve the new standard of 25 changes per hour (Department of Health 2007). It is simple to calculate the air change rate: a room that is 60 m³ supplied with 1200 m³ of air per hour has an air change rate of 1200 ÷ 60, which is 20 air changes per hour.

Conventional filters of Grade EU 7 should clean the air provided by the air-handling unit. HEPA (high-efficiency particulate air) filters are neither clinically justified nor cost-effective for conventional theatres. Economies concerning the use of theatre ventilation can be made, as the ventilation system can safely be turned off or the ventilation rate reduced (generally known as 'setback') when the theatre is not in use as long as the system is returned to a fully operational level from a reduced flow a minimum of 15 minutes before a procedure (or 30 minutes if the system is completely switched off) (Hoffman *et al.* 2002).

Laminar flow theatres

Some theatre suites have spaces that are designated as ultra-clean ventilated theatres. Also known as laminar flow theatres, in these rooms highly filtered air that is free from particles (and therefore bacteria) is passed down from a canopy in a unidirectional manner over the centre of the theatre, rapidly removing any contamination generated by the operating team and preventing air from outside the canopy from contaminating the area. The evidence for the use of filtered air for high-risk surgery dates from the 1980s (Lidwell *et al.* 1983), however much of the evidence relates to particle counts and bacteriological measurements rather than infection rates. More recent studies have found no difference in infection rates between surgery performed under laminar flow and conventional ventilation (Brandt *et al.* 2008). Although, therefore, the evidence base is inconclusive, most guidelines have adopted a pragmatic

Section 2

approach to the use of laminar flow and recommend the use of this form of ventilation for high-risk surgery when an implant is used.

Commissioning and validation

Although there is no internationally agreed standard on methods of sampling and limits that are tolerable (Dharan and Pittet 2002), regardless of whichever system of ventilation is present, all installations require commissioning to nationally acceptable standards prior to being put into use for patients. This validation process will include an estimation of the air change rate, warning systems for ventilation failures and indications of correct function and whether the system is on 'setback'. Visual checks of flow direction are made using smoke, which can also highlight areas of turbulence, for example around ceiling-mounted lighting or medical gas supplies.

Following successful commissioning, theatres are subject to an annual validation process at the time of servicing. This should also be carried out after any major repair work concerning the ventilation system (Hoffman *et al.* 2002).

Staff Movement within the Perioperative Environment

As with many other aspects of theatre practice (Woodhead *et al.* 2002), a high level of discipline with regard to staff movements will greatly reduce risks to vulnerable patients. It has long been established and accepted that bacterial counts that have been measured during surgery do fluctuate and are raised when large numbers of people are present during surgery or when there is an increase in activity levels (Ford *et al.* 1967). The levels of bacteria present in the air are at their peak during the initial phase of the procedure, where turbulence occurs as the patient is brought in and positioned (Ayliffe 1991). Staff movement around the theatre during the procedure also produces further turbulence, which affects the cleanliness of the air. Most good practice guides recommend the minimisation of staff movements during surgery (Association for Perioperative Practitioners 2011).

Cleaning and Ventilation for 'Dirty' or Infected Cases

If the ventilation is fully functional a theatre may be returned to use as soon as the local cleaning policy has been implemented, as a sufficient number of air changes will have taken place in approximately 30 minutes in the majority of theatre settings. The products used for cleaning after cases classed as 'dirty' or 'infected' will be detailed in local policies, which should always be adhered to. Special regard should be paid to dilution and reconstitution of any specialised disinfectant solutions to ensure that the effective concentration is achieved, and when applied the solution should remain in contact with surfaces for the recommended contact time.

Cleaning Routines

The inanimate environment that does not come into contact with patients presents little risk. Floors may be effectively cleaned using detergent and hot water at the end of each session and the use of sticky mats is unwarranted and undesirable. Any spillage of blood or body fluids should always be removed as speedily as possible. Wall washing is frequently performed in theatres, however this is for visual purposes and not infection control. Although cleaning is performed routinely in theatres at the end of each session, a periodic 'deep clean' where equipment that is more difficult to access without a degree of dismantling is good practice.

Aseptic Technique

Asepsis has been defined as the prevention of transmission of microorganisms, both to and from wounds, from healthcare workers' hands and other susceptible sites (Hill and Millward 2009). The maintenance of asepsis in the perioperative setting encompasses a range of procedures and actions, including the preparation of the patient, the cleansing of hands, the use of sterile instruments and the maintenance of the sterile field.

Surgical hand preparation and scrub

Hand hygiene has long regarded as one of the key constituents of any infection prevention and control strategy. Traditional surgical scrub techniques, where those involved in the surgical procedure ensure that hands, nails and parts of the forearm are lathered and scrubbed have been a standard practice for many years. Recent evidence suggests that the traditional ritual of scrubbing can be replaced by a more succinct, less ritualistic method. In a large study involving six surgical specialties and over 4000 consecutive patients who underwent clean and clean-contaminated surgery, there was no significant difference in the rate of surgical site infection regardless of whether the operator used a hand rub technique with 75% aqueous alcohol or a hand scrub protocol using either povidone–iodine or chlorhexidine.

Another key finding was that the alcohol rub solution was better tolerated and this was linked with improved compliance with the chosen protocol.

Theatre Attire

Although there is no evidence that theatre attire (generally known as scrubs) affects infection rates if gowning procedures and products are correctly used, it is considered good practice to remove personal clothing and to change into clean theatre attire. It is also recommended that sufficient supplies of scrubs are available to enable staff to change should they become soiled (Advisory Committee on Dangerous Pathogens 2005).

Surgical gowns

After a comprehensive review, the NICE Guideline Development Group (National Collaborating Centre for Women's and Children's Health 2008) found that is no evidence that any specific form of surgical attire reduces the risk of surgical site infection for patients. However, from a commonsense and practical point of view the recommendation was made that all persons within the operating team should wear a sterile gown during the procedure. The most important aspect of any gown is that it should be impervious to fluids, thus protecting both the patient, and importantly the staff who are at risk of body fluid exposure. There is no evidence as to whether single-use or reusable gowns present differing risks of infection, however as all surgical gowns and drapes are classed as medical devices, the ability of local reprocessing services to maintain compliance with modern standards such as BS EN13795 (European Committee for Standardization 2002) at each use of the items has meant that many organisations have converted to single-use systems.

Surgical gloves

Gloves are the barrier that separate the operators from contamination by blood and body fluids present in the operative field and the patient from bacterial flora present on the skin of those undertaking the procedure. The majority of gloves in use at the present time are composed of latex, which is increasingly being linked with allergic reactions. Other alternative materials of a suitable quality are now becoming available. All gloves used by the scrub team should be single-use and demonstrably sterile.

There has been much interest in double gloving as a method of reducing the risk of punctures, placing the patient and wearer at risk (Tanner and Parkinson 2006), however no study to date has demonstrated a reduction in the rate of surgical site infection when comparing single with double gloving. The NICE Guideline Development Group (National Collaborating Centre for Women's and Children's Health 2008) chose to adopt a pragmatic view when making recommendations with regard to double gloving and stated that operators should consider using two pairs of gloves where there is an increased risk of perforation (for example when using power tools or where the hands cannot be visualised) and where the consequences of any cross-contamination arising from glove perforation would be serious.

The Area of Sterility (the Sterile Field)

Following the completion of hand antisepsis and the donning of the sterile gown and gloves the Association for Perioperative Practitioners Standards recommend that scrubbed personnel should consider that the area between the gloved hands and forearms and the area between the nipple to the waist to be understood to be the area of sterility or sterile field (Association for Perioperative Practitioners 2011). Hands should never fall below the waist nor rise above the shoulder line and it is good practice to ensure that the hands of scrub staff remain visible at all times in order to prevent accidental contamination occurring.

Setting the Instrument Trolley

The instrument trolley is a critical area on which sterile instruments are placed prior to, during and after use in the operation. Laying up the trolley and the preparation of the instruments is a skilled procedure. The principles of asepsis must be adhered to during the setting of the trolley. For the practitioner undertaking these actions, the surgical procedure effectively begins at this point. A designated area that has sufficient space in which to open packs that are wrapped to maintain sterility should be used for this procedure. The area should have the same number of air changes that the case to be performed has and so if the case is to be undertaken in an ultra-clean theatre the instruments should be opened and set within the canopy area.

The same principles of limited staff movement also apply to minimise the risks of contamination (Association for Perioperative Practitioners 2011). Key principles are listed in Box 5.1.

Sharps Safety

Each year over 100 000 sharps injuries are recorded in the NHS (Trim and Elliott 2003) with attendant risks of the transmission of bloodborne infection to the injured party.

Section 2

> ## BOX 5.1
>
> ### Key principles of setting a trolley (Association for Perioperative Practitioners 2011)
>
> - All sterile packs should be checked for expiry date, integrity and sterility by both the scrub and the circulating practitioner.
> - Instrument packs should be opened as close as is possible to the time of use. The Association for Perioperative Practitioners do not recommend the pre-preparation of sterile trolleys with a sterile sheet cover due to the risk of contamination.
> - Trolleys should be covered with a minimum of two layers of sterile sheets that meet regulatory requirements.
> - All staff should be aware of the correct method of opening a sterile pack for presentation to the scrubbed person.
> - When the circulating person opens the external wrapping, the furthermost flap should be opened first and the nearest wrap last. Outer wraps should be held back or otherwise secured in order to prevent contamination when presenting a sterile item to the scrubbed person.
> - When the circulating person opens the inner wrapping the pack is opened towards themselves initially and then away from the body to avoid contamination.
> - Items to be passed to the scrubbed person should always be passed at the edge of the sterile field and should be passed in a way that prevents contamination of the sterile gloves by external wrappings.
> - Items should always be passed and never dropped onto the sterile field.
> - When solutions are poured, the receiving container should either be placed on the trolley edge or be held by the scrubbed person. Once a container has been opened, the edge of the container should be considered to be contaminated and sterility can no longer be guaranteed.
> - Sharps should always be opened into a container in order to reduce the risk of sharps injury or damage to the drapes.
> - Should any item be considered to have been at risk of contamination, for example by hanging over the sterile field it should not be brought back into the sterile field.
> - If there has been any break in asepsis this must be reported immediately. The contaminated item(s) should immediately be removed without compromising the sterility of the rest of the equipment and re-gloving and re-draping carried out as necessary.

Despite information on these risks being widely disseminated, the number of injuries that go unreported is substantial, with one study looking at surgeon reporting of sharps injury noting that over 50% of surgeons questioned had experienced an injury but had not reported it (Kerr *et al.* 2009). Worryingly, this study also found that only 15% of surgeons were consistently adopting all of the three principles of sharps safety and prevention of percutaneous contamination: double gloving, face shields and a hands-free technique.

The hands-free technique, in which sharps are passed in a neutral zone (often a designated tray), has been demonstrated to reduce sharps injuries and associated percutaneous contamination by 60% (Stringer *et al.* 2002), yet these authors found that this technique was only used in 42% of operations.

All organisations will have detailed policies and procedures that are intended to protect staff from sharps injury, yet these polices are not adhered to. One study showed that seniority seemed to be a factor in adherence to policy, with 93% of consultants, 67% of junior medical staff and 13% of other perioperative practitioners not complying with local protocols (Adams *et al.* 2010). The two main reasons cited for the lack of compliance were given as the length of time it takes to do so (48%) and a low perception of risk of infection from the patient (78%). Local procedures should take these factors into account in order to increase compliance with policies that are intended to protect the health of staff and all perioperative practitioners should familiarise themselves with local procedures.

Patient Preparation

The purpose of patient preparation prior to an operative procedure is to reduce the risk of endogenous skin flora contaminating the surgical field with infection as a consequence. Prior to any surgical procedure it is good practice to wash the skin with soap and water (preferably in the form of a shower), as the effects of the soap are to remove dirt and break down skin oils before an antiseptic solution is applied. There is also a growing body of literature that suggests that there are benefits to showering with an antiseptic soap preparation with iodine (Finkelstein *et al.* 2005) or chlorhexidine gluconate (Milstone *et al.* 2008) in the immediate preoperative period and even the period prior to admission, as chlorhexidine has been demonstrated to have a cumulative and persistent effect on the skin (Edmiston *et al.* 2008). The optimal duration and frequency of preoperative showering is as yet unknown (Jakobsson *et al.* 2011).

Organism-specific risk assessment and patient preparation

Although many patients are now screened for specific organisms such as MRSA (methicillin-resistant *Staphylococcus aureus*), it should be remembered that these tests are for screening purposes and are not 100% specific or sensitive. All patients undergoing surgery should be risk-assessed for the potential for carriage of certain organisms. For example, a risk assessment for MRSA should include: number of healthcare contacts (for example, frequent admissions to hospital), nursing/care home residency, presence of chronic wounds and other long-term indwelling medical devices (for example, urinary catheters). If emergency surgery is required, the results of the screening test may not be available. The risk assessment should ensure that appropriate and effective antibiotic prophylaxis is given and that specific transmission-based measures, for example contact precautions, are implemented throughout the patient's journey through the perioperative area.

Antiseptic preparations for the skin

Although the skin can never be sterilised, immediately before the surgery commences, the skin is normally cleansed with an antiseptic solution. Lister's pioneering work with antiseptics in this area (Lister 1867) enabled complex and time-consuming surgery to be undertaken with a greatly reduced risk of infection as a postoperative complication (which at the time normally resulted in the death of the patient as no treatments were available).

The purpose of the antiseptic solutions used to prepare the skin surface is to eradicate organisms in skin fissures and crevices that would not easily be removed by using soap and water. Both iodine and chlorhexidine have been found to be effective in reducing skin flora to a level that minimises the risk of infection and each of these antiseptics has historically had its champion groups of users. Iodine has the advantage of tinting the skin, enabling the person applying the solution to check that all areas have been covered, but chlorhexidine has the considerable advantage of having a demonstrably persistent effect, prolonging the effectiveness of the solution. Both are available in either aqueous or alcoholic preparations, although alcohol-based solutions have been the subject of hazard reports when excessive amounts of the solution have been used and allowed to pool underneath the patient, presenting a fire hazard when diathermy is used.

Until relatively recently there has been a lack of robust studies that have looked at the comparative efficacies of iodine and chlorhexidine in reducing infection rates. Dairouiche and colleagues (2010) performed a study of the effectiveness of alcoholic chlorhexidine when compared with aqueous povidone–iodine, reporting findings that demonstrated a significant reduction in the infection rate when the chlorhexidine solution was used. Although this study would have been improved by comparing alcohol-based solutions of both antiseptics, the authors took a pragmatic approach to the study by comparing the most widely used skin preparations in order to improve acceptance of the findings. The study has been considered of sufficient merit to have been included in a number of surgical guidelines, including those produced by the English Department of Health's 'Saving Lives' care bundle programme (Department of Health 1999).

Skin preparation procedures

The area to be covered by the skin preparation should always cover the area of the incision and a significant area around this, ensuring that all of the skin areas exposed when the drapes are applied have been covered. Care should be taken to ensure that any additional or anticipated incisions or sites that may be used for wound drainage are also treated. Solutions should not be allowed to pool or to contaminate other items of equipment, for example tourniquet cuffs, diathermy electrodes or other patient-monitoring equipment.

If the skin is intact, the actual incision site should be prepped first, moving outwards to the other areas. The most contaminated areas should be prepared last. The chosen solution should be in contact with the skin surface for the time period recommended by the manufacturer, as any antiseptic is effective when the correct dilution is used for the correct contact time. All prepped areas should reach the contact time before any drapes are applied.

Preoperative hair removal

Hair removal is occasionally necessary in order to be able to gain unhindered access to the operative field, although it is recognised that sometimes hair is removed because of a perception that it presents an increased risk of infection. Shaving has until recently been the traditional method of hair removal, however this procedure can damage the skin and such injury may cause increased risk of infection by producing microscopic infected abrasions to the skin surface that can become colonised by organisms not normally found at the site by the time the operative procedure takes place.

The relative effects of different methods of hair removal have long been described; for example, a seminal study in the 1970s reported an infection rate of 2.3% in shaved patients and a lower rate (1.7%) in patients who had their hair clipped (Cruse and Foord 1973). Patients who were not clipped or shaved had the lowest infection rate of all of the groups under study (0.9%). Prior to that study, others had also reported an infection rate of 5.6% in shaved patients, whereas in unshaved patients or where depilation was used the rate was 0.6% (Seropian and Reynolds 1971).

The timing of hair removal is also significant (Alexander *et al*. 1983). A lower infection rate has been reported in patients who had hair removal by clipping on the morning of surgery as opposed to the night before both at discharge and 30 days follow-up.

These methods have been subject to a systematic review of the published studies, which concluded that should hair removal be absolutely necessary, clippers are the preferred method (Tanner *et al*. 2006). Interestingly, even though most guidelines now recommend using chemical hair removal, followed by clipping with a single-use device or clipper head as close to the operation as possible, the NICE Guideline Group (National Collaborating Centre for Women's and Children's Health 2008) reported that opportunities for research still remain, as they found no studies that compared clipping with no hair removal or compared clipping with chemical hair removal.

> **BOX 5.2**
>
> **NICE Recommendation: category 1**
>
> Only the area to be incised needs to be shaved, and if this cannot be done by depilatory cream the day before operation, it should be done in the anaesthetic room immediately preoperatively, using clippers rather than a razor. Shaving brushes should not be used.
>
> - Avoid shaving if at all possible
> - Use depilatory cream, if this is not possible, then use clippers
> - Only shave if other options are not possible

Drapes and their application

Surgical drapes are medical devices (European Committee for Standardization 2002) that are used primarily as a barrier to separate the operative field from the rest of the patient and the theatre environment. They allow a discrete area to be effectively prepared aseptically prior to surgery commencing and facilitating the maintenance of the integrity of this area during the procedure. This area is commonly known as the 'sterile field'. In addition to the patient, this field may also cover the furniture and other equipment, for example Mayo tables and other tables used to lay instruments on.

The drapes also have the effect of protecting the staff undertaking the procedure from contamination with blood and body fluids and, like gowns, they should be made of fluid-repellent materials. In the early days of surgery all drapes were simply white sheets. The change to green as the most predominant colour for drapes can be traced back to Berkley Moynihan (later to become Lord Moynihan), who wrote a letter to the *Lancet* stating:

> For the last two and a half years I have used towels and sheets of green colour instead of white. Green is a restful colour, offers no sharp contrast to the colours of the wound surfaces, and allows ligatures and sutures to be clearly seen against it. (Moynihan 1915)

He went on to have his theatre walls and floors painted in the same colour.

The evidence base as to whether drapes are effective at all and the relative merits of disposable vs. reusable drapes is particularly poor. No study has demonstrated a significant difference between reusable and single-use drapes, however the complexities of organisations maintaining compliance with BS EN 13795 (European Committee for Standardization 2002), where the reprocessor effectively becomes a manufacturer who must be able to demonstrate compliance with the standard at each use has meant that there has been a widespread switch to disposable drapes. Where reusable drapes are used, there should be a system that enables the tracking of the number of uses of each item, as continual washing and sterilisation will cause the patency of the material to deteriorate. Some materials may take up to 75 washes for this to occur, whereas untreated materials may become porous after only 30 cycles (Association for Perioperative Practitioners 2011).

The tests that are carried out to demonstrate compliance with the European Standard are comprehensive and have to be achieved in order for products to be awarded the essential CE mark.

There may be other desirable aspects of drapes that should be considered when selecting the most appropriate drape. Maintenance of body temperature during the procedure, glare reduction, ease of use, conformability, fire retardancy and antistatic features are all desirable features of surgical drapes.

> **BOX 5.3**
>
> **Tests to demonstrate compliance with EN 13796**
>
> - Cleanliness: microbial and particulate matter
> - Resistance to microbial penetration: wet and dry
> - Burst strength: wet and dry
> - Tensile strength: wet and dry
> - Resistance to liquid penetration
> - Lint production
> - Adhesion

> **BOX 5.4**
>
> **Desirable properties of incise drapes**
>
> - Allow an incision to be made with ease
> - Impermeable to bacterial ingress
> - Good adherence to the skin for the duration of the operation
> - Hypo-allergenic
> - Flexible to allow movement of the patient and skin during surgery
> - Transparent to allow the skin to be visualised
> - Permeable to water vapour, allowing the skin to breathe
> - Impregnated with iodophors to prevent recolonisation of the skin margins

Incise drapes

Additional to the use of general drapes, incise drapes may be used to further enhance this effect. Incise drapes are adhesive films that are used to cover the site of the incision, providing a barrier to the remaining skin. The theory behind this is to reduce the risk of contamination of the operative field by flora recolonising the patient's skin around the procedure site. Although some studies have noted that the use of non-antiseptic impregnated incise drapes slightly increase the risk of infection, this risk is mitigated by the use of iodophor-impregnated films and these have been recommended by the NICE Guideline Group (National Collaborating Centre for Women's and Children's Health 2008). If an iodophor-impregnated film is to be used, the potential allergic status of the patient should be ascertained prior to its application.

The draping procedure

Draping takes place following the positioning of the patient on the theatre table. The following principles should be followed when applying drapes:

- The team applying the drapes should have a detailed understanding of the procedure and have planned the application of drapes before the procedure is commenced.
- The drapes are applied after the skin has been prepared.
- The drapes must be sterile and intact at the time of draping.
- Drapes should be folded over the gloved hand in order to prevent contamination of the glove by touching a patient.
- Drapes should be placed with a minimum disturbance to the air; they should not be shaken, as this may result in abnormal air currents and lint (fibres from the material that the drape is made from) production and dispersal.

- Drapes are first applied to the operative area and then the surrounding areas are covered.
- Once placed, a drape should not be removed by scrubbed staff. If this is necessary, a circulating person may undertake this and then the area should be re-draped by the scrub team.
- Penetrating towel clips should not be removed until the end of the procedure.
- If there is ever any doubt as to the sterility of a drape it should not be used.

Once the drapes have been applied and the sterile field defined, only scrubbed persons should work in this area. The drapes should remain in place until the sterile postoperative wound dressing has been applied or a sealed wound has been achieved. The scrub practitioner has been recommended as the person of choice to dispose of all drapes into the appropriate bags for disposal or reprocessing while they are still gloved and gowned (Association for Perioperative Practitioners 2011).

References

Adams S, Stojkovic SG and Leveson SH (2010) Needlestick injuries during surgical procedures: a multidisciplinary online study. *Occupational Medicine* 60(2): 139–144.

Advisory Committee on Dangerous Pathogens (2005) *Biological Agents: Managing the risks in laboratories and healthcare premises*. London: Health and Safety Executive.

Alexander JW, Fischer JE, Boyajian M, Palmquist J and Morris MJ (1983) The influence of hair-removal methods on wound infections. *Archives of Surgery* 118(3): 347–352.

American Institute of Architects (2006) *Guidelines for Design and Construction of Health Care Facilities*. Washington, DC: American Institute of Architects Committee on Architecture for Health.

Association for Perioperative Practitioners (2011) *Standards and Recommendations for Perioperative Practice*. Harrogate: AfPP.

Ayliffe GA (1991) Role of the environment of the operating suite in surgical wound infection. *Reviews in Infectious Disease* 13(Suppl 10): S800–804.

Brandt C, Hott U, Sohr D, Daschner F, Gastmeier P and Ruden H (2008) Operating room ventilation with laminar airflow shows no protective effect on the surgical site infection rate in orthopedic and abdominal surgery. *Annals of Surgery* 248: 695–700.

Cruse PJ and Foord R (1973) A five-year prospective study of 23,649 surgical wounds. *Archives of Surgery* 107(2): 206–210.

Darouiche RO, Wall MJ, Jr., Itani KM *et al.* (2010) Chlorhexidine-alcohol versus povidone-iodine for surgical-site antisepsis. *New England Journal of Medicine* 362(1): 18–26.

Department of Health (1999) *Saving Lives: Our healthier nation*. http://www.dh.gov.uk/en/Publicationsandstatistics/Publications/PublicationsPolicyAndGuidance/DH_4008701 (accessed March 2012).

Department of Health (2007) *Health Technical Memorandum 03-01: Specialised Ventilation for Healthcare Premises. Part A: design and validation*. London: Department of Health, Estates and Facilities Division.

Dharan S and Pittet D (2002) Environmental controls in operating theatres. *Journal of Hospital Infection* 51(2): 79–84.

Edmiston C, Krepel C, Seabrook G, Lewis B, Brown K and Towne J (2008) Preoperative shower revisited: can high topical antiseptic levels be achieved on the skin surface before surgical admission? *Journal of the American College of Surgeons* 207(2): 233–239.

European Committee for Standardization (2002) *BS EN 13795-1 Part 1: Surgical Drapes, Gowns and Clean Air Suits Used as Medical Devices for Patients, Clinical Staff and Equipment*. Brussels: CEN.

Finkelstein R, Rabino G, Mashiah T *et al.* (2005) Surgical site infection rates following cardiac surgery: the impact of a 6-year infection control program. *American Journal of Infection Control* 33(8): 450–454.

Ford CR, Peterson DE and Mitchell CR (1967) Microbiological studies of air in the operating room. *Journal of Surgical Research* 7(8): 376–382.

Health and Safety Executive (2005) Control of substances hazardous to health. The Control of Substances Hazardous to Health Regulations 2002 (as amended). *Approved Code of Practice and Guidance* L5, 5th edn. London: Health and Safety Executive, HSE Books.

Hill D and Millward S (2009) Prevention of infection in wards and outpatient departments. In Fraise AP and Bradley C (eds) *Ayliffe's Control of Healthcare-Associated Infection*. London: Hodder Arnold.

Hoffman PN, Williams J, Stacey A *et al.* (2002) Microbiological commissioning and monitoring of operating theatre suites. *Journal of Hospital Infection* 52(1): 1–28.

Humphreys H (1993) Infection control and the design of a new operating theatre suite. *Journal of Hospital Infection* 23(1): 61–70.

Humphreys H and Taylor EW (2002) Operating theatre ventilation standards and the risk of postoperative infection. *Journal of Hospital Infection* 50(2): 85–90.

Jakobsson J, Perlkvist A and Wann-Hansson C (2011) Searching for evidence regarding using preoperative disinfection showers to prevent surgical site infections: a systematic review. *Worldviews on evidence based nursing/Sigma Theta Tau International, Honor Society of Nursing* 8(3): 143–152.

Kerr HL, Stewart N, Pace A and Elsayed S (2009) Sharps injury reporting amongst surgeons. *Annals of the Royal College of Surgeons of England* 91(5): 430–432.

Lidwell OM, Lowbury EJ, Whyte W, Blowers R, Stanley SJ and Lowe D (1983) Airborne contamination of wounds in joint replacement operations: the relationship to sepsis rates. *Journal of Hospital Infection* 4(2): 111–131.

Lister J (1867) On the antiseptic principle in surgery. *Lancet* 2: 353–356.

Milstone AM, Passaretti CL and Perl TM (2008) Chlorhexidine: expanding the armamentarium for infection control and prevention. *Clinical Infectious Diseases* 46(2): 274–281.

Moynihan B (1915) A green background for the operation area. *Lancet* Sept 11th: 595.

National Collaborating Centre for Women's and Children's Health (2008) *Clinical Guideline 74: Surgical Site Infection.* London: National Institute for Health and Clinical Excellence.

Seropian R and Reynolds BM (1971) Wound infections after preoperative depilatory versus razor preparation. *American Journal of Surgery* 121(3): 251–254.

Statutory Instruments (2002) *Control of Substances Hazardous to Health Regulations.* Health and Safety Executive. London: The Stationery Office.

Stringer B, Infante-Rivard C and Hanley JA (2002) Effectiveness of the hands-free technique in reducing operating theatre injuries. *Occupational and Environmental Medicine* 59(10): 703–707.

Tanner J and Parkinson H (2006) Double gloving to reduce surgical cross-infection. *Cochrane Database of Systematic Reviews* 3: CD003087.

Tanner J, Woodings G and Moncaster K (2006) Preoperative hair removal to reduce surgical site infection. *Cochrane Database of Systematic Reviews* 3: CD00412.

Trim JC and Elliott TS (2003) A review of sharps injuries and preventative strategies. *Journal of Hospital Infection* 53(4): 237–242.

Woodhead K, Taylor EW, Bannister G, Chesworth T, Hoffman P and Humphreys H (2002) Behaviours and rituals in the operating theatre. A report from the Hospital Infection Society Working Party on Infection Control in Operating Theatres. *Journal of Hospital Infection* 51(4): 241–255.

Section 2

CHAPTER 6

Introduction to Decontamination and Sterilisation

Wayne Spencer

What is Decontamination and Sterilisation

Decontamination is defined as the combination of processes (including cleaning, disinfection and sterilisation) used to make a reusable item safe for further use on service users and for handling by staff (Department of Health 2010). The unfortunate term 'service users' (a product of the quoted document's need to reflect the wider social care context of the intended audience) can, in the context of this book, be taken to mean 'patients'. In past years decontamination has been taken to mean the cleaning element alone but the term is now almost universally taken to mean the whole cycle of making a used surgical instrument or medical device fit for use on subsequent patients.

Cleaning, as the first step in both the definition and most processes, is widely accepted as the removal of contamination from an item to the extent necessary for its further processing (and in the case of some low-risk medical devices for its intended subsequent use). *Disinfection* is defined in the relevant European standard for washer–disinfectors as a reduction of the number of viable microorganisms on a product to a level previously specified as appropriate for its intended further handling or use (ISO BS EN ISO 15883; International Standards Organization 2009). *Sterilisation*, however, has a much more rigidly described definition. Within the European standard for sterility it defines sterile as being of a state free from viable microorganisms (British Standards Institute 2001).

In practice these three distinct processes are often applied sequentially in combination with the ultimate aim of producing a sterile instrument. In some cases the first two stages alone (cleaning and disinfection) may be sufficient. The decision as to which of these processes is the final one is often made on the basis of the Spaulding Classification. The system is based on the patient's risk for infection that various types of intervention can create. A modified form has been adopted by the Medicines and Healthcare products Regulatory Agency (MHRA) in their guidance from their Microbiology Advisory Committee, commonly called the MAC manual (MHRA 2010) (Table 6.1).

Manual of Perioperative Care: An Essential Guide, First Edition. Edited by Kate Woodhead and Lesley Fudge.
© 2012 John Wiley & Sons, Ltd. Published 2012 by John Wiley & Sons, Ltd.

Table 6.1   Classification of infection risk associated with the decontamination of medical devices (Spaulding 1972).

Risk	Application of item	Recommendation
High	• In close contact with a break in the skin or mucous membrane • Introduced into sterile body areas	Sterilisation
Intermediate	• In contact with mucous membranes • Contaminated with particularly virulent or readily transmissible organisms • Prior to use on immunocompromised patients	Sterilisation or disinfection required Cleaning may be acceptable in some agreed evidence-based situations
Low	• In contact with healthy skin • Not in contact with patient	Cleaning

The Need for Decontamination and Sterilisation

Decontamination is an issue of public health importance due to both concerns about preventing healthcare-associated infection and the increased focus on healthcare standards. The MHRA recently issued a device alert stating that it had received a coroner's report which found that a patient death was caused by a failure to decontaminate a laryngoscope handle appropriately between each patient use. This led to cross-infection and subsequently septicaemia (MHRA 2011). There are undeniable links between failures in decontamination processes and patient infection.

The key to the need for decontamination lies within the definition used earlier. It says 'make a reusable item safe for further use' and it is this safety for reuse that drives the need. If we are to ensure that one patient's microorganisms (no matter how benign) are not passed to another then successful decontamination is essential. In recent times minimising the risk of iatrogenic transmission of variant Creutzfeldt–Jakob disease (vCJD) has brought the cleaning part of the decontamination regime into sharp focus. In 1999 the Department of Health issued a circular stating that cleaning is of the utmost importance in minimising the risk of transmitting this agent via surgical instruments (Department of Health 1999).

A Brief History of Decontamination and Sterilisation

In 1878 Robert Koch demonstrated the usefulness of steam for sterilising instruments, and by 1880 Charles Chamberland had built the first autoclave using steam under pressure. By 1960 vacuum sterilisers had become readily available, although their use for surgical instruments did not become widespread until later in the decade.

Until the mid 1960s instruments and dressings were often sterilised separately, with dressings and gowns being processed in a large dressings steriliser and instruments sterilised at the point of use and often within boiling water sterilisers. At this stage the cleaning process was manual and undertaken in a multipurpose sink. Bowie *et al.* (1963) published a paper describing a combined dressing and instrument tray system which they named the Edinburgh Pre-set Tray System. This is still in use in many hospitals today although most have moved to a system of pure instrument trays, with consumables and textiles supplied separately as pre-sterile items. Only a few years previously an article by Allison (1960) had outlined the work that had been undertaken in Belfast in developing a full central sterilised supply department that reprocessed everything from dressings and syringes to composite packs of theatre instruments and drapes. This became the blueprint for the future. At this stage, however, the reprocessing of single theatre instruments and bowls was still advocated within the theatre area.

By the early 1990s many hospitals had also moved the reprocessing of the remaining theatre instruments to centralised departments and had adopted the use of automated wash processes. With the publication of Health Technical Memorandum (HTM) 2030 (Department of Health 1997), the validation of cleaning and disinfection processes came to a level equivalent to that of the steriliser.

The Legislative Framework

European Directives (MDD) and the Consumer Protection Act

The European legislative framework regarding reusable surgical instruments and their reprocessing is the Medical Devices Directive MDD93/42/ECC (European Community 1993). This covers the placing on the market (not necessarily for sale or reward) of any medical devices within Europe. A number of amendments have since been introduced, the most recent being Directive 2007/47/EC (European Community 2007). The Medical Device Regulations implement the directives in UK law. The regulations have been enacted under the Consumer Protection Act 1987 and therefore there is a direct link between the reprocessing of a medical device and consumer protection. The Medical Device Directives have little technical content other than essential requirements. These make it clear that devices must not compromise the health or safety of the patient, user or any other person. The CE mark that appears on a medical device or on its packaging means that the device satisfies the relevant essential requirements and is fit for its intended purpose as specified by the manufacturer.

The Role of the Medicines and Healthcare products Regulatory Agency in sterilisation

The Directive sets out a role in each European member state called the Competent Authority. The Competent Authority is the body responsible for implementing the requirements of the Directives in each country. In the UK, this is the MHRA. Their role is to ensure that manufacturers comply with the regulations and to evaluate adverse incident reports received from manufacturers of medical devices. Any hospital decontaminating a surgical instrument (which is a medical device) which makes that instrument available to another organisation to use would, in most cases, need to be registered with the MHRA as a manufacturer of a medical device.

Harmonised European standards

European standards that are accepted as meeting the essential requirements of the Directive are referred to as harmonised standards. Medical devices reprocessed in line with such standards will generally be presumed to comply with the relevant essential requirements in the Directive. Since the application of harmonised standards is voluntary, somebody reprocessing a surgical instrument may choose alternative methods of demonstrating compliance. For example, they may use international, national or in-house standards. Within the UK, where a robust system of national guidance around sterilisation exists, an organisation sterilising instruments may decide to use that guidance as its route to demonstrating compliance with the essential requirements. However if it does so then it should satisfy itself that the guidance does address the requirements in full.

National Standards and Compliance

Code of Practice on Healthcare Associated Infection and its impact on decontamination

In 2006 the Health Act passed into UK legislation and with it came the 'Code of Practice for the Prevention and Control of Health Care Associated Infections'. Since renamed the 'Code of Practice on the prevention and control of infections and related guidance' (Department of Health 2010), it sets out a series of core requirements providing the National Framework for decontamination regulation. It stipulates that an organisation must have a lead for decontamination and for there to be a decontamination policy. It also requires that:

- decontamination of reusable medical devices takes place in appropriate facilities
- appropriate procedures are followed for the acquisition, maintenance and validation of decontamination equipment
- staff are trained in decontamination processes and hold appropriate competences for their role and
- a record-keeping regime is in place to ensure that decontamination processes are fit for purpose and use the required quality systems.

Importantly, it contains the following paragraph:

> Reusable medical devices should be decontaminated in accordance with manufacturers' instructions and current national or local best practice guidance. This must ensure that the device complies with the 'essential requirements' provided in the Medical Devices Regulations 2002 where applicable. This requires that the device should be clean and, where appropriate, sterilised at the end of the decontamination process and maintained in a clinically satisfactory condition up to the point of use.

The key point here is the link to the essential requirements of the MDD regardless of any mention of placing on the market or registration with the MHRA. Therefore whether a hospital sees itself as a supplier to other organisations or not, it should still meet the requirements of the Directive.

Regulation regimes including the Care Quality Commission role

The Regulated Activities Regulations 2010 (Department of Health 2010) set out the requirements for registration of a Health or Social Care provider. The Care Quality Commission, as the regulator, has the responsibility for making sure that the care that people receive meets essential standards of quality and safety. Regulation 16 (Safety, availability and suitability of equipment) requires that organisations make suitable arrangements to protect patients and others who may be at risk from the use of unsafe medical devices. The CQC have powers of enforcement to bring about improvement in poor services, or to prevent a hospital from carrying out regulated activities.

Locations for Decontamination and Sterilisation

Role of centralised departments, local decontamination, on-site/off-site

Most decontamination of invasive surgical instruments is undertaken within purpose-designed centralised departments. These departments exist with a variety of names such as centralised sterile supply departments, hospital sterilisation and disinfection units and, more recently, sterile service departments. Occasionally some hospitals may have a sterile services department located just for operating theatres and these are often called theatre sterile supply units. The abbreviation SSD is used within this chapter to mean all of these.

In general, these departments process a mixture of theatre trays, supplementary instruments and other more general packs for wards and departments. Whereas 15 years ago most departments still provided a composite tray containing a mix of instruments, swabs and consumables, the current trend is for trays to contain instruments only (with other supplies being provided either by the SSD as separately packaged pre-sterile supplies or direct by the theatre).

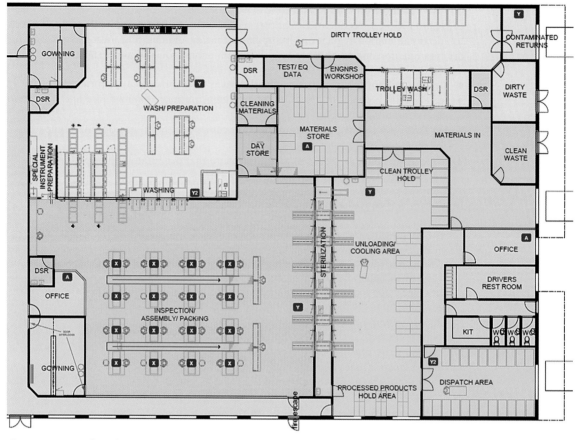

Figure 6.1   Typical sterile services department production area layout.

In 2002 the Department of Health in England embarked on a modernisation programme for decontamination (National Decontamination Programme 2003) whereby large off-site centres were procured that were operated by the private sector. These centres were typically located away from the hospital and served between 2 and 12 hospitals. They have become known as supercentres. The *Theatre Support Pack* (National Decontamination Programme 2009) provides advice on using an off-site service.

Local decontamination of invasive instruments has gradually been reduced to very low levels within hospitals although bench-top sterilisers remain in some small treatment centres and are used widely in dentistry. Most flexible endoscopes are processed within small local facilities typically adjacent to the endoscopy suite, although there is a current trend to create larger endoscopy reprocessing departments and to transport the endoscopes to the point of use in specially designed trolleys.

Decontamination facility requirements

The Department of Health published a design guide to SSDs called Health Building Note (HBN) 13 (Department of Health 2004). The document sets out the rooms required, suggests a typical floor layout and offers advice as to the mechanical services (including ventilation) required. A typical sterile services production area layout is shown in Figure 6.1. The key features are:

- a work and staff flow that avoids cross-contamination with segregated clean and dirty work areas

- an ISO Class 8 (BS EN ISO 14644; International Standards Organisation 1999) controlled and monitored inspection, assembly and packing (IAP) room
- a dedicated wash room with pass-through washer–disinfectors that exit their load into the IAP room
- either double-door pass-through sterilisers or single-door sterilisers with a loading area separated from the IAP room and
- gowning rooms for both the wash and IAP rooms.

Whether medical devices are processed in a purpose-designed SSD or the smallest dental practice, a key objective for the facility must be the segregation of dirty from clean processes and a workflow through the room/facility that avoids crossover. Decontamination should never be undertaken within patient treatment areas.

Decontamination/Sterilisation Methods

The lifecycle approach

The decontamination life cycle (Figure 6.2) is a graphical means of representing each stage of the decontamination process. At all stages, the following issues need to be considered:

- management of processes
- location for decontamination activities
- activity at each location
- facilities and equipment at each location
- validation, testing and maintenance of equipment
- policies and procedures
- training.

Section 2

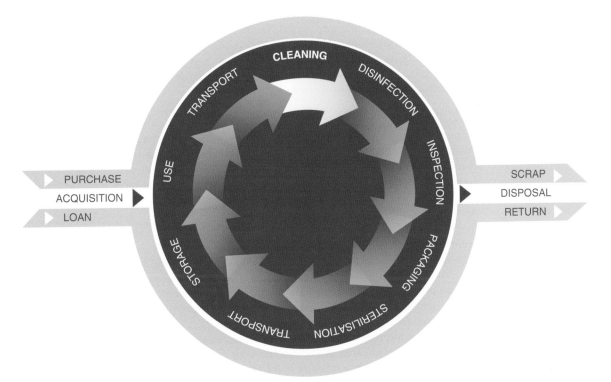

Figure 6.2 Decontamination lifecycle.

HBN 13 (Department of Health 2004) suggests a number of key postulates for successful decontamination. They include the following:

- Effective management control systems should be in place covering all aspects of the life cycle.
- Instruments should be decontaminated using automated and validated processes.
- Equipment requires planned preventative maintenance and calibration to ensure it operates to the same parameters as those set up when it was commissioned.
- Validated processes require monitoring of the critical variables of each cycle and this should be independent of the controller.
- Processes that require validation should only be carried out using automated equipment to ensure reproducibility, including cleaning.
- Decontamination processes should be segregated and environmental conditions under which devices are prepared should be controlled to prevent adventitious contamination.
- Surgical instruments should be tracked through the decontamination processes and to the patients on whom devices have been used.
- Appropriate dedicated facilities should be provided.

Washing/cleaning methods

Thorough cleaning of instruments before sterilisation is of the utmost importance to reduce the risk of transmission of infectious agents. There are four basic types of wash process used to clean surgical instruments and flexible endoscopes. These range from basic manual cleaning methods, through ultrasonic baths, thermal washer–disinfectors to the most complex automatic endoscope reprocessors. As can be seen from the postulates for successful decontamination, the Department of Health recommends automated methods over manual ones. Cleaning needs to be validated where possible and it is difficult to validate a manual process. However there are some instruments that due to their construction or materials of manufacture cannot be processed in an automated washer–disinfector. Flexible endoscopes, for example, should always be manually pre-cleaned before processing in an automated endoscope reprocessor.

Manual cleaning

Manual cleaning should be carried out in accordance with the Protocol for the Local Decontamination of Surgical Instruments issued by the Department of Health (2001). Manual cleaning should be by one of two methods: immersion or non-immersion. To minimise the risk to personnel, splashing and the creation of spray must be avoided at all times. Staff carrying out manual cleaning should wear personal protective equipment at all times.

Automated methods: thermal washer–disinfectors

A thermal washer–disinfector is a purpose-designed washing machine for processing surgical instruments and other medical devices. Versions are available for instrumentation, hollowware, anaesthetic accessories and non-invasive medical devices. They utilise a mechanical cleaning action in combination with a detergent. The pass-through double-door option is the preferred model.

Washer–disinfectors should be purchased against an appropriate specification and be capable of being validated in accordance with the relevant European standard. NHS Supply Chain operates a procurement framework which allows purchasers to pick from a pre-selected range of models without having to undertake a full tender exercise. There are a number of different models of washer–disinfector that meet current standards. The size, model and type to be chosen should be considered against workload and throughput requirements, together with the availability of space.

Logbooks and records should be kept by the designated 'user'. Records should include a description of any loads processed, cycle parameters and any independent monitoring records, together with details of routine testing and maintenance.

Automated methods: automatic endoscope reprocessor

Automatic endoscope reprocessors (AERs) are a type of washer–disinfector designed to process flexible endoscopes. They have a lower operating temperature than generic washer–disinfectors and their disinfection action is usually achieved by chemical rather than thermal action. They incorporate additional connections and pipework to enable the water, detergents and disinfectants to flow through the lumens of the endoscope. There should be a method of checking the flow of liquids through the channels (called channel patency testing) and a means of leak-testing the endoscope. These machines are available in both single-door/lid and pass-through models.

As with washer–disinfectors, AERs should also be purchased against an appropriate specification and be capable of being validated to European standards. Similarly NHS Supply Chain also operates a procurement framework. Selection of these machines is a little more complex than that of a standard thermal washer–disinfector as compatibility with the endoscope (via connectors for the channels) and the disinfectant also needs to be considered.

Appropriate record-keeping as discussed for the thermal washer–disinfector should also be made.

Ultrasonic cleaners

These are often the simplest of all cleaning machines. At their most basic they consist of a tank with a single ultrasonic transducer mounted on the bottom and a timer. More complex models include an interlocked lid, a drain and a timer linked to cycle control. At the top end of the range they often have attachments for irrigating lumen devices. They work well with instruments with joints or multiple components that are difficult to clean manually. Ultrasonic cleaners are not recommended for cleaning certain items, in particular rubber products which will absorb the ultrasonic waves.

Ultrasonic cleaners may be of the standalone ultrasonic bath type or may be part of larger washer–disinfectors. Many bath types do not incorporate a disinfection stage. Within an SSD setting they are often intended for use as a pre-cleaning process before final cleaning and disinfection in a washer–disinfector for surgical instruments. It is important with an ultrasonic bath that the tank is emptied as a minimum, every 4 hours, or when the water is visibly soiled.

A flowchart to demonstrate cleaning choices is shown in Figure 6.3.

Inspection

All items that have been through the cleaning processes should be inspected for cleanliness using a visual check as part of the decontamination process. All non-conforming items (for example items that are dirty, wet or stained) should be rejected and returned for a rewash before continuing to be packaged or sterilised. Instruments with cutting edges should be checked for sharpness.

Section 2

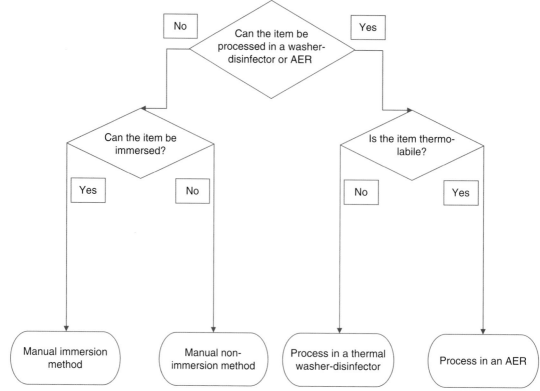

Figure 6.3 Choice of cleaning process.

Packaging Types

Most instruments supplied by an SSD will be wrapped or supplied within sterilisation containers. However in some cases instruments may not have been wrapped before being sterilised. In areas such as primary care practices or community dentistry when certain types of sterilisers are used (such as non-vacuum bench-top sterilisers), packaging is not recommended as this may impede sterilisation. Where packaging is used, it should comply with the BS EN ISO 11607 (International Standards Organization 2006) series. The packaging materials must be compatible with the sterilisation process and may be of either a rigid or flexible material. Flexible endoscopes are not wrapped after processing in an AER and are normally stored in drying cabinets or used within 3 hours of reprocessing.

Common packaging types include:

- paper wrap systems using disposable wraps in two layers
- single paper wrap systems using a disposable paper two-layer bonded wrap
- reusable barrier fabric wraps in two layers
- reusable barrier fabric outer wrap combined with a paper inner wrap
- rigid sterilisation containers with filters or valves
- peel pouch wraps with paper/film.

Most packaging systems incorporate a colour change indicator (either printed on the package itself or as a label) that provides reassurance that the item has been through an appropriate sterilisation process. A tray or instrument should never be used if this indicator has not changed to the appropriate colour.

Sterilisation Methods

Successful sterilisation requires all surfaces of the instruments and devices to be in contact with a sterilising agent. Selection of an appropriate agent to achieve sterility depends primarily upon the nature of the item to be sterilised, their materials of manufacture and the way it is packaged. Every sterilisation process will have a number of key parameters that need to be achieved and/or monitored for it to be deemed successful. When a product can be used after inspection of these parameters alone then the process is said to be verified by parametric release. In the case of some low-temperature and chemical sterilisation processes it is not possible to verify all these parameters during the cycle and a biological indicator must be placed within the load. In these cases, before the item can be used, the results of the biological challenge must be known. This system is called biological release. HTM 01-01 (Department of Health 2007) recommends the use of an independent authorising engineer (decontamination) for signing off validation records and providing advice to healthcare professionals on decontamination. NHS Supply Chain operates a procurement framework which allows purchasers to pick from a pre-selected range of models without having to undertake a full tender exercise.

Logbooks and records should be kept by the designated 'user'. Records should include a description of any loads processed, cycle parameters and any independent monitoring records together with details of routine testing and maintenance.

Steam sterilisers (autoclaves)

These are by far the most common type of steriliser found within hospitals. They rely upon pressurised steam for their killing action. Within an SSD facility they are usually of a high-vacuum type called porous load and have an active air removal system using a series of vacuum pulses. They are suitable for processing wrapped items such as trays and instruments in containers and lumen devices as well as plain instruments. Dental clinics, primary care practices and some theatre departments may have a type without active removal called downward displacement, flash or gravity sterilisers. These are for unwrapped non-lumen instruments only. Their use within the theatre environment as an alternative to reprocessing within an SSD is discouraged.

Low-temperature sterilisation

There are several different types of low-temperature sterilisation process available, with the most common types being vaporised hydrogen peroxide system (with or without gas plasma) and ethylene oxide sterilisers. Many hospitals are now investing in vaporised hydrogen peroxide sterilisers in order to reprocess and sterilise items that cannot withstand the temperatures associated with steam. Ethylene oxide sterilisers are now less common but many organisations use this process from commercial suppliers.

Transport and Distribution

It is important that the transport and storage of sterilised trays and surgical instruments does not compromise sterility. If transport includes movement of used trays from one location to another via a public highway then the requirements of the carriage of Dangerous Goods by Road Regulations (ADR) should be taken into account (Economic Commission for Europe, Committee for Inland Transport 2010). Secure, leak-proof trolleys and tote-style boxes should be used for transporting surgical instruments and trays (Figures 6.4 and 6.5). Specialist carts using trays and liners are available for endoscopes.

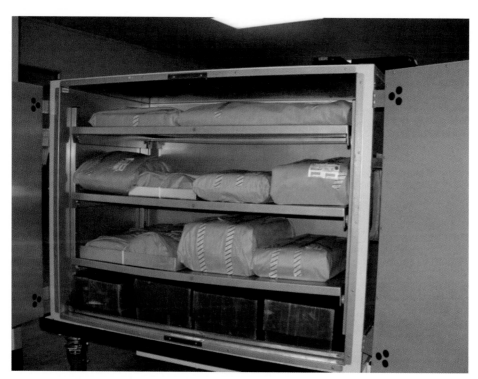

Figure 6.4   Typical distribution trolley loaded with paper-wrapped trays.

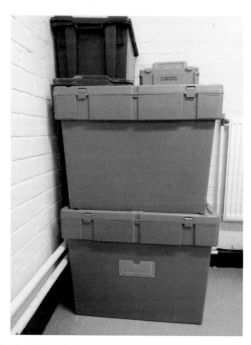

Figure 6.5   Tote-style box for distribution of supplementary instruments.

To prepare used instruments for return, all sharps, swabs or other clinical waste should be disposed separately and the trays should be reassembled, ensuring that all instruments are placed back in the correct tray. Instrument trays should either be returned wrapped in their original packaging or packaged in a plastic disposable bag (as required by the SSD) and any additional wraps should be disposed of. Used supplementary items and trays should then be placed in the transport containers for collection. The trolleys should be loaded to ensure the safety of staff and protection of the instruments.

Storage

Theatre stores should:

- be dedicated for the purpose
- have appropriate, easy-clean shelving with room for air to circulate and designed to prevent damage to packs
- allow trays to be stored above floor level away from direct sunlight and water in a secure, dry and cool environment.

Heavier trays should be easily accessible and not placed on top of lighter ones.

Most organisations apply a use-by date on their sterile products. This should always be checked before using the tray. However the preservation of sterility is event based and rough handling can cause damage to the product and compromise sterility. Before using any sterile product it should be checked to ensure that the packaging is intact.

New Instruments and Manufacturers Reprocessing Instructions

Compliance with the MDD requires a manufacturer of a reusable medical device to provide validated, written reprocessing instructions detailing how the item should be cleaned and if appropriate, sterilised. New instruments should be purchased according to a specification. Those responsible for purchasing must ensure that the manufacturer's reprocessing instructions are available and that the instrument can be appropriately reprocessed by the equipment that is available.

Prion Disease and vCJD

The emergence of vCJD and the discovery of the prion protein has dramatically affected the approach taken to the cleaning of surgical instruments. There are several key points to bear in mind:

- Prions do not behave the same way as microbiological diseases and are resistant to standard sterilisation techniques.
- There are significant sums of money being invested into research in this area. It is likely that new decontamination processes will be developed that are more effective.
- The current advice is that cleaning in an automated washer–disinfector is the best defence against the spread of prions via surgical instruments.
- Patient diagnosis cannot be confirmed until post mortem and therefore patients are classified as possible and/or at risk.
- The distribution of prions within the body means that procedures undertaken on 'at risk' or 'probable' patients are classified into high-, medium- and low-risk procedures corresponding to tissue infectivity.
- Instruments used during high- or medium-risk procedures on patients at risk of having the disease or with a possible diagnosis should be quarantined until the diagnosis is either confirmed or ruled out.

Section 2

The Department of Health has published guidance on the quarantining of surgical instruments in such cases (Advisory Committee on Dangerous Pathogens 2011).

Tracking and Traceability

It is essential to be able to trace products through their reprocessing cycle and also to the patient on whom they have been used. This enables corrective action to be taken when required and products to be recalled. With the advent of vCJD, the ability to look back at the history of an instrument and to trace previous patients who had been exposed to it became important. There are many systems on the market that facilitate this and electronic ones are better than paper versions.

Should I Use the Instrument?

The process by which a sterilised item is released to the theatre store in a safe manner is called product release. But good product release does not stop at the exit to the SSD. In deciding to use an instrument or tray the theatre practitioner is also taking a product release decision. It is the responsibility of the theatre practitioner to ensure that the equipment he or she intends using is 'fit for purpose'. In the Theatre Support Pack mentioned earlier, the Association for Perioperative Practice recommends the following:

- The condition of items should be checked to ensure that the packaging is fit for purpose.
- Before opening sets within theatres, the outer container/wrap should be checked to ensure its integrity as well as the presence of valid labelling and external sterility indicators.
- Once opened, the contents should be checked to ensure there is no residual moisture; internal sterilisation monitors are present and valid; and there are no visual signs of contamination. Any non-conformances should be reported.
- The contents should be checked against the tray checklist and then signed by the circulator undertaking the check. Any discrepancies should be noted, documented on the checklist and reported as a non-conformance. At the end of the case, a further check of the set should be undertaken and the checklist signed by the scrub practitioner.
- Any broken/missing instruments or instruments requiring attention, such as sharpening, should also be documented on the checklist.

References

Advisory Committee on Dangerous Pathogens (2011) *Transmissible Spongiform Encephalopathy Agents: Safe Working and the Prevention of Infection: Annex E.* London: Department of Health.

Allison VD (1960) Hospital central sterile supply departments. *British Medical Journal* 2(5201): 772–778.

Bowie JH, Gillingham J, Campbell I and Gordon R (1963) Hospital sterile supplies. *British Medical Journal* 2(5368): 1322–1327.

British Standards Institute (2001) *CEN. BS EN 556–1:2001 Sterilisation of medical devices. Requirements for medical devices to be designated 'STERILE.' Requirements for terminally sterilized medical devices.* s.1. London: British Standards Institute.

Department of Health (1997) *Washer–disinfectors.* Health Technical Memorandum 2030. London: Department of Health.

Department of Health (1999) *HSC 1999/178: Variant Creutzfeldt–Jakob disease (vCJD): minimising the risk of transmission.* http://www.dh.gov.uk/en/Publicationsandstatistics/Lettersandcirculars/Healthservicecirculars/DH_4004969 (accessed 3 October 2011).

Department of Health (2001) *Protocol for the Local Decontamination of Surgical Instruments*. London: Department of Health.
Department of Health (2004) *Health Building Note 13, Sterile Service Department*. London: Departrment of Health.
Department of Health (2007) *Health Technical Memorandum 01-01: Decontamination of reusable medical devices - Part A (Management and environment)*. Estates and Facilities Division. London: Department of Health.
Department of Health (2010) *The Health and Social Care Act 2008: Code of Practice for health and adult social care on the prevention and control of infections and related guidance*. London: Department of Health.
Economic Commission for Europe, Committee for Inland Transport (2010) *European Agreement concerning the International Carriage of Dangerous Goods by Road*. Geneva: United Nations, 2010.
European Community (1993) Council Directive 93/42/EEC of 14 June 1993 concerning medical devices. *EUR LEX*. http://eur-lex.europa.eu/LexUriServ/LexUriServ.do?uri=CELEX:31993L0042:EN:HTML (accessed 3 October 2011).
European Community (2007) Directive 2007/47/EC of the European Parliament and of the Council. *Official Journal of the European Union*. s.1.
International Standards Organization (1999) *BS EN ISO 14644 Cleanrooms and associated controlled environments Part 1: Classification of air cleanliness*. London: British Standards Institute.
International Standards Organization (2006) *BS EN ISO 11607 Packaging for Terminally Sterilized Medical Devices*. s.1. London: British Standards Institute.
International Standards Organisation (2009) *BS EN ISO 15883 Washer-disinfectors – Part 1: General requirements, terms and definitions and tests*. s.1. London: British Standards Institute.
MHRA (Medicines and Healthcare products Regulatory Agency) (2010) *Sterilisation, Disinfection and Cleaning of Medical Equipment: Guidance on Decontamination from the Microbiology Advisory Committee to Department of Health, Part 1*. London: Department of Health.
MHRA (2011) *Medical Device Alert: Reusable laryngoscope handles – all models and manufacturers (MDA/2011/096)*. http://www.mhra.gov.uk/home/groups/dts-bs/documents/medicaldevicealert/con129221.pdf (accessed March 2012).
National Decontamination Programme (2003) *Strategy for Modernising the Provision of Decontamination Services*. London: Department of Health.
National Decontamination Programme (2009) *Theatre Support Pack*. London: Department of Health.
Spaulding EH (1972) Chemical disinfection and antisepsis in the hospital. *Journal of Hospital Research* 9: 5–31.

Further Readings

Medicines and Healthcare products Regulatory Agency. *Directive Bulletin No 8*. London: Department of Health.
Medicines and Healthcare products Regulatory Agency. *Directive Bulletin 13*. London: Department of Health.

CHAPTER 7

Wound Healing and Surgical Site Infection

Melissa Rochon

Introduction

Successful surgical wound healing relies on the careful apposition of the wound edges and the prevention of infection. Surgical healing is supported by haemostasis, careful handling and management of the tissues, prudent diathermy use and exacting tension at closure. The surgeon's technique and expertise will determine how well aligned the wound margins are. It is important all members of the multi-disciplinary team actively apply safe and consistent practices to help reduce the risk of surgical site infection (SSI).

Although wound infections can involve fungus (for instance the yeast *Candida*) (Modrau *et al.* 2009), protozoa (Wolcott *et al.* 2009) or viruses associated with skin lesions (for instance herpes simplex) (Patel *et al.* 2009), it is bacteria (outlined in Box 7.1) that are generally responsible for incidences of SSI (Collier 2004). This chapter provides an overview of the wound-healing process, bacteria and wound infections before introducing key measures in preventing SSI.

Principles of Wound Healing

Wound healing refers to the processes following injury, trauma or incision which restore the integrity and function to the epithelial surface and the tissue beneath. Generally, with good conditions, tissue perfusion and oxygenation (which are supported by normothermia), acute wounds heal quickly. Although the three phases of wound healing may be described as overlapping and non-linear (Figure 7.1), chronic wounds arise when the healing process becomes stalled within one of the phases.

Phases of wound healing

Inflammatory phase
At the time of injury, the sympathetic nervous system and wound hormones are stimulated and the inflammatory phase of healing is initiated (Walsh 2004).

Manual of Perioperative Care: An Essential Guide, First Edition. Edited by Kate Woodhead and Lesley Fudge.
© 2012 John Wiley & Sons, Ltd. Published 2012 by John Wiley & Sons, Ltd.

BOX 7.1

Bacteria

Bacteria are ubiquitous single-cell microorganisms (living cells) whose coexistence with humans is usually mutually beneficial. Bacteria called normal or commensal flora (which are present on the skin and in the upper respiratory tract, the intestinal tract and vagina) have a protective role as they compete with other harmful bacteria for space and nutrients.

Under certain circumstances during surgery, if particularly virulent bacteria get into the wound, or if commensal bacteria are inadvertently transferred from where they naturally reside (conditional pathogens), or usually harmless bacteria bind to unhealthy/damaged or breached tissue in a vulnerable patient (opportunistic pathogens), then bacteria may cause a wound infection.

Such bacteria are termed pathogens if they are able to cause disease; this chapter focuses on their ability to cause SSI. Pathogens possess virulence factors, which determine how easily they can cause structural or functional damage to cells and host.

In response to a critical load of bacteria, the body's inflammatory response is frequently responsible for the classic signs of infection.

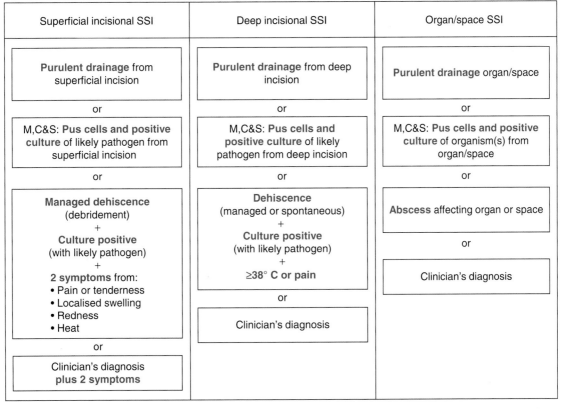

Superficial incisional SSI	Deep incisional SSI	Organ/space SSI
Purulent drainage from superficial incision	**Purulent drainage** from deep incision	**Purulent drainage** organ/space
or	or	or
M,C&S: **Pus cells and positive culture** of likely pathogen from superficial incision	M,C&S: **Pus cells and positive culture** of likely pathogen from deep incision	M,C&S: **Pus cells and positive culture** of organism(s) from organ/space
or	or	or
Managed dehiscence (debridement) + **Culture positive** (with likely pathogen) + **2 symptoms** from: • Pain or tenderness • Localised swelling • Redness • Heat	**Dehiscence** (managed or spontaneous) + **Culture positive** (with likely pathogen) + ≥38° C or pain	**Abscess** affecting organ or space
	or	or
or	Clinician's diagnosis	Clinician's diagnosis
Clinician's diagnosis **plus 2 symptoms**		

Figure 7.1   Surgical site infection: definition and classification adapted from Health Protection Agency protocol. Adapted from HPA protocol (2011).

Vascular response   Following the creation of a wound, the body seeks to rebalance itself (return to homeostasis). The aim of the microvascular response is to stop the bleeding (haemostasis) and to protect the area against foreign material or the ingress of harmful bacteria.

This is achieved via attributes of the blood vessel walls (the endothelium) as well as properties of the blood. Blood vessels constrict or narrow, which reduces blood flow to the area. Platelets (small cell fragments) gather together at the site. Chemical signals direct vascular and cellular activities to create a mesh of plasma proteins – predominantly fibrin and fibronectin – which trap red blood cells, resulting in coagulation (clotting) to stop the bleeding (Bale 2004). In addition, the clot provides a rudimentary barrier to bacteria and forms a basic structure upon which the cellular response will build (Benbow 2005).

After haemostasis, further microvascular events serve to dilute any toxins in the area and to facilitate the cellular response:

- The blood vessels dilate – arteriolar smooth muscle relaxes so that the blood flow to the small blood vessels (the capillaries and venules) is increased.
- Mild hyperaemia (an increase in haemoglobin or red blood cells) results – this brings oxygen, warmth and protective cells to the injured area (Woolf 2000, Collier 2004). The hyperaemia accounts for the heat and redness observed at the wound site.
- The permeability of small vessels increases – intercellular pores expand in order to create temporary gaps in the endothelium (Walsh 2004). Together, the increased blood flow (which causes pressure on the small vessels and fluid to escape into the tissue) and the increased permeability of the blood vessels account for the oedema (swelling) and pain at the wound site.
- Pain is stimulated either by the direct trauma or swelling due to the increase in tissue tension, and/ or the release of chemical stimulants (Walsh 2004).
- When of sufficient magnitude, both swelling and pain may result in what may be considered the fifth sign of inflammation – loss of function.

Cellular response   The tissue injury and the clotting factors stimulate the inflammatory cells, cytokines and other proinflammatory substances (such as prostaglandin, bradykinin and histamine) (Benbow and Stevens 2010). In order to coordinate their efforts, inflammatory cells need to send signals to each other and they do this by releasing cytokines (molecules which attract and stimulate cells).

Facilitated by the vascular response, a restorative and protective exudate of fluid, colloid particles and larger molecules of the immune defences (antibodies and complement) can then move out of the vessel and into the local tissue (Benbow and Stevens 2010). The clearance of exudate, dead tissue, debris and bacteria is reliant on phagocytosis, which is the engulfment and destruction of the microbe by inflammatory cells (Male 2007). Phagocytosis is performed by white blood cells (WBCs).

WBCs may reside in the tissue (polymorphonuclear leukocytes or 'polymorphs') or they may circulate in the system and are mobilised to areas of acute inflammation (neutrophils and monocytes – monocytes later change into macrophages). The purposeful movement of phagocytic cells towards the site is called chemotaxis. The presence of bacteria attracts more neutrophils to the area than would the creation of the wound (Woolf 2000).

In a wound healing by primary intention, this phase is usually completed in 3 days. However, heavy bacterial contamination, impaired immunity, underlying illness, poor vascularity or perfusion may all prolong the inflammatory process.

Proliferative or reconstructive phase

Lakhani and Dogan report that 'the process of repair requires many different cell types to proliferate and synthesize proteins necessary for restoring integrity and strength to the tissue' (Lakhani and Dogan 2004, p. 322). Two to four days after surgical incision, as the clearance of bacteria and debris finishes, macrophages attract fibroblasts (connective tissue cells) and myofibroblasts to the area to deposit collagen (Gould and Brooker 2000). The different types of collagen (the main supportive protein in the

> **BOX 7.2**
>
> **Moist wound healing**
>
> Moist wound healing (MWH) proposes that an optimal wound environment with an interactive dressing will promote healing for cells of the epidermal layer so healing is ameliorated (Winter 1962).
>
> It has been noted that the evidence for MWH is based on older, smaller, non-blinded studies. More recent studies have demonstrated that surgical wounds, unlike wounds healing by secondary intention, do not necessarily benefit from (nor are they adversely affected by) MWH. Conventional dry dressings may be as efficient and as acceptable to the patient as alternative dressings, as well as being more cost effective (Wynne *et al.* 2004, Vogt *et al.* 2007, Ubbink *et al.* 2008, Shinohara *et al.* 2008).
>
> Whichever dressing is selected, until the wound is sealed it is still vulnerable and aseptic technique is required (Wilson 2003).

body) and extracellular substances provide the framework (extracellular matrix) for new tissue and angiogenesis (the creation of new blood vessels) to take place.

Granulation tissue, made up of inflammatory cells and fibroblasts, fills the wound from the base upwards and is usually not evident in wounds healing by primary intention; this process is more laborious and of a larger scale in wounds healing by second intention (Woolf 2000, Vuolo 2010).

The vascularity of the area produces bright red, granular tissue which bleeds easily because of the newly formed capillaries present (Lakhani and Dogan 2004).

The wound margin or border will be pulled together, which reduces the overall size of the wound; however contraction is minimal in wounds healing by primary closure (Bryant and Nix 2007). Concurrently, cells migrate and proliferate to cover over the wound. Within 24 hours epithelial cells are present on clean surgical wounds (Mercandetti and Cohen 2005), although healing will still be taking place below (Sheperd 2009). It should be noted epithelial cells will not form over eschar or necrotic tissue.

The new epithelial cells are white/pink in appearance and are vulnerable to shear forces.

Maturation phase

During this phase, the wound becomes less vascular. Over time, the structure and strength of the new tissue is improved (Gould and Brooker 2000).

Types of Wound Closure

The type of suture/closure material, the use and type of needle delivery system and suturing technique (method and stitch size) all depend on where the suture is placed, the features of the closure material and the condition of the patient. Sutures may be placed in a variety of manners, for instance using continuous or interrupted (e.g. knotted) methods such as the 'interrupted mattress', 'percutaneous' or 'transdermal' techniques, or using the more complex figure of eight or subcuticular techniques (NICE 2008).

Wound healing by primary intention

Wounds healing by primary intention have their incisions closed directly following the operation, with sutures, staples or adhesives (Table 7.1). This type of closure is applied in instances where there is little tissue loss and the wound edges can be brought together. Such wounds generally result in minimal oedema, gaping and serous discharge (Gottrup

Table 7.1 Wound closure materials.

Absorbable	Non-absorbable
Natural	Natural
Synthetic	Surgical silk
Coated vicryl	Synthetic
Monocryl	Nylon
Polydioxanone (PDS) II	Polypropylene (Prolene)
	Tissue adhesive (e.g. Dermabond®, Bioglue®)
	Tapes/strips (e.g. Steri-strip®)

Table 7.2 Surgical wounds.

	Recommendation	Comment
Incisions	The incision is protected by dressing and /or sealant	The skin should be allowed to seal and resume its natural protective role against bacterial ingress – only a minority of pathogens can penetrate intact skin (Roitt et al. 1993). Edward-Jones (2010) notes microbes rarely penetrate intact skin, and if they do the resultant infection is likely to be systemic rather than local wound infection
	Compression may be required to reduce bleeding, exudate, oedema or haematoma formation	Fold a sterile surgical pad or layers of gauze into a narrow strip (which provides extra height area – to improve the mechanism for pressure) over the original wound dressing and either encircle with a crepe bandage (50% overlap) or apply an adhesive dressing stretched over and onto the skin (David et al. 2010). If bleeding is not stemmed, continue to apply firm pressure on dressing/ additional padding and seek surgical advice
		After approximately 72 hours, the presence of serous exudate is no longer contributing to the healing process (Wilson 2003). Wound management choices should avoid both frequent dressing changes and maceration of the surrounding skin/ tissue breakdown. Seek advice from tissue viability nurse or surgeon (Sheppard and Wright 2006)
		Wound margins under strain may benefit from additional suture or adhesive tape (for instance Steristrips) (NICE 2008) but equally re-suturing, support resources (e.g. cough lock, bras for females with sternal wounds), appropriate fluid balance management and counter-gravity measures (e.g. elevating the affected limb) may be appropriate
Dressings	Dressings which allow the wound to be viewed, and offer good conformability, patient comfort and which do not requiring frequent changing (allowing the patient to shower with the dressing remaining intact) are ideal (NICE 2008)	The dressing application must allow for postoperative oedema (either of the wound and/or general) and patient movement otherwise the skin may blister (Pukki et al. 2010)
		Dressings with a favourable vapour transmission rate and which promote moist wound healing (see Box 7.2) should be selected (NICE 2008)
Drains	Surgical incisions may have drains (e.g. Redivac, Bellovac) placed distally through a separate incision	This is to reduce the risk of complications including dehiscence due to pressure on the suture line and to improve healing by countering dead space and haematoma formation (Gruendemann and Mangum 2001). Drain entry sites need to be managed aseptically to reduce introduction of bacteria. Output from the drains should be monitored and reported and the drains should be removed as soon as their purpose has been served

> **BOX 7.3**
>
> **Gram-negative and Gram-positive bacteria**
>
> Most bacteria can be distinguished by a staining technique, the Gram stain, used in laboratories giving rise to the classification of Gram-positive or Gram-negative species. Those that cannot be determined by Gram staining are considered acid-fast bacteria (Trounce 2002).
>
> Most bacteria have a layer of peptidoglycan in the cell wall which protects them from mechanical and osmotic damage. Gram-negative bacteria have a plasma membrane bounded by a thin layer of peptidoglycan, a middle space called the periplasmic space and a further outer membrane which includes lipopolysaccharide (LPS) (Weston 2010). In contrast, the structure of Gram-positive bacteria wall is made up of a plasma membrane surrounded by a thick layer of peptidoglycan. Its structure is less complex and less protective than that of the Gram-negative cell wall.
>
> Examples of Gram-positive bacteria are: *Staphylococcus* and *Streptococcus* species, *Clostridium*, *Bacillus* and *Corynebacterium*.
>
> Examples of Gram-negative bacteria are: *Enteroccocus* species (*Proteus*, *Pseudomonas*, *Klebsiella*, *Escherichia coli*), *Acinetobacter* and *Bacteroides*.

et al. 2005). Table 7.2 provides further comment. This method is suitable for clean, clean-contaminated or traumatic wounds if thorough cleansing/debridement of the wound is achieved (Gould and Brooker 2000).

Wounds healing by secondary intention

Wounds healing by secondary intention do not have their incisions closed directly, rather they are left to heal 'from the bottom up'. These are usually wounds left open either due to significant epithelium and tissue loss and/or bacterial contamination. Granulation, contraction and re-epithelialisation are significant features of this type of wound (Sheperd 2009). Such wounds should be managed with tissue viability specialist input (NICE 2008).

Delayed primary closure (tertiary intention)

Some surgical incisions benefit from a period of time before the final surgical closure of the wound occurs. Before definitive or staged closure, the wound may be packed and the skin may be sutured or a material may be used to protect the wound in the interim.

Delayed closure may be used when there has been heavy bacterial contamination, or due to the presence of excessive exudate or oedema (Hess 2002), or in surgeries where the organ needs to stabilise before closure, as may be the case with some cardiac or bowel surgery.

The wound closure type and care plan for the wound should be clearly communicated at handover. Continuous assessment is important so that if required, reinforcement (tension sutures) or staged removal (e.g. remove intermittent clips) may be undertaken.

Wound Infection

Conservative estimates suggest that 5% of patients having surgery develop a SSI arising from bacteria (see Box 7.3 for classification of bacteria). The associated high costs to the individual in terms of mortality, morbidity and quality of life as well the impact on hospital resources are well documented (NICE 2008; Scottish Intercollegiate Guidelines Network 2008).

Sources of infection

It has been suggested that approximately 95% of wound infections are from endogenous sources of bacteria (arising from the host, e.g. patient's skin, hollow viscera) acquired at the time of operation (Weston 2010). In contrast, cross-infection may arise when transient bacteria are transferred to the patient from exogenous sources (outside of the host). Exogenous spread may be via contact include direct contact or indirect contact (e.g. hands of healthcare workers or medical equipment) or airborne spread (e.g. of droplets or squamous epithelial cells) from infected individuals or from aerosol-generating or air management systems (Elliott *et al.* 2000).

Risk of infection

The development of infection is believed to rely on three factors: the virulence of the bacteria, number of bacteria present and host immunity.

Virulence factors

Few bacteria are pathogenic; those that are possess a variety of mechanisms or bacterial products (including toxins and toxic components) which facilitate entry, attachment and spread of the organism, which result in pathophysiological changes in the host. Toxins may be either exotoxins or endotoxins:

- Exotoxins are mainly secreted by Gram-positive bacteria and can interfere with or damage cell structure and/or function.
- Endotoxins may be released from the cell walls of Gram-negative bacteria when they divide or when they break up and die (cell lysis). Endotoxins can direct macrophages to release cytokines, which may evoke overwhelming inflammatory and immune responses. In the bloodstream, the presence of endotoxins may result in septicaemia, a life-threatening illness caused by infection of the (usually sterile) blood. Bacteraemia is the transient presence of microbes in the blood (usually cleared by the liver or spleen but may require clinical treatment).

Virulence factors, such as antibiotic resistance, can be passed vertically (e.g. from mother to daughter cells) or may rapidly spread via horizontal transmission (by exchange of genetic material between microbes which may not necessarily of the same strain) (Galbraith *et al.* 1999).

Recall that bacteria of low virulence, such as coagulase-negative staphylococci (which are present in normal skin flora), may become pathogenic if transferred to another body site: in the UK, a 2009 outbreak of prosthetic valve endocarditis was linked to a surgeon who had unknowingly become infected with the resistant strain of *Staphlycoccus epidermis*, a coagulase-negative staphylococci (National Patient Safety Agency 2011).

Number of organisms

Bacteria grow and divide (binary fission). Under optimal conditions a bacterium such as *E. coli* has a doubling rate around of 20 minutes – so one cell could produce over 10^8 progeny within a day (Smith *et al.* 2000). Under good conditions, the normal defences of a healthy individual can effectively manage a reasonable micro-burden – indeed there will always be some bacteria in the wound (Young 2010). However, as Hranjec *et al.* (2010) highlight, $>10^5$ microorganisms/g of tissue will affect healing regardless of the organism.

Importantly, the risk of infection may be just as great in the presence of a very small number of pathogens if ischaemic tissue, foreign material (for instance prosthetic material, plastic tubing or implant device such as a pacemaker), haematoma or exudate are

> **BOX 7.4**
>
> **Risk factors for developing SSI (adapted from Risk factors for developing SSI, SIGN 2008, p. 6)**
>
> - Poor nutrition
> - Extremes of age
> - Underlying illness such as diabetes, cancer, genetic defects, AIDS
> - Immunosupresssion: Medication, radiotherapy or chemotherapy
> - Remote infection (e.g. infection elsewhere in the body) or bacterial colonisation
> - Lifestyle – obesity, excessive smoking or drinking
> - Hypothermia (Hulse 2011)

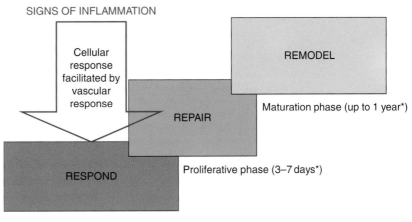

Figure 7.2   Response to trauma, foreign material, wound breakdown and infection.

present (Gottrup *et al*. 2005). Biofilms are described as a proliferating poly-microbial mass which adheres to inanimate objects (fomites). Biofilms appear to be more resistant to the immune response and antibiotic treatment (Salyers and Whitt 2005).

Host immunity

Host immunity is provided by the physical, cellular and chemical defences of the immune system (Salyers and Whitt 2005). The immune system has non-specific defences (skin, mucosal surfaces and normal flora) as well as specific blood and tissue defences (called acquired or specific immunity provided by complement and antibodies). Host factors that lower resistance are listed in Box 7.4. Smith *et al*. (2000) point out there are still gaps in knowledge as to how microorganisms cause wound infection in the host, as many of the SSIs which develop post discharge do not reflect these risk factors.

Definition of Surgical Site Infection

This section refers to the definition and classification of wound infection proposed by the Health Protection Agency (HPA) (Figure 7.2) as it evidences the role of bacteria in its criteria for SSI: either the likely pathogen is identified along with the host's

---

BOX 7.5

Microscopy, culture and sensitivity (MC&S)

- *Microscopy*: The sample is allowed to dry before it is fixed onto a slide and Gram stained. The slide is then examined under a microscope. This is a non-culture method of identifying the species of bacteria based on its shape (e.g. rod-shaped, spherical, helical). A counterstain may be applied to examine the sample for evidence of pus cells. Not all samples are tested for the presence of pus cells; this may need to be requested.
- *Culture*: Microbes grown in a nutrient medium (such as blood agar) on a plate. Once material from patient is inoculated (added) into sterile medium and incubated overnight, evidence of bacterial colonies may become visible to the unaided eye.
- *Sensitivity*: Prior to incubation, antibiotic discs are arranged on the plate for the bacterial culture. The growth of the bacteria is either inhibited (sensitive to the antimicrobial) or unimpeded (resistant to the antibiotic).

Key points
- The labs use a selection of media which favour or inhibit specific microbes. The responsible pathogen may not be identified if the lab did not have enough information to choose best possible media.
- When reviewing wound swab results, resident bacteria will always be present to some degree. However, the presence of transient bacteria in a wound indicates practice has not been optimal.
- Some labs do not routinely report resident bacteria, or report these as 'possible contaminants' unless a specific request is made or the clinical details are suggestive that bacteria such as CNS may be the responsible organism. Clinical details (such as whether the patient has positive blood cultures or pyrexia) are fundamental to the tests performed and results issued by the lab.
- Record any antibiotics the patient is on to avoid false negatives, as this will impact on patient management and safety.

---

inflammatory response, or the symptoms are so linked with a clinician's review as to likely point to SSI (rather than to mechanical breakdown of the wound or to delayed healing), or the clinician/radiographer observes infection that is not specific to the incision, but related to the space and/or organ manipulated during the operation.

The HPA definition can be applied across a broad range of surgery types; and it allows for early identification and appropriate treatment of wound infection (Aziz and Isalska 2010). Nevertheless, the definition was designed to facilitate a dichotomous outcome (yes/no), and as such it does not capture data on patient management and impact of the infection on the patient and/or resources.

Microscopy, culture and sensitivity (MC&S)

Sometimes pus cells (reported as WBC, or polymorphs) are reported by microbiology. After the initial wound-healing phase, their presence is indicative of either delayed wound healing or infection. Box 7.5 describes MC&S testing and provides some key points on this criterion of infection. Although wound infection cannot arise without bacteria, the presence of bacteria does not necessarily indicate infection (Gottrup *et al.* 2005). Meaningful MC&S results rely on accurate, detailed request forms and samples obtained using aseptic technique (see Chapter 19). Even with these considerations, positive swab results may not yield the causative pathogen (agent responsible for infection).

Equally, negative swab results do not necessarily mean the absence of infection. The pathogen may simply not be present in the sample, or the pus/exudate may have dried and the bacteria have died in the interim before testing (Gould and Brooker 2000). Also, the bacterial cell wall may not be distinguishable, destroyed either by antibiotics or phagocytosis.

Purulent drainage

At times confusion may arise between pus and slough. Pus is a mobile, easy to remove fluid (e.g. 'drains' following palpation of the area, or due to the build-up in pressure exerted on the surrounding tissue as the body tries to contain or wall off the infection). Certain pathogens elicit a strong neutrophil response, subsequently pus appears opaque because of the number of cells present in the fluid (Woolf 2000). In contrast, slough is a moist material that appears as part of the wound matrix and its presence in the wound is typically longer than that observed in pus. Slough may appear to extend to the wound margin and can sometimes be difficult to remove. Slough would not be observed in a wound healing by primary intention unless there was some wound gaping or dehiscence.

Dehiscence

Dehiscence may be described as managed dehiscence, meaning mechanical opening of the incision as in sharp debridement, or spontaneous dehiscence where the wound opens due to wound breakdown (failure to heal due to host condition), poor technique (e.g. incorrect suturing) or infection. Many pathogens release collagenase which digests collagen fibers and thus reduces the strength of the new tissue (Gould and Brooker 2000, p. 167) which can result in dehiscence.

Heat, redness, pain, heat and clinician's diagnosis

These symptoms should be set into context.

- What operation did the patient have? For instance, operations involving the joints may have more pronounced swelling or redness for a longer period of time.
- Where is the wound? Wound disturbances (e.g. positive culture or gaping) may arise from the location of the wound rather than to overt infection.
- What postoperative day is it? Inflammation is normal on day 2, but would be suspect on, for example, day 7.
- What is the patient's skin like? Does the patient have any underlying conditions that may slow healing? Does the patient report usually healing well?
- Is the pain increasing over time rather than reducing?
- Redness and swelling should be specific to the incision and extend beyond the wound margins. Distinguish from haemotomas (which may be precursors to infection and so also should be noted).
- Is fever related to another cause (e.g. chest or urinary tract infection)?
- An agreed definition and classification of SSI ensures consistent and impartial reporting of SSI.

Surgical Site Infection Surveillance Schemes

Proactive, unbiased, accurate and continuous surveillance is recommended to monitor and feedback on SSI rates. In the UK, participation in the Health Protection Agency (HPA) surveillance scheme is mandatory in orthopaedic surgery and currently voluntary for its other modules.

The advantage of the HPA definition is it allows for national benchmarking as well as participation in broader agencies such as Hospitals in Europe Link for Infection Control through Surveillance (HELICS), thus contributing to the framework of clinical governance as well as to evidence-based practice (Pellowe *et al.* 2004).

Saving Lives Care Bundle to Reduce Surgical Site Infection

Box 7.6 lists the evidence-based practices which have been demonstrated to reduce incidences of SSI. At its core are principles aimed to improve host immunity and reduce the number of pathogens from endogenous and exogenous sources.

Downie (2010) points out clinical guidelines must be viewed as credible and workable if they are going to be implemented. Unfortunately, knowledge generated by randomised controlled trials (RCTs) is sometimes restricted by a theoretical problem: quantitative findings may be perceived as being rigid and inflexible (Paley 2005) when actually the aim of the research is to extend or generalise the finding to a larger population (Cormack 2003). Bear in mind that the care bundle is not designed to be imposed in cases where the element it is not practical, such as seeking normothermia in cardiac

---

BOX 7.6

Care bundle to prevent surgical site infection (adapted from Department of Health 2008)

Preoperative phase

- *Screening and decolonisation*: Patient has been screened for MRSA (methicillin-resistant *Staphylococcus aureus*) using local guidelines. If found positive they have been decolonised according to the recommended protocol prior to surgery.
- *Preoperative showering*: Patient has showered (or bathed/washed if unable to shower) preoperatively using soap.
- *Hair removal*: If hair removal is required, it is removed using clippers with a disposable head (not by shaving) and timed as close to the operating procedure as possible.

Intraoperative phase

- *Skin preparation*: Patient's skin has been prepared with 2% chlorhexidine in 70% isopropyl alcohol solution and allowed to air dry. (If the patient has a sensitivity, povidone–iodine application is used.)
- *Prophylactic antibiotics*: Appropriate antibiotics were administered within 60 minutes prior to incision and only repeated if there is excessive blood loss, a prolonged operation or during prosthetic surgery.
- *Normothermia*: Body temperature is maintained above 36 °C in the perioperative period.
- *Incise drapes*: If incise drapes are used they are impregnated with an antiseptic.
- *Supplemented oxygen*: Patient's haemoglobin saturation is maintained above 95% (or as high as possible if there is underlying respiratory insufficiency) in the intra- and postoperative stages (recovery room).
- *Glucose control*: A glucose level of <11 mmol/L has been maintained in diabetic patients. (This tight blood glucose control is not yet considered relevant in non-diabetic patients.)

Postoperative phase

- *Surgical dressing*: The wound is covered with an interactive dressing at the end of surgery and while the wound is healing.
- *Interactive wound dressing* is kept undisturbed for a minimum of 48 hours after surgery unless there is leakage from the dressing and need for a change.
- The principles of *asepsis* (non-touch technique) are used when the wound is being redressed.
- *Hand hygiene*: hands are decontaminated immediately before and after each episode of patient contact using the correct hand hygiene technique. (Use of the World Health Organization's '5 moments for hand hygiene' or National Patient Safety Agency's 'Clean your hands campaign' is recommended.)

cases where hypothermia is intentionally sought (in fact this category is excluded from the care bundle). Instead there are other ways to use the findings – for instance reviewing patient comfort measures on the ward and in recovery; or using the care bundle to support new equipment (e.g. thermometers) or resources (e.g. blankets). This approach ensures that are bundles are not applied in isolation, but rather used in conjunction with expert input so as to produce best practice for patient care.

Summary

This chapter focuses on the basic anatomical and physiological principles of wound healing and infection in order to draw out the general reasoning behind measures to reduce SSI. The types of wound closure are described and the aetiology, identification and treatment of wound infections are outlined.

References

Aziz AM and Isalska B (2010) Sternal wound infections: improvements made to reduce rates. *British Journal of Nursing* 19(20): S20–29.

Bale S (2004) Wound healing. In *Nursing Practice Hospital and Home. The Adult*, 2nd edn. London: Churchill Livingstone.

Benbow M (2005) *Evidence Based Wound Management*. London: Whurr.

Benbow M and Stevens J (2010) Exudate, infection and patient quality of life. *British Journal of Nursing* 19(20): S30–41.

Bryant R and Nix D (2007) *Acute and Chronic Wounds Current Management Concepts*, 3rd edn. London: Mosby.

Collier M (2004) *Recognition and Management of Wound Infections*. www.worldwidewounds.com/2004/january/Collier/Management-of-Wound-infections.html (accessed 7 April 2010).

Cormack D (ed.) (2003) *The Research Process in Nursing*. Oxford: Blackwell Publishing.

David M, Gogi N, Roa J and Selzer G (2010) The art and rationale of applying a compression dressing. *British Journal of Nursing* 19(4): 235–236.

Department of Health (2008) *Clean, Safe Care: Reducing Infection and Saving Lives*. London: HMSO.

Downie F (2010) NICE clinical guideline: prevention and treatment of SSIs – is it enough? *Wounds UK* 6(4): 102–110.

Edward-Jones V (2010) Science of infection. *Wounds UK* 6(2): 86–93.

Elliott T, Hastings M and Desselberger U (2000) *Lecture Notes on Medical Microbiology*, 3rd edn. Oxford: Blackwell Science.

Galbraith A, Bullock S, Manias E, Hunt B and Richards A (1999) *Fundamentals of Pharmacology*. London: Pearson Prentice Hall.

Gottrup F, Melling A and Hollander DA (2005) An overview of surgical site infections: aetiology, incidence and risk factors. http://www.worldwidewounds.com/2005/september/Gottrup/Surgical-Site-Infections-Overview.html (accessed 20 April 2011).

Gould D and Brooker C (2000) *Applied Microbiology for Nurses*. London: Macmillan Press.

Gruendemann BJ and Mangum SS (2001) *Infection Prevention in Surgical Settings*. London: W.B. Saunders Co.

Hess TC (2002) *Clinical Guide: Skin and Wound Care*, 6th edn. London: Lippincott Williams & Wilkins.

HPA (Health Protection Agency) (2011) *Protocol for the Surveillance of Surgical Site Infection Version 5. Surgical Site Infection Surveillance Service*. http://www.hpa.org.uk/web/HPAwebFile/HPAweb_C/1194947388966 (accessed 10 May 2011).

Hranjec T, Swenson BR and Sawyer RG (2010) Surgical site infection: how we do it. *Surgical Infections* 11(3): 289–294.

Hulse M (2011) *Forced Air-warming: an effective tool in fighting SSI*. http://www.infectioncontroltoday.com/articles/2011/03/forced-air-warming-an-effective-tool-in-fighting-ssi.aspx (accessed 23 April 2011).

Lakhani SR and Dogan A (2004) Wound healing. In Kirk RM and Ribbans WJ (eds) *Clinical Surgery in General*, 4th edn. London: Churchill Livingstone.

Male D (2007) *Immunology*. Cambridge: The Open University.

Mercandetti M and Cohen AJ (2005) Wound Healing: Healing and Repair. *Emedicine.com* http://emedicine.medscape.com/article/1298129-overview (accessed 20 April 2011).

Modrau IS, Ejlersten T and Rasmussen BS (2009) Emerging role of Candida in deep sternal wound infection. *Annals of Thoracic Surgery* 88(6): 1905–1909.

National Patient Safety Agency (2011) *Outbreak of Prosthetic Valve Endocarditis. National Reporting and Learning Service*. http://nrls.npsa.nhs.uk/resources/type/signals/?entryid45=130186 (accessed 22 April 2011).

NICE (National Institute for Health and Clinical Excellence) (2008) *Surgical Site Infection: Prevention and treatment of surgical site infection*. http://tinyurl.com/35zeekf (accessed 02 March 2011).

Paley J (2005) Error and objectivity: cognitive illusions and qualitative research. *Nursing Philosophy* 6: 196–209.

Patel AR, Romanelli P, Roberts B and Kirsner RS (2009) Herpes simplex virus: a histopathologic study of the depth of herpetic wounds. *International Journal of Dermatology* 48(1): 36–40.

Pellowe CM, Pratt RJ, Loveday HP, Harper P, Robinson M and Jones SRLJ (2004) The EPIC project. Updating the evidence-base for national evidence-based guidelines for preventing healthcare-associated infections in NHS hospitals in England: a report with recommendations. *British Journal of Infection Control* 5(6): 10–16.

Pukki T, Tikkanen M and Halonen S (2010) Assessing Mepilex® Border in postoperative wound care. *Wounds UK* 6(1): 30–40.

Roitt I, Brostoff J and Male D (1993) *Immunology*, 3rd edn. London: Mosby.

Salyers AA and Whitt DD (2005) *Bacterial Pathogens: A Molecular Approach*. Washington, DC: ASM Press.

Scottish Intercollegiate Guidelines Network (SIGN) (2008) *Antibiotic Prophylaxis in Surgery: A National Guideline 104*. Edinburgh: SIGN.

Sheperd A (2009) The role of the surgical technologist in wound management. *Surgical Technologist* June: 255–261.

Sheppard M and Wright M (2006) *Principles and Practice of High Dependency Nursing*. London: Baillière-Tindall.

Shinohara T, Yamashita Y, Satoh K *et al.* (2008) Prospective evaluation of occlusive hydrocolloid dressing versus conventional gauze dressing regarding the healing effect after abdominal operations: randomized controlled trial. *Asian Journal of Surgery* 31(1): 1–5.

Smith JMB, Payne JE and Berne TV (2000) *The Surgeon's Guide to Antimicrobial Chemotherapy*. London: Arnold.

Trounce J (2002) *Clinical Pharmacology for Nurses*, 16th edn. London: Churchill Livingstone.

Ubbink DT, Vermeulen H, Goosens A, Kelner RB, Schreuder SM and Lubbers MJ (2008) Occlusive vs gauze dressings for local wound care in surgical patients: a randomized clinical trial. *Archives of Surgery* 143(10): 950–955.

Vogt KC, Uhlyarik M and Schroder TV (2007) Moist wound healing compared with standard care of treatment of primary closed vascular surgical wounds: a prospective randomized controlled study. *Wound Repair and Regeneration* 15(5): 624–627.

Vuolo J (2010) Hypergranulation: exploring possible management options. *British Journal of Nursing* 19(6): S4–S7.

Walsh TS (2004) The metabolic response to injury. In Garden JO, Bradbury AW and Forsythe J (eds) *Principles and Practices of Surgery*, 4th edn. London: Churchill Livingstone.

Weston D (2010) The pathogenesis of infection and immune response. *British Journal of Nursing* 19(16): S4–11.

Wilson J (2003) *Infection Control in Clinical Practice*. London: Ballière Tindall.

Winter GD (1962) 'Formation of the scab and the rate of epitheliasation of superficial wounds in the skin of the young domestic pig. *Nature* 193: 293–294.

Wolcott RD, Gontcharova V, Sun Y and Dowd SE (2009) Evaluation of the bacterial diversity among and within individual venous leg ulcers using bacterial tag-encoded FLX and titanium amplicon pyrosequencing and metagenomic approaches. *BMC Microbiology* 9: 226.

Woolf N (2000) *Cell, Tissue and Disease: The basis of pathology*, 3rd edn. London: W.B. Saunders Co.

Wynne R, Botti M, Stedman H *et al.* (2004) Effect of three wound dressings on infection, healing comfort, and cost in patients with sternotomy wounds: a randomized trial. *Chest* 125: 43–49.

Young T (2010) Managing the 'at risk' patient: minimizing the risk of wound infection. *British Journal of Nursing* 19(20): S1–11.

Section 3

Patient Safety and Managing Risks in Perioperative Care

CHAPTER 8

Preoperative Care

Mark Radford and Ross Palmer

Prior to any surgical intervention, the perioperative journey involves a period of assessment and optimisation to ensure that the patient is physically and psychologically prepared for their procedure. The preoperative period is therefore vital in a number of areas to ensure patients receive timely and appropriate surgical care (García *et al.* 2009). This chapter will examine the key aspects of care during this phase from the ward admission, management of presurgical anxiety, clinical optimisation and safe transfer to the operating theatre.

Models of Surgical Care

The specialisation of surgery through technology, pharmacology and refined techniques has seen a radical shift in the organisation of surgical care. Soreide (2009) highlights that day-case/short-stay, inpatient, emergency and trauma surgery have all developed significantly in recent years with an integrated model of surgery as outlined in Figure 8.1. This has resulted in the development of surgical models that require healthcare professionals to deliver care to patients in different environments and modalities (Soreide 2009). However, the majority of preoperative care is common and should be applied to all patients irrespective of their surgical pathway and will be discussed in this chapter.

Day-Case and Short-Stay Facilities

The modern surgical facility has evolved to manage patients by pathway and acuity (Thomas and Senninger 2008). Day units are often self-contained wards and theatre units (Figure 8.2) designed around efficiency of patient admission, treatment and discharge. Preoperative care focuses on ensuring that a thorough preoperative assessment is completed, risk factors (clinical, social and psychological) are identified and managed prior to surgery. Day-case surgery has evolved with some units including those patients who require a shorter stay of 23 hours or less although follow a similar preoperative process.

Manual of Perioperative Care: An Essential Guide, First Edition. Edited by Kate Woodhead and Lesley Fudge.
© 2012 John Wiley & Sons, Ltd. Published 2012 by John Wiley & Sons, Ltd.

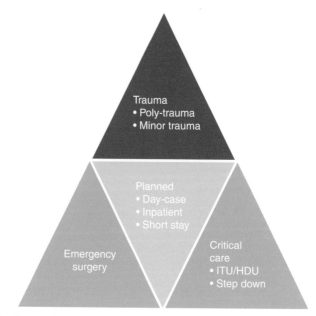

Figure 8.1   Models of surgical care. Adapted from Soreide (2009).

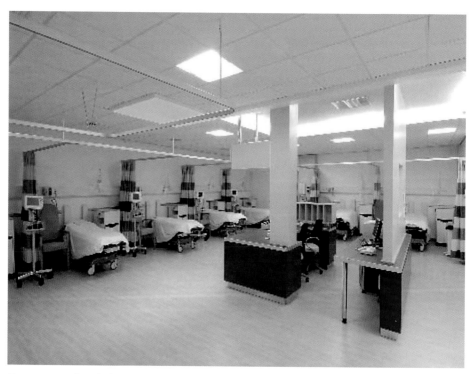

Figure 8.2   A day-of-admission unit facility.

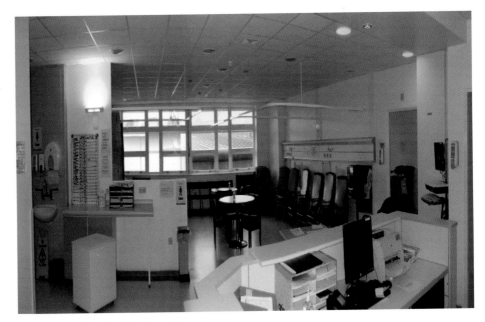

Figure 8.3 A day-of-admission unit.

Inpatient Surgery and Day of Admission

The majority of inpatients arrive in the hospital on the day of surgery after being preassessed and optimised prior to their admission. Day-of-surgery admission areas have developed to provide an environment away from busy wards, where pre-procedure checks can be undertaken and patients and their relatives can wait, which reduces anxiety and stress (Kulasegarah *et al.* 2008, Ortiga *et al.* 2010). Same-day admissions units (Figure 8.3) also provide the hospital with the ability to improve patient scheduling for surgery, provide a central area for clinicians to see patients on the day and improve communication with patients and their relatives. Once prepared, patients are then often walked from the unit to the operating theatre.

The Intensive Care Society (ICS) has highlighted a classification system for patient acuity that also indicates their place of care (Table 8.1). Acuity and dependency are important factors to understand the required staffing ratios on wards as outlined in the Association of United Kingdom University Hospitals (AUKUH) guidance, developed from the work of Hurst (2005). The AUKUH system highlights the acuity level, criteria and the types of care likely to be needed for the patient. An adapted table is outlined in Table 8.1, which also includes possible staffing levels to care for the patient.

Classification of Surgery Urgency and Implications for Care

There is a requirement to risk-stratify surgery to ensure that the correct priority and preoperative care can be assigned to patients and ensure that they are operated on within a clinically appropriate timeframe. The UK system, instituted by the National Confidential Enquiry into Patient Outcome and Death (NCEPOD) in 2004 (NCEPOD 2004), identifies four main surgical priorities, as outlined in Table 8.2.

Table 8.1 Adapted levels of dependency for wards and departments.

Levels	Definition	Criteria	Guidance on care	Environment and staffing
Level 0	Patients whose needs can be met on a normal ward in hospital	Elective admissions, routine post-diagnostic/surgical procedure care. May have underlying medical condition requiring on-going treatment, patient awaiting discharge	Routine post-op care (including half-hourly obs until stable), regular observations 2–4 hourly, ECG monitoring to establish stability, fluid management, patient-controlled analgesia, oxygen therapy 24–40%	Normal surgical ward/day-case unit or short stay facility. Staffing range: 1 trained nurse for 6–8 patients
Level 1a	Increased acuity. This identifies patients who are acutely ill or have the potential to deteriorate (such as fluctuating vitals signs)	Observation and therapeutic intervention. 'Step down' from level 2 care, post-op care following emergency or complex surgery, or following perioperative event. Deteriorating condition or fluctuating vital signs	Instability requiring continual observation/ invasive monitoring, support of outreach team but NOT higher level of care. O$_2$ greater than 40% ± chest physiotherapy 2–6 hourly. Arterial blood gas analysis – intermittent. 24–48 hours following tracheostomy, insertion central lines/ epidurals/chest drains	A surgical step down facility. Staffing levels: 1 trained to 4 patients
Level 1b	Increased dependency. This identifies patients who require intensive therapeutic intervention or more nursing input but are not necessarily acutely unwell	Severe infection, sepsis, complex wound management. Compromised immune system. Psychological support/preparation. requires continual supervision. Spinal instability/mobility difficulties	Complex drug regimes, patient and/or carers require continued support owing to poor disease prognosis or clinical outcome. Completely dependent on nursing assistance for all activities of daily living. Constant observation due to risk of harm	
Level 2	Patients requiring more detailed observation or intervention including support for a single failing organ system or postoperative care and those stepping down from higher levels of care	Deteriorating/compromised single-organ system, post-op management following major surgery, postoperative optimisation/ extended post-op care. 'Step down' from level 3 care. Uncorrected major physiological abnormalities	Patients requiring non-invasive ventilation/ resp. support. Requires a range of therapeutic interventions including: greater than 60% O$_2$, continuous ECG and invasive pressure monitoring, vasoactive drug infusions, haemodynamic instability. Pain management: IV analgesic infusions, CNS depression of airway and protective reflexes, neuro monitoring	Surgical or general high-dependency. Staffing levels: 1 trained to 2 patients
Level 3	Patients requiring advanced respiratory support alone or basic respiratory support together with support of at least two organ systems. This level includes all complex patients requiring support for multi-organ failure.	Monitoring and supportive therapy for compromise or collapse of two or more organ systems	Respiratory or CNS depression/compromise requires mechanical/invasive ventilation, invasive monitoring, vasoactive drugs, treatment of hypovolaemia/haemorrhage/ sepsis or neuroprotection	Intensive care unit. Staffing levels: 1 trained to 1 patient

Reproduced with kind permission of Association of UK University Hospitals Classification of Surgery Urgency and implications for care.

Table 8.2 NCEPOD system of surgical classification.

Code	Category	Description	Time target	Example
1	Immediate	Immediate (A) lifesaving or (B) limb or organ-saving intervention. Resuscitation simultaneous with surgical treatment	Within minutes of decision to operate	Ruptured aortic aneurysm Major trauma to abdomen or thorax Fracture with major neurovascular deficit Compartment syndrome
2	Urgent	Acute onset or deterioration of conditions that threaten life, limb or organ survival; fixation of fractures; relief of distressing symptoms	Within hours of decision to operate and normally once resuscitation completed	Compound fracture Perforated bowel with peritonitis Critical organ or limb Ischemia Perforating eye injuries
3	Expedited	Stable patient requiring early intervention for a condition that is not an immediate threat to life, limb or organ survival	Within days of decision to operate	Tendon and nerve injuries Stable and non-septic patients for wide range of surgical procedures Retinal detachment
4	Elective	Surgical procedure planned or booked in advance of routine admission to hospital	Planned	Encompasses all conditions not classified as immediate, urgent or expedited.

Reproduced with kind permission of National Confidential Enquiry into Patient Outcome and Death (NCEPOD, 2004).

Admission to the Ward or Department

The admissions process is designed to ensure that the patient is prepared safely. This process starts at the preassessment phase with a structured approach that incorporates the patient's specific surgical and holistic needs. Prior visits to surgical units or orientation on the day can aid explanation of equipment such as nurse call-bells, bedside televisions or which staff to ask for help during their stay.

Preoperative Care Assessment

Patients are likely to have been assessed prior to admission, but an assessment of care needs is required when they arrive on the ward. These pre-procedure checks give a baseline from which risk assessments and subsequent care plans can be drawn.

For example, the risks associated with developing tissue damage due to pressure in a mobile patient before the procedure may be low, however post procedure this may increase greatly. The baseline assessment needs to be completed, with a proactive care plan identified. Examples of common care assessments include:

- tissue viability – measures risk of developing pressure damage
- VTE (venous-thrombo-embolism) – measures risk of developing thrombo-emboli and associated risk of pulmonary emboli
- nutrition – particularly important aspect of surgical care as good recovery is highly dependent on nutritional status
- falls – increased risk of falls can occur postoperatively due to anaesthesia-induced disorientation, post blood loss, hypotension and unrealistic patient expectation.

The care assessment completed on admission should consider all aspects of the patient, their health needs, personal preferences, lifestyle choices and social circumstances. Consideration should be particularly given to surgical history and co-morbidities as this may impact directly on the care that they receive. A patient's dietary preferences are also important, for example if they are a strict vegetarian and do not wish to have gelatine-based medicine capsules. Further to this, aspects of personal choice such as faith may also impact on the care delivered. For example, in caring for a Sikh patient undergoing limb amputation or Jehovah's witnesses and blood transfusions.

The patient is central to these assessments and in the majority of cases information will be gathered from the patient themselves. Some patients may not be able to discuss these issues independently and therefore the role of the patient's caregiver needs to be taken into consideration. When nursing a patient with dementia or learning disabilities, behavioural challenges may exist that the carer has developed mechanisms to cope with. During the care assessment it is ideal to document these so that all staff involved in caring for that patient are aware and can utilise these strategies.

Preparing for Discharge

Discharge needs to be discussed at the earliest opportunity and involve a multidisciplinary approach to the process. This should include all aspects of the discharge from medication needs to referral to external agencies for home care. The discharge process is a time for assessment and an opportunity to listen to the patient's concerns with an aim to reduce anxiety and stress. Advice plays a key role in the process.

Contemporary Modalities in Preoperative Care

Evidence in the literature highlights that traditional practices of surgery are often outdated, leading to the development of enhanced recovery programmes (ERP). An ERP is a systematic approach to planning and implementing a patient's journey through elective surgery using evidence-based techniques and care protocols (Kehlet and Wilmore 2001) (Table 8.3). An ERP aims to minimise morbidity and mortality while promoting early mobilisation and normal function. These will, in turn, result in shorter lengths of stay and increased efficiency. This preoperative phase of care is seen as increasingly important in improving the patient's perioperative care.

Table 8.3 Principles of enhanced recovery after surgery.

Preoperative	Improved patient information and expectation
	Optimisation of clinical condition prior to surgery
	Modern fasting and nutritional management prior to surgery
	Same-day admission
	Carbohydrate loading prior to intestinal surgery
Intraoperative	Perioperative haemodyamic management
	Analgesic optimisation
	Minimal Invasive techniques where appropriate
Postoperative	Early mobilisation
	Early nutritional approach post surgery
	Revised use of drains, tubes and catheters
	Supported discharge

Improved Patient Information and Expectation

The effectiveness of an ERP depends on changing patients' expectations for their hospital stay. Modern perioperative techniques have significantly improved outcomes and reduced lengths of stay and patients should be prepared for this. To achieve a full and consistent explanation of each part of the perioperative journey it should be backed up with clear, easy-to-understand written material which helps to manage patients' expectations. The result of this provides the patient with a better understanding of their journey, potential challenges, an achievable goal in terms of improvement and length of stay. This will also reduce the anxiety that many patients experience before surgery.

Understating the Causes of and Management of Preoperative Anxiety

McClean and Cooper (1990) suggest that anxiety begins as soon as the surgical procedure is planned and increases in intensity until it reaches maximum levels on admission (Pritchard 2009, Lee and Gin 2005). Anxiety has a number of sources including fear of the unknown, concern about pain, nausea and safety, concerns about recovery and even fears of death and dying. The impacts of this have been linked to increased need for analgesia and incidence of postoperative nausea (Moerman *et al.* 1996). Therefore, recognising and treating anxiety can have a great impact on the patient's care.

The Amsterdam Preoperative Anxiety and Information Scale (APAIS) (Moerman *et al.* 1996) was designed to assess the source of preoperative anxiety and develop a tool for alerting professionals to an individual's risk of developing anxiety (Table 8.4).

This scale highlights that information and knowledge need to be addressed in managing preoperative anxiety. Pritchard (2009) discussed how preoperative anxiety can be managed through increasing levels of information being given to the patient. A different view was considered by Kiyohara *et al.* (2004) and Ivarsson et al. (2005) and by combining the two aspects of anxiety, Moerman's scale allows for a more patient-defined management plan. Pritchard (2009) suggests multi-modal strategies, such as allowing family members to be present, reorganising investigations such as blood tests so that they are completed when patients are sedated, or using distraction techniques such as music, books and therapeutic conversation.

Section 3

Table 8.4   The Amsterdam Preoperative Anxiety and Information Scale.

	1 Not at all	2	3	4	5 Extremely
I am worried about the anaesthetic					
The anaesthetic is on my mind continually					
I would like to know as much as possible about the anaesthetic					
I am worried about the procedure					
The procedure is on my mind continually					
I would like to know as much as possible about the procedure					

Adapted from the Amsterdam Preoperative Anxiety and Information Scale (Moerman *et al.* 1996).

Table 8.5   Table outlining preoperative optimisation strategies in acute and chronic disease.

Surgical urgency	Acute preoperative optimisation considerations	Chronic disease preoperative optimisation considerations	
		New onset/exacerbation	Long-term conditions
Immediate	Optimisation is primarily to treat the surgical condition simultaneously with resuscitation, e.g. fluid resuscitation for massive haemorrhage, severe sepsis, other infections and pain control	Long-term conditions may require active treatment as a result of their deterioration and/or surgical/trauma insult; e.g. cardiac ischemia, diabetes, chronic renal insufficiency	
Urgent	Optimisation aims to stabilise the surgical condition prior to surgery taking place, e.g. fluid resuscitation for haemorrhage, shock, sepsis, other infections and pain control	Condition is actively treated and improved leading up to surgery. A delay of hours only can be required if an improvement that reduces risk can be achieved	Maintain normal treatment regime, unless contraindicated by surgery or acute optimisation
Expedited	Pain control, hydration, haematological and biochemical conditions and gastrointestinal (bowel prep and GORD)	Condition is actively treated and improved leading up to surgery. Delay can be required if an improvement that reduces risk can be achieved, e.g. chest infection, AF, UTI	Maintain normal treatment regime, unless contraindicated by surgery or acute optimisation
Elective	Pain control, hydration, nutritional and gastrointestinal (bowel prep and GORD)	Consideration is given to delay surgery (if appropriate) until condition has stabilised	Conditions such as asthma, hypertension, diabetes are often optimised by preoperative assessment services prior to operation. Maintain normal treatment regime, unless contraindicated by surgery to acute optimisation

Optimisation of Clinical Condition Prior to Surgery

Clinical optimisation prior to surgery is essential and determined on the urgency of surgery and clinical condition of the patient. With immediate surgery, the options to delay to improve condition are limited. Optimisation may occur at the same time as surgery (e.g. blood loss during an aortic aneurysm repair of trauma case). In urgent surgery, an optimisation window is present where conditions can be improved to reduce risks. There are two main foci of optimisation: acute and chronic condition optimisation which need to be managed inline with the current clinical condition and concurrent treatment of the patient (Table 8.5).

Medication Management Prior to Surgery

As outlined above, optimisation of a patient's condition will require the management of a range of medications in the preoperative phase. As Young and Thompson (2011) highlight, several specific considerations applying to medications including:

- the effects on drug therapy of fasting before surgery and altered gastrointestinal function postoperatively
- the effects of surgery and anaesthesia on coexisting illnesses
- the effects of anaesthesia and surgery on drug action, metabolism and elimination.

In most cases, drugs required for chronic diseases should be continued up to the day of surgery and restarted as soon as possible unless cancelled by the surgeon or anaesthetist. However, evidence highlights that as patients are often 'nil by mouth', these medications are omitted prior to surgery, which can have serious consequences. A range of other medications should be routinely reviewed prior to surgery because of their interactions with anaesthetic agents or potential complications for surgery (Table 8.6).

Modern Fasting and Nutritional Management Prior to Surgery

Patients are routinely fasted prior to surgery to reduce the risk of aspiration during induction of anaesthesia. Evidence has highlighted that prolonged starvation times can impact on the clinical condition of the patient, and fasting advice has been updated to reflect best practice. In the elective adult patient it is recommended (Royal College of Nursing, Association of Anaesthetists of Great Britain and Ireland) that patients refrain from taking:

- solid food 6 hours before surgery
- clear fluids 2 hours before surgery (including water, tea and coffee).

For children, the same rules apply, with the addition that breast milk can be given 4 hours before surgery. Chewing gum can also be taken up to 2 hours before surgery.

Many units practice staggered admission times for patients arriving at the unit, to improve efficiency and comfort. This requires good communication with patients to advise them of fasting guidance. It is important to note that changes to the operating list or delays may require reassessment of the patient to ensure adequate hydration. Further water intake (250 mL) can be given if the patient's operation is scheduled later than 2 hours.

Table 8.6 Medication management in the preoperative phase.

Drug group	Drugs	Management
Anticoagulants	Warfarin, heparin	Management will depend on the balance of risks between bleeding and thromboembolism. INR test will determine if the patient should stop and/or converted to heparin. Prophylactic low molecular weight heparin is given the evening prior to surgery
Antiplatelets	Aspirin, clopidogrel	Requires a thorough risk assessment by anaesthetist, surgeon and cardiologist prior to stopping, often 5–10 days before surgery
Steroids	Prednisolone	Steroids should not be stopped abruptly as this may precipitate serious complications. It is often a requirement for patients to have steroid cover intraoperatively
Antiarrhythmics	Digoxin	An ECG should show whether the ventricular rate is well-controlled (<100). U&Es are needed to exclude hypokalaemia
Monoamine oxidase inhibitors (MOAIs)	Phenelzine, isocarboxazid, tranylcypromine	These drugs can have serious interactions with anaesthetic and analgesic drugs. They are routinely stopped before surgery
Oral contraceptives		Oestrogen-containing combined pills are procoagulant with an increased risk of DVT. Patients about to undergo major surgery, surgery to the legs, hips or pelvis should stop the oral contraceptive pill one month before surgery and be given alternative contraceptive advice
Insulin and oral hypoglycaemic agents	Glicazide	All diabetes will require close monitoring of blood glucose levels. Oral agents are usually omitted on the day of surgery, and restarted postoperatively. Depending upon the patients' diabetic control and type of surgery, they may require a sliding scale to control blood glucose
Herbal remedies	Ephedra, garlic, ginkgo, ginseng, kava and St. John's wort, etc.	Ideally should be stopped 2 weeks before surgery

Immediate and urgent patients are also routinely fasted prior to surgery. Patients with abdominal conditions (appendicectomy, bowel obstruction) will have a degree of reduced gut motility and gastric emptying. The use of opiates preoperatively can also slow gastric emptying, leading to increased risk of aspiration. In emergency and trauma surgery the anaesthesia technique is adjusted to further reduce the risk of aspiration through the rapid sequence induction technique (RSI).

ERP has also highlighted that improved outcomes for intestinal surgery have been demonstrated by improving pre- and postoperative nutritional intake. In the preoperative phase, carbohydrate loading has been advocated with the use of carbohydrate drinks in the days and hours leading to surgery. Clear, non-particulate carbohydrate drinks have been developed that can be given 2 hours before surgery and cause no complications. This is followed by rapid introduction of carbohydrate drinks, oral fluid and solid food postoperatively.

Fluid and Electrolyte Management Prior to Surgery in the Elective and Emergency Patient

It is important that fluid and electrolyte management are considered in all preoperative patients. For day-case and 23-hour-stay patients, this will be addressed by short fasting times, rapid recovery and early fluid intake postoperatively. For other planned, expedited and urgent patients, intravenous fluids will be an important consideration when they are having more complex surgery, have been delayed getting to the operating theatre, have required preparation that will cause fluid loss (e.g. bowel prep) or their chronic condition requires close fluid management (chronic renal failure or insulin sliding scale). The choice of fluid will be directed by the condition of the patient, with particular attention being applied to their electrolyte tests, acute and chronic disease processes and fluid balance recordings.

Safe Transfer to the Theatre Environment

Following a patient's admission and optimisation on the ward, he or she will then require transfer to the operating theatre suite. In all types of surgery, this will require a number of processes that are designed to ensure that safety and efficiency are maintained.

Pretransfer ward checks

Prior to a patient leaving the ward, it is imperative that a system of checks is instituted to minimise the possibility of procedural error occurring. Patient checklists have been devised to deliver this, and map across to preanaesthetic checks in the operating theatre. Those checks aim to ensure that the patient is fully prepared for theatre (Box 8.1).

Transfer methods to the operating theatre

There are several methods by which patients can be transferred to the operating theatre, which will be determined by the clinical assessment on the ward, urgency of surgery and patient choice. Increasingly these days patients walk to the operating theatre (Ball *et al.* 2006). Evidence suggests that this approach is both accepted by patients and advocated by staff as an efficient system (Nagraj *et al.* 2006). These patients should be preselected based upon physical ability, the lack of an underlying exercise-induced comorbidity (e.g. angina), no medication that may cause sedation such as opiates and benzodiazepines or dizziness. Alternatively patients are transferred via trolley or wheelchair (Figure 8.4).

Patient transfer trolleys have specific design features to provide comfort for the patient (mattress, semi-recumbent/sitting position), safety (head tilt, oxygen, suction and cot sides) and also a degree of multifunctional use (including induction of anaesthesia and recovery).

The high-risk patient assessment and transfer to theatre

Emergency patients can deteriorate prior to transfer to the operating theatre and may require stabilisation on the ward or department, prior to transfer to theatre. Transferring such patients can be challenging, requiring significant skills, resources and coordination.

> ### BOX 8.1
>
> ## Ward and pre-theatre clinical and safety check prior to transport and procedure
>
> - The patient is wearing an identification band
> - The patient is wearing theatre attire
> - The operation site is marked correctly
> - The patient is accompanied by the correct documents, including relevant nursing documentation/prescription sheet
> - A completed consent form/preoperative checklist
> - Any hard copy X-rays/photographs relating to procedure being undertaken
> - The patient has fasted
> - Jewellery is removed and retained in a safe place on the ward
> - All internal prostheses, metalwork, pacemakers and defibrillators are noted on the checklist
> - Relevant infections are noted on the checklist (e.g. MRSA, C. diff., Hep B/C, HIV, CJD)
> - Allergies including drugs, latex and foods are noted
> - Preoperative observations and test results are recorded
> - Makeup and nail varnish removed
> - Any potential communication difficulties and interpreting requirements noted
> - VTE assessment and management plan completed

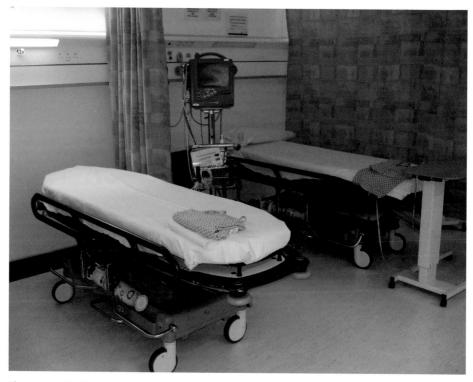

Figure 8.4   Multi-purpose patient transfer trolley.

BOX 8.2

Pre-transfer checklist for unstable patients requiring theatre

A – Airway maintenance with care and control of a possible injury of cervical spine
- Is the airway controlled?
- Is the airway likely to deteriorate during transfer?
- What method has been used?
- Is the cervical spine stable?

B – Breathing control or support
- Is there good gas exchange?
- Has PaO_2 $PaCO_2$ been measured via arterial blood gas?
- What oxygen level is needed to support above?
- Does the patient need sedating, ventilating or paralysis?
- What type of ventilation/pressure support is required?

C – Circulation control and support
- Is the patient haemodynamically stable?
- Perfusion status assessed (urine output)
- Blood loss vs. fluid replaced
- Inotropes utilised

D – Disability
- Neurologically stable (AVPU, Glasgow Coma Scores)
- Other injuries (chest, long bones, etc.)
- Co-morbid condition prior to injury/illness
- Mode of analgesia

E – Exposure
- Is the patient hypothermic?
- Will this be exacerbated during transfer?

Unstable patients must be escorted by qualified staff who have the skills and knowledge to manage any potential complications during transfer.

Prior to any transfer, clinical optimisation must be achieved; a modified assessment protocol ABCDE is a useful guide for assessing condition (Radford 2005). The questions asked will vary according to clinical condition, and reason for transfer (Box 8.2).

The equipment should be light, compact, user-friendly and easy to clean and disinfect. Battery-powered equipment should allow 2 hours of continuous use with additional spare batteries carried by the team (Figure 8.5).

Transfer of care to the operating theatre staff and ensuring patient safety

The transfer of care from ward to theatre is a critical time. Patients are at their most anxious and practitioners require skills to ensure they reassure patients (and relatives) as well as focusing on the handover of information. A number of procedural checks are required in this phase to ensure that handover is completed and to provide the opportunity to discuss optimisation or changes in clinical condition (see Box 8.1).

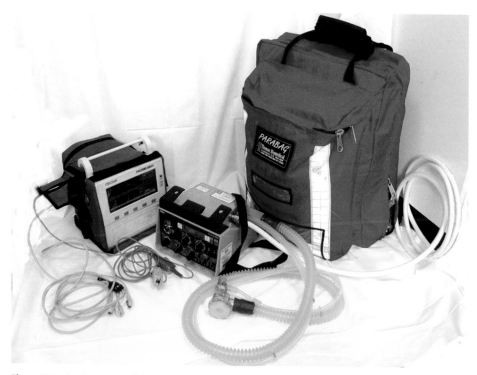

Figure 8.5   Equipment used during transfer for critical care patients.

World Health Organization Surgical Checklist

An additional safety check has been implemented in the UK based upon the work of the WHO 'Safe Surgery Saves Life' campaign. The National Patient Safety Agency (NPSA) has implemented a checklist (Figure 8.6) which contains three points at which additional checks can be performed to improve safety in the operating theatre.

Conclusion

The preoperative phase of the perioperative journey is an important time for patients, their families and practitioners to prepare for surgery. This chapter has outlined a number of key principles of perioperative care that are delivered within the preoperative period. First, a diversity of complex skills are required on the part of the healthcare practitioner in a number of challenging clinical scenarios from day-case assessment to the transfer of unstable surgical patients to the operating theatre. Second, the preoperative period is of crucial importance in the continued assessment and optimisation of surgical patients prior to their procedure. Third, patient safety must be a continued focus of healthcare practitioners throughout the journey to ensure safe and effective care is delivered. However, it is important to understand that further study and experience would be required to care for patients in such settings.

WHO Surgical Safety Checklist

(adapted for England and Wales)

NHS

National Patient Safety Agency

National Reporting and Learning Service

SIGN IN (To be read out loud)

Before induction of anaesthesia

Has the patient confirmed his/her identity, site, procedure and consent?
- [ ] Yes

Is the surgical site marked?
- [ ] Yes/not applicable

Is the anaesthesia machine and medication check complete?
- [ ] Yes

Does the patient have a:

Known allergy?
- [ ] No
- [ ] Yes

Difficult airway/aspiration risk?
- [ ] No
- [ ] Yes, and equipment/assistance available

Risk of >500ml blood loss (7ml/kg in children)?
- [ ] No
- [ ] Yes, and adequate IV access/fluids planned

PATIENT DETAILS

Last name:

First name:

Date of birth:

NHS Number:*

Procedure:

*If the NHS Number is not immediately available, a temporary number should be used until it is.

TIME OUT (To be read out loud)

Before start of surgical intervention
for example, skin incision

Have all team members introduced themselves by name and role?
- [ ] Yes

Surgeon, Anaesthetist and Registered Practitioner verbally confirm:
- [ ] What is the patient's name?
- [ ] What procedure, site and position are planned?

Anticipated critical events

Surgeon:
- [ ] How much blood loss is anticipated?
- [ ] Are there any specific equipment requirements or special investigations?
- [ ] Are there any critical or unexpected steps you want the team to know about?

Anaesthetist:
- [ ] Are there any patient specific concerns?
- [ ] What is the patient's ASA grade?
- [ ] What monitoring equipment and other specific levels of support are required, for example blood?

Nurse/ODP:
- [ ] Has the sterility of the instrumentation been confirmed (including indicator results)?
- [ ] Are there any equipment issues or concerns?

Has the surgical site infection (SSI) bundle been undertaken?
- [ ] Yes/not applicable
  - Antibiotic prophylaxis within the last 60 minutes
  - Patient warming
  - Hair removal
  - Glycaemic control

Has VTE prophylaxis been undertaken?
- [ ] Yes/not applicable

Is essential imaging displayed?
- [ ] Yes/not applicable

SIGN OUT (To be read out loud)

Before any member of the team leaves the operating room

Registered Practitioner verbally confirms with the team:
- [ ] Has the name of the procedure been recorded?
- [ ] Has it been confirmed that instruments, swabs and sharps counts are complete (or not applicable)?
- [ ] Have the specimens been labelled (including patient name)?
- [ ] Have any equipment problems been identified that need to be addressed?

Surgeon, Anaesthetist and Registered Practitioner:
- [ ] What are the key concerns for recovery and management of this patient?

This checklist contains the core content for England and Wales

www.npsa.nhs.uk/nrls

0861 January 2009

Figure 8.6 WHO Surgical Safety Checklist. Adapted for the UK from the WHO 'Safe Surgery Saves Lives' campaign by the National Patient Safety Agency.

References

Ball DR, Clark M and Clark M (2006) Which patients would prefer to walk to theatre? *Annals of the Royal College of Surgeons of England* 88(2): 172–173.

García M, Serrano Aguilar and López B (2009) Preoperative assessment. *The Lancet* 362(9397): 1749–1757.

Hurst K (2005) Relationships between patient dependency, nursing workload and quality. *International Journal of Nursing Studies* 42(1): 75–84.

Ivarsson B, Larsson S, Luhrs C and Sjoberg T (2005) Extended written pre-operative information about possible complications of cardiac surgery: do the patients want to know? *European Journal of Cardio-thoracic Surgery* 28(3): 407–414.

Kehlet H and Wilmore DW (2001) Multimodal strategies to improve surgical outcome. *American Journal of Surgery* 183(6): 630–641.

Kiyohara LY, Kayano LK and Oliviera LM (2004) Surgery information reduces anxiety in the pre-operative period. *Revista do Hospital das clinicas* 59(2): 51–56.

Kulasegarah J, Lang EE, Carolan E, Viani L, Gaffney R and Walsh RM (2008) Day of surgery admission – is this safe practice? *Irish Medical Journal* 101(IP-7): 218–219.

Lee A and Gin T (2005) Educating patients about anaesthesia: effects of various modes on patients' knowledge, anxiety and satisfaction. *Current Opinion in Anaesthesiology* 18(2): 205–208.

McClean GJ and Cooper R (1990) The nature of preoperative anxiety. *Anaesthesia* 45(2): 153–155.

Moerman N, Van Dam FS, Muller MJ and Oosting H (1996) The Amsterdam preoperative anxiety and information scale (APAIS). *Anaesthesia and Analgesia* 82(3): 445–451.

Nagraj S, Clark CI, Talbot J and Walker S (2006) Which patients would prefer to walk to theatre? *Annals of the Royal College of Surgeons of England* 88(6): 607–608.

NCEPOD (National Confidential Enquiry into Patient Outcome and Death) (2004) *The NCEPOD Classification of Intervention.* London: NCEPOD.

Ortiga B, Capdevila C, Salazar A, Viso MF, Bartolome C and Corbella X (2010) Effectiveness of a surgery admission unit for patients undergoing major elective surgery in a tertiary university hospital. *BMC Health Services Research* 10(12): 23.

Pritchard MJ (2009) Identifying and assessing anxiety in pre-operative patients. *Nursing Standard* 23(51): 35–41.

Radford M (2005) Surgery in specialised settings. In Woodhead K and Wicker P (eds) *Brigdens Textbook of Perioperative Practice.* Edinburgh: Elsevier.

Soreide K (2009) Trauma and the acute care surgery model – should it embrace or replace general surgery? *Scandinavian Journal of Trauma, Resuscitation and Emergency Medicine* 17(1): 4.

Thomas W and Senninger N (2008) *Short Stay Surgery.* London: Springer.

Young S and Thompson J (2011) Perioperative pharmacological optimisation. In Radford M, Evans C and Williamson A (eds) *Preoperative Assessment and Perioperative Management.* Keswick: M&K publishing.

Section 3

CHAPTER 9

Anaesthetic Care

Russell Chilton and Ross Thompson

The word 'anaesthesia' comes from the Greek and translates to mean 'without feeling' (Williams and Smith 2008) and this is the objective of the anaesthetic process; to render the patient insensitive to pain, so that a procedure may take place, be that awake, sedated or under a general (unresponsive) anaesthetic.

The anaesthetic does not start when the patient comes through the anaesthetic room door, it begins when the patient comes for the preoperative assessment, which establishes his or her fitness for anaesthesia and surgery (Hughes and Mardell 2009). The National Institute for Health and Clinical Excellence (NICE) has devised a set of criteria that grade the type of surgery, in line with the ASA (American Society of Anesthesiologists) score, which is the assessment of a patient's fitness before surgery (Carlisle 2006). This information, coupled with a pre-anaesthetic assessment and the nature of the procedure, will guide the anaesthetist to the most appropriate plan for the patient. This plan is communicated to the supporting practitioner prior to or on the day of the procedure.

Principles

The rationale for using anaesthesia is to provide the best possible set of conditions for surgery to take place (Oakley and Van Limburgh 2005). There are a number of techniques used to produce the ideal circumstances for the surgical team: general, regional and local anaesthesia or sedation (Wicker and O'Neil 2006, p. 243). A combination of these techniques can also be deployed. The state of the patient is accomplished by using a range of specialised drugs, commonly referred to as the 'triad of anaesthesia', a term introduced by Rees and Gray in 1950. It may prove difficult to maintain a balance during anaesthesia, so the 'triad' can be manipulated by the administration of further medicines, depending upon which aspect requires attention. This results in the triad transforming into the 'star of anaesthesia' (Figure 9.1).

Manual of Perioperative Care: An Essential Guide, First Edition. Edited by Kate Woodhead and Lesley Fudge.
© 2012 John Wiley & Sons, Ltd. Published 2012 by John Wiley & Sons, Ltd.

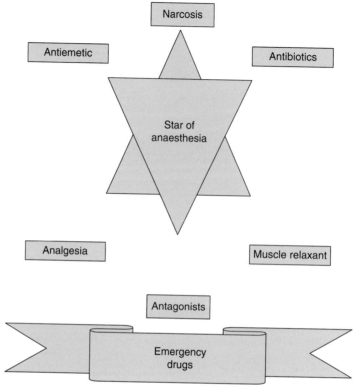

Figure 9.1 The star of anaesthesia.

Traditionally, anaesthesia is viewed as being in four stages and the object is to obtain the third stage as quickly and smoothly as possible:

- Stage 1 – Disordered consciousness. This is now known as 'induction', and is the stage at which the patient passes from analgesia without amnesia to analgesia with amnesia, leading to unconsciousness.
- Stage 2 – Excitement. This is characterised by uncontrolled muscular movement, altered vital signs, pupil dilation, vomiting and possibly laryngeal spasm.
- Stage 3 – Surgical anaesthesia. This is achieved when the patient loses the ability to consciously respond to stimuli and reflexes serving muscle control become relaxed. It is at this stage a patient under a general anaesthetic will require support to maintain their airway via an appropriate airway adjunct.
- Stage 4 – Overdose. This stage is when a potential increased risk is present. If the anaesthetist does not titrate the level of anaesthetic to the surgical stimulation, this will cause an adverse impact upon the patient. Originally this was described as the 'law of diminishing resistance'.

Staffing

Wherever anaesthesia is commenced, the anaesthetist must have exclusive and qualified assistance (AAGBI 2010, p. 10). This assistance typically takes the form of an anaesthetic practitioner, who can be either a registered nurse (RN) or an operating department practitioner (ODP). These assistants have two fundamental functions: to provide support

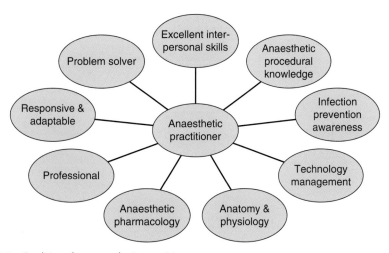

Figure 9.2 Qualities of an anaesthetic practitioner.

to the anaesthetist and to support the patient, acting as advocate (Hughes and Mardell 2009). A third person should also be available to help support the patient and assist with any unforeseen occurrences.

Training

Any anaesthetic practitioner must comply with the National Occupational Standards (NOS) (AAGBI 2010, p. 11). The RN is required to achieve additional professionally recognised and approved training before taking on the duties of an anaesthetic practitioner.

All relevant professional bodies acknowledge and positively encourage a programme of continuing professional development (CPD) for all anaesthesia practitioners. This will enable the practitioner to remain both vigilant and effective, thus maintaining a safe environment and delivery of the best quality care to the patient (Wicker and O'Neil 2006, p. 243). CPD forms the basis of employer reviews and professional registration compliance.

A clear function of the anaesthetic practitioner is to promote the wellbeing of the patient, to act as advocate and provide a professional approach to their duties. This is achieved by using sound, patient-centred, evidence-based practice and critical thinking, supported by a positive, reflective attitude. The application of a range of professional and personal skills is necessary to function as part of the anaesthetic multi-disciplinary team (MDT). Particular proficiencies must be evident in the form of preparation of the environment, maintaining health and safety, preparation of medical devices, undertaking vital signs monitoring, supporting the patient's cardiovascular requirements and airway management (College of Operating Department Practice 2009).

The role of the anaesthesia assistant

The guiding principle for any practitioner working in anaesthetics is to ensure that the patient's safety is maintained at all times (Younger 2000, p. 148). In order to achieve the best possible outcome for the patient, the knowledge base of the practitioner is continually advancing with core skills (Figure 9.2).

Many practitioners will evolve how they practice and will develop habits based upon their experiences; however this must be underpinned by best practice. Wicker and O'Neil (2006) argue that the basis of the anaesthetic practitioner's role is to:

- prepare the environment
- prepare appropriate equipment

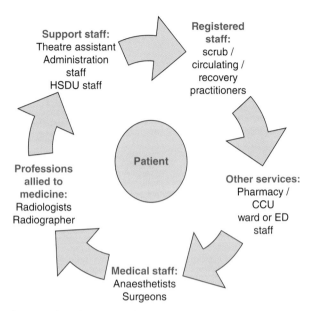

Figure 9.3   Immediate interdisciplinary team for surgical patients (from Hughes and Mardell 2009).

- ensure the safety checklist is completed
- support the patient as their needs dictate
- support the chosen method of anaesthesia
- work as part of a multi-disciplinary team (MDT)
- attach appropriate monitoring
- communicate any potential problems to relevant members of the MDT
- ensure documentation is accurate and complete.

When consultant anaesthetists are asked 'What makes a good anaesthetic practitioner?', a common response is 'Someone who has what I need before I know I need it!' While this is true, it only comes with exposure to a wide range of differing situations.

A critically important component in the operating department is communication. We must recognise our potential barriers, including gender, ethnicity, prejudices, professional rivalry, own limitations or organisational confusion to be able to overcome them. Gopee and Galloway (2009) suggest that clear and effective communication/information given to the patient preoperatively:

- improves the patient's outcomes
- improves patient's expectations
- requires less postoperative analgesia and
- reduces the patient's length of stay in hospital.

The act of communication is a two-way meaningful process, not a rudimentary non-rhetorical remark or gesture (Russell 2005). To support the patient or member of the MDT an effective practitioner will adjust how, when and at what level there is a need to communicate (Figure 9.3). The NHS Institute for Innovation and Improvement (2009) advocates a framework referred to as 'SBAR' (situation, background, assessment, recommendation).

Environment

The size and layout of an anaesthetic room is guided by many factors, usually by recommended good practice through to statute intervention, such as the Association for Perioperative Practice (AfPP) (2011), Health and Safety Executive (HSE), Health and Safety at Work Act 1974 and NHS Estates (2005). The layout of the anaesthetic room should follow a logical sequence of when and where the practitioner needs to access items; for example, suction close to the anaesthetic machine, syringes close to needles, and so on. It should also be in close proximity to appropriately stocked stores.

The anaesthetic practitioner will develop his or her own way of working. Ideally, a routine should be established. Some may use the patient journey process – preparing monitoring first, then cannulae, airway equip, etc. Some may check their room in a clockwise manner. It does not matter which approach is used so long as it leads to nothing being forgotten or overlooked. Students and newly qualified practitioners should consider writing their 'routine' down so that they can refer to and adapt it.

Equipment

An essential aspect for any anaesthetic practitioner is the sound knowledge base regarding the equipment they will be expected to use. All medical devices are governed by the Medicines and Healthcare Regulatory Agency (MHRA), by the Medical Devices Regulations (MHRA 2002) plus subsequent amendments. Further regulation and guidance is taken from professional bodies, especially the AfPP (2011) and Association of Anaesthetists of Great Britain and Ireland (AAGBI 2004). The main tenets revolve around:

- not using unfamiliar equipment
- not using out of serviceable date
- following manufacturers instructions
- not using faulty equipment
- reporting faulty equipment as per the local protocol.

The primary guidance for checking anaesthetic equipment is issued by the AAGBI, which states that it is the responsibility of anaesthetists to be satisfied that checks have been carried out correctly. It is common practice for the anaesthetic practitioner to undertake initial checks. The AAGBI state that it is a mandatory activity to check anaesthetic equipment at the beginning of each session of use, and in the event of any changes to the current set-up (AAGBI 2004). These checks cover all aspects associated with the administration of anaesthesia, including the gas supply pipelines, the anaesthetic machine, filters, circuits, airway adjuncts, ventilators, suction, monitoring and ancillary equipment. A record of these checks should be kept with the anaesthetic machine (AAGBI 2004). A copy of the checklist produced by the AAGBI should be attached permanently to the anaesthetic machine.

The following advice is predominantly taken from the guidance issued by the AAGBI document entitled *Checking Anaesthetic Equipment 3* (AAGBI 2004).

Anaesthetic machine

Most anaesthetic machines may be described simply as a box which draws in a medical gas (i.e. O_2), the option to mix it with an anaesthetic agent and deliver a specific quantity of this gas/mixture to the patient via a circuit. Usually anaesthetic machines are connected directly to the mains electrical supply. Although other equipment can be

Section 3

connected into it, multi-socket extension leads must not be used with these devices. In essence, the anaesthetic machine is a collection of medical devices assembled in a convenient, transportable trolley.

In the event of machine failure an alternative method of effective oxygen supply is required. This can be via self-inflating bag or a circuit coupled with an oxygen cylinder. These items must be present in the anaesthetic room and checked appropriately.

Medical gas supplies

The anaesthetic practitioner should identify and note which gases are being supplied by pipeline and note that each pipeline is correctly inserted into the appropriate gas supply terminal. The use of size-specific connections should prevent cross-connection.

All machines have an oxygen failure alarm; testing this may involve disconnecting the oxygen pipeline on some machines. Repeated disconnection of gas hoses may lead to premature failure of the Schroeder socket and probe. As a result of this, a 'tug' test to confirm correct insertion of each pipeline into the appropriate socket is sufficient. If a gas master switch is present that should be used instead. In addition to these checks, the oxygen failure alarm must be checked on a weekly basis by disconnecting the oxygen hose while the oxygen rotameter/flowmeter is turned on. A written record must be kept. In addition to sounding an alarm which must sound for at least 7 seconds, oxygen failure warning devices are also linked to a gas shut-off device.

All gas pressure gauges for pipelines connected to the anaesthetic machine should indicate between 400 and 500 kPa.

Adequate supplies of any other gases intended for use must be available and connected as appropriate. All reserve cylinders should be securely seated and turned off after checking their contents.

Where fitted to an anaesthetic machine, the operation of rotameters/flowmeters must be checked, ensuring that each control valve operates smoothly and that the bobbin spins freely. If nitrous oxide is to be used, the anti-hypoxia device should be tested by first turning on the nitrous oxide flow and ensuring that at least 25% oxygen also flows. The oxygen flow should then be turned off and a check made that the nitrous oxide flow also stops.

Vaporisers

These units hold specific anaesthetic agents, such as Sevoflurane™ and Isoflurane™. They are used to either induce or maintain anaesthesia (Oakley and Van Limburgh 2005). The vaporiser(s) must be fitted correctly to the anaesthetic machine and secured to the back bar and the control knobs rotated. They should be kept upright at all times and not overfilled. Reference should be made to local policy with regard to the appropriate filling method, although COSHH regulations require that it should take place in a fume cupboard, unless fixed to the delivery unit, when filling should be carried out in isolation.

Humidifiers

Humidifiers are used to protect the patient's respiratory tract and to counter the 'drying out' effect of anaesthetic gases. They also act as a barrier to potential microbiological bacteria. They are placed between the catheter mount and the breathing circuit.

Anaesthetic gas scavenging system

This system assists in the removal of anaesthetic gases. The anaesthetic practitioner must ensure that the system is switched on, connected to the machine and working correctly.

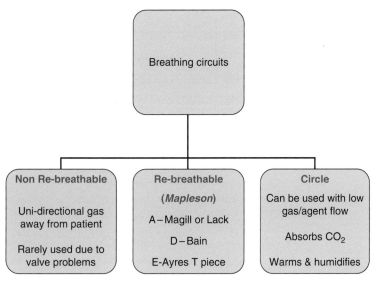

Figure 9.4   Breathing circuits.

Circular absorption of carbon dioxide

Many modern anaesthetic machines have an absorption facility using modified soda lime crystals. This should be checked to ensure it is airtight and not exhausted. This process can produce caustic fluid, so glove-wearing is essential when changing the crystals and cleaning.

Breathings systems

A breathing circuit is required to enable the delivery of anaesthetic mixtures from the anaesthetic machine to the patient via a facemask, laryngeal mask airway (LMA) or an endotracheal tube (ETT) (Oakley and Van Limburgh, 2005). There are three main types of circuit: non-rebreathable, rebreathable and circle (Figure 9.4). Rebreathable systems are subdivided into the 'Mapleson classifications', which are either open, semi-open or semi-closed. These are the most commonly used circuits in anaesthetics today (Hughes and Mardell 2009).

All circuits should be inspected manually for correct configuration and assembly before each use and changed as appropriate. The connections are secured by 'push and twist' motion. The practitioner should ensure that there are no leaks or obstructions in the reservoir bags or breathing system. A 'dead cap' should protect the patient end when not in use to prevent the intrusion of foreign bodies.

A new single-use bacterial/viral filter and angle piece/catheter mount must be used for each patient. It is important that these are checked for patency and flow, both visually and by ensuring gas flow through the whole assembly when connected to the breathing system.

Ventilators

On many anaesthetic machines, ventilators are inbuilt and undertake a self-check. However, if not, they need to be checked separately. The ventilator and tubing must be securely connected and the controls set for use ensuring that adequate pressure is generated during the inspiratory phase. The disconnection alarms should be checked for correct function.

Size	Colour	Purpose	Picture
14G	Orange	Rapid fluid administration	
16G	Gray	Fluid therapy, inc	
18G	Green	Blood	
20G	Pink	Intermittent drug	
22G	Blue	administration	
Note: Flow rate for 22G = 40ml/min approx & 14G = 270 – 300ml/min			

Figure 9.5   Cannulae comparison. Image of BD Venflon TM Pro Safety IV cannula reproduced with kind permission of BD UK Ltd.

Suction

Suction is required for rapid response to aspiration, regurgitation or vomiting by the patient during anaesthesia. The check should comprise confirmation function and connection security and also a test for the rapid development of an adequate negative pressure, done by occluding the tubing.

Cannulation

Intravenous access is a prerequisite for anaesthesia to be undertaken and is achieved by insertion of a cannula. Its placement in a blood vessel is for a variety of uses: administration of medicines, fluids or nutrition, invasive monitoring or haemodialysis (Wolverson 2008). In exceptional circumstances (e.g. babies or a needle-phobic patient), the patient can be induced without this access but it is established at the earliest opportunity.

In anaesthetics, the most common use is for the administration of anaesthetic medicines, usually via a peripheral vein.

Cannulae come in a range of sizes (Figure 9.5), the choice of which is dependent upon the size of vein and its use. The siting of peripheral cannulae can be into any viable vessel, though the most common are the back of the hand, forearm or antecubital fossa. A convention exists in the UK relating to the gauge size and specific colours. Once inserted, they must be secured with an appropriate transparent dressing. This is to enable the site to be observed for any potential signs of infection, reaction or haemorrhage. The size, location, time and date are recorded on patient documentation.

The use of invasive monitoring via an arterial cannula is only justified in certain circumstances when a severe change in blood pressure is expected. The uses of arterial lines include continuous/precise blood pressure monitoring or repeated arterial blood gases (ABG). An arterial line is usually sited in the radial artery, on the non-dominant hand side, though where peripheral access is difficult, the brachial or femoral arteries may be used on a short-term basis (Wolverson 2008). There are increased risks of bleeding, haematoma, ischaemia and infection when arterial lines are used, so great care is required when they are being inserted, secured, connected to and removed. The cannula is connected to a transducer, which converts the signal into a blood pressure reading. The transducer must be placed approximately level with the heart and 'zeroed' to atmospheric pressure (Hughes and Mardell 2009).

Central venous lines via the internal jugular, subclavian or femoral veins are used for monitoring central venous pressure (CVP), administration of medicines, infusions, nutrition, and long-term access or if there is poor peripheral access. They are typically inserted using the Seldinger technique (Wolverson 2008).

Monitoring equipment

Pre, peri and post anaesthesia the patient needs to be monitored effectively (AAGBI 2007). Direct clinical observations are a vital and effective form of monitoring and should be utilised as such (Thompson 2009) although advances in technological monitoring devices have increasingly become more sophisticated to help with this task. All apparatus must be functionality checked before use.

Monitoring devices must be attached before induction of anaesthesia and their use continued until the patient has recovered from the effects of anaesthesia (AAGBI 2007). Particular attention must be paid to ensuring that all devices used are clean, fit for purpose and free from obstruction.

Induction and maintenance of anaesthesia

The following are required for the induction and maintenance of anaesthesia:

- pulse oximetry – for measuring the circulating level of oxygen saturation, as well as heart rate (Oakley and Van Limburgh 2005)
- non-invasive blood pressure via a cuff attached externally to the patient.
- electrocardiograph
- fresh inspired and end-tidal gases and anaesthetic agents
- airway pressure – to avoid barotraumas and ensure adequate ventilation is taking place.

A nerve stimulator (whenever a neuromuscular blocking agent is used) and a way of measuring the patient's temperature should also be available.

Patients who undergo an 'operative procedure' under either a regional technique or sedation must have a minimum of the following monitoring devices:

- pulse oximeter
- non-invasive blood pressure monitor
- electrocardiograph.

Thermoregulation

NICE defines hypothermia as a core temperature of below 35.0 °C and recommends that patients should be maintained as 'comfortably warm' (between 36.5 °C and 37.5 °C), pre and post operatively.

From an anaesthetic viewpoint, effective management of thermoregulation revolves around monitoring before and during the procedures. The patient's temperature should be measured and documented before induction of anaesthesia and then every 30 minutes until the end of surgery.

It is noteworthy that hypothermia can be used to manage a patient during their operation (especially in neurological and cardiac surgery) after resuscitation or in the intensive care unit. This can be achieved via cooling catheters, cooling blankets, vests and leg wraps.

Airway adjuncts

There are five main categories associated with these devices (Figure 9.6):

- facemasks,
- oropharyngeal (OP airway)
- nasopharyngeal (NP airway),
- laryngeal mask airway (LMA)
- endotracheal (ET) tubes.

Section 3

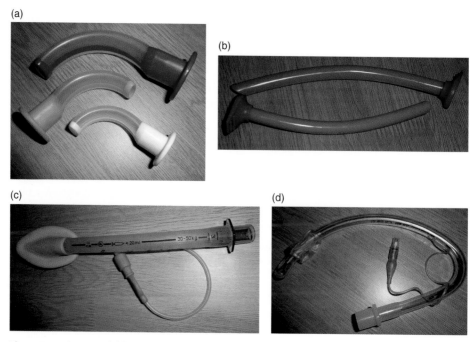

Figure 9.6   A range of different airways.

For each device there are a range of versions, some reusable, most disposable, along with some developmental advances (e.g. Proseal™ and iLMA™). Combined use of devices is not uncommon (e.g. OP airway with an ET tube upon extubation). All practitioners should ensure that all appropriate sizes of relevant adjuncts and connectors are available. The devices should only be prepared for use and checked for patency at the point of use as this will avoid contamination, unnecessary wastage and possible confusion of size. Each device must be correctly sized and practitioners must know how it is inserted, in case of an emergency.

Ancillary equipment

A check should be made that all ancillary equipment, including intubating forceps (Magill's), bougies, nerve stimulators etc. are present and working. The patient trolley/bed/operating table should be able to be rapidly tilted head-down in the event of an emergency. All syringes must have a colour-coded label that conforms to the national standard (AAGBI 2003). A stethoscope must always be available (AAGBI 2007).

A laryngoscope should be present with a variety of blade sizes. This enables the anaesthetist to examine the larynx and introduce an ET tube and/or nasogastric tube. Its functionality needs to be tested; spare batteries and lamps (if not fibreoptic) must also be readily available. Specialist laryngoscope (e.g. McCoy's, fibreoptic laryngoscope or paediatric) attachments should be readily available within the department.

Techniques

The following section is a broad overview of the common techniques related to supporting the anaesthetist. The patient's journey will be used as a guide to give the techniques logic, each progressing from a basic start point and ranging through to increased complexity, covering a range of anticipated situations. It is in the interests of the patient that the practitioner considers the potential consequences of any treatment regime, anatomical anomaly or reactive condition, and is prepared.

It is essential that the anaesthetic practitioner attends the team briefing, to absorb the knowledge held by the surgeon and anaesthetist. Enquiries at this stage may include significant allergies, body dimension, including obesity, communication and learning difficulties and any expected complications that may impact on care provision.

Once the patient arrives and has been checked into the theatre by the registered practitioner, monitoring is applied and the next stage is venous cannulation. All equipment must be available a cannula tray ready, containing a range of cannulae, approved fixative dressings, swabs, and disposable disinfection wipes for skin.

Peripheral cannulation

Cannulation of the peripheral veins is a skilled activity, usually carried out by the anaesthetist assisted by the theatre assistant, who compresses the forearm tissues sufficiently to obstruct venous return distal to the placement of his or her hands (in circumference around the arm) but not to obstruct arterial supply. This will facilitate filling of the veins and enable safe and quick cannulation and reduce patient anxiety. The patient should be told what is going to happen before it occurs as cannulation can be uncomfortable. As the patient's advocate, the theatre assistant could offer to get more experienced assistance if the inserter is struggling. In most cases, cannulation is achieved quickly and a dressing applied and reinforced, if necessary.

It is imperative to know the drugs that are in common use in the anaesthetic/post-anaesthetic care of the patient, plus those needed for any emergency situations.

Central venous catheterisation

Central venous catheters are used to measure returning blood flow pressure to the right side of the heart, provide access to central veins for fluid augmentation and allow access for the delivery of drugs. The catheter is usually inserted aseptically into either the internal or external jugular vein. The patient is tilted head-down, with the head turned to the left. The skin is prepared and disposable drapes applied. A sterile field is created on a trolley and the equipment placed on it. The catheter is introduced using the Seldinger method, using a wire through the needle, which is then removed and a larger dilator is threaded over the wire to increase the diameter of the lumen. Once the aperture is created, the catheter is introduced over the wire. The lumen(s) of the catheter are flushed and attached to a transducer. When the device is in situ it is secured by suturing and then covered with a transparent dressing.

Arterial cannulation

Arterial cannulation is carried out to provide accurate monitoring of blood pressure. The cannula is introduced in a similar method to the central venous catheter. Securing is of paramount importance, as the patient can lose a large volume of blood if the cannula comes out under the drapes. A small volume of fluid is given continually to keep the distal tip of the cannula clear. Once removed, a pressure dressing must be applied to prevent haemorrhage.

Basic airway management

The anaesthetist must ensure that all equipment is checked, so will usually check the anaesthetic delivery device/machine in accordance with guidelines prior to commencing the list. Where the anaesthetic device is checked by the anaesthetic practitioner, the permanent record is signed. The practitioner should inform the anaesthetist of the equipment that they have checked and whether there are any issues such as shortages or unavailability of items and discuss specific plans for each patient on the operating list.

The practitioner should prepare the airway trolley with the following items available:

- a range of appropriately sized, single-patient use silicone facemasks
- appropriate sizes of disposable oropharyngeal and nasopharyngeal airways
- patient-appropriate LMA – re-usable or disposable
- syringes for cuff inflation and water-based lubricant jelly
- Magill's forceps, securing tapes, pads and tape for the eyes, if that is the preferred method.

The patient should be pre-oxygenated. As the patient is given the hypnotic agent, they will lose consciousness. Their airway can become compromised, as the tongue fills the oropharynx. The practitioner is required to concentrate on the anaesthetist's actions, both in induction and airway management. Remember that they are a knowledgeable observer so should be noticing drug doses and the effect of the drug. Once the airway has been controlled, the practitioner should be prepared to hand out an oro- or naso-pharyngeal airway, having been taught how to size these, to ensure correct fitting and reduce airway obstruction. Before the anaesthetist indicates that they wish to insert the LMA, all of the necessary items must be checked to ensure that they are close to hand. The practitioner must be ready to open the airway to assist the insertion, by performing a jaw thrust and extending the airway entry. Once it is confirmed that the LMA is in place, the cuff is inflated, only with the recommended volume of air, and then secured with a cotton tie or adhesive tape (as long as the patient is not allergic). Some anaesthetists prefer to leave the LMA unsecured.

Once the airway is in place, an appropriate method is used to cover the eyes. This may be gauze pads, preformed dressings or simple tape.

Once the eyes are taped, the anaesthetist will be ready to move the patient to the theatre suite. Monitoring is disconnected; the anaesthetic circuit being the last to be separated from the airway. The anaesthetist should ensure that medical gases and vaporisers are turned off, as well as ventilators, if used.

Advances to basic airway management

The procedure highlighted above is for a routine, elective patient undergoing a minor or intermediate procedure. The patient may on the other hand, present with:

- an underlying medical condition, such as COPD
- an anatomical defect (e.g. hiatus hernia)
- having shared airway surgery or dual-life
- being an emergency
- another reason.

Definitive control of the airway requires insertion of an endo/nasotracheal tube. One of the key issues with preparing the tube is the length, which is usually indicated on the device, but can be guided by the anaesthetist, who will have met the patient. It is important to ensure, once the tube has been cut, that the circuit connector is inserted fully into the tube so that there is no gap. The tube tie may catch in the gap and pull the tube out of the trachea, or push it in and cause an obstruction. The tube must be fully tested prior to use for patency, cuff inflation, pilot line and cuff inflation valve. The remainder of the equipment required for intubation should be laid out within easy reach and be checked for function and cleanliness. The following items may be required:

- two fully working laryngoscopes with a long blade available
- appropriate sized gum-elastic bougies
- Magill's forceps, size dependent on patient type (i.e. small for a child or baby)
- range of syringes to inflate cuff
- full set of oropharyngeal and/or nasopharyngeal airways – dependent on patient/ surgery type
- tube ties, tape or preformed devices and products to secure airway
- anaesthetic swabs, not white, but may have X-ray detectable line through them
- lubricating gel
- a range of tube sizes and/or different styles – dependent on surgery/patient.

The tube is passed through the upper airway passages, under direct vision, using the laryngoscope. The distal tip of the ET tube is passed through the vocal cords and sits in the space externally identified as the suprasternal notch (Pattnaik and Bodra 2000). The cuff is then inflated. An overpressurised ET tube cuff can cause disruption to the mucociliary escalator and may lead to necrosis of the tracheal tissues (Al-Shaikh and Stacey 2007). It is worth noting here that the cuff pressure can rise during the procedure due to increase in air temperature (21–37 °C) and the diffusion of N_2O, if used. The cuff should be monitored and assessed during long cases or if the patient is repositioned.

Additional airway management

So that individual lungs can be deflated (unilateral ventilation) to allow surgical procedures to be carried out, it is important that any devices that are inserted into the lungs have features to ensure an airtight seal. Endobronchial (EB) tubes are tubes which have extended length, they do not require cutting, and they have two cuffs, one normal-sized proximal cuff and a smaller distal cuff, which sits in the smaller main bronchus. The endobronchial tubes come in a kit, complete with all of the connections. The tubes need to be put together in the correct manner, tested and prepared for intubation. The techniques for insertion are the same as for the ET tube, but the individual passageways within the tube must be tested to ensure they are patent and will allow one lung to deflate while ventilating the other.

Longer suction catheters must also be available for EB tubes. A tube clamp is employed when using EB tubes. This is used to clamp off the fresh gas supply line prior to opening the exhaust/suction port.

Spinal anaesthesia

Used as an alternative to, and sometimes in conjunction with, a general anaesthetic, spinal anaesthesia involves the insertion of a needle into the spinal space distal to the termination of the spinal cord at L2. Through the needle a combination of drugs can be given to induce a total block of all sensations, usually from the umbilicus and below. The patient usually sits upright, in an arched-back position, supported on a pillow with a member of support staff in front of them to provide communication and positional support. The procedure is carried out under strict aseptic technique. The anaesthetist will scrub and don gown and gloves. The skin is prepared with a non-irritant solution (e.g. chlorhexidine with tint 2% isopropyl alcohol). The anaesthetist selects a location to insert the needle, usually around L3/L4. The patient's position should encourage the vertebra to part, making insertion of the needle easier. The skin is anaesthetised with local anaesthetic, followed by deeper infiltration.

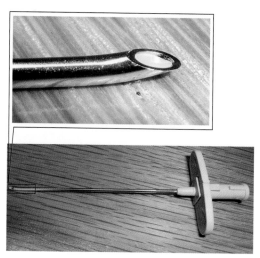

Figure 9.7 Tuohy needle.

The spinal needle is extremely thin and flexible to prevent it being manoeuvred within the tissue plains of the back, so it needs to be almost fully withdrawn before reinserting in a different angle, if required. Proper insertion is achieved when the anaesthetist feels the needle 'pop' through the ligamentum flavum and into the spinal space. The indication that the needle is in the correct space is a flow of cerebral spinal fluid (CSF) back along the needle, until it drips out of the proximal hub. The practitioner should observe the CSF and also note its turbidity as it mixes with the local anaesthetic prior to injection. The fluid should be clear. The CSF fluid can be tested with a blood glucose monitor to confirm that it is CSF; it should show as positive for glucose (approximately equal to plasma concentration). Once the needle is positioned, the anaesthetist 'fixes' the position by holding the needle firmly and then injecting either a high concentration local anaesthetic (e.g. Heavy Marcain™) or a combination of normal local anaesthetic with diamorphine.

Because of the size of the needle bore, the hole self-seals when the needle is withdrawn. The skin can be sprayed with a dressing spray or an adhesive dressing applied to capture any leakage. Gradually, paralysis takes effect and the patient will lose sensation below the waist. The patient is usually then laid down, possibly requiring some manual handling that should be coordinated by the anaesthetist to ensure no patient or staff risk. The patient should be communicated with throughout the procedure, ensuring comfort and response to any questions. Elderly patients or those with hearing deficiencies may require the anaesthetist's instructions to be repeated by the member of staff supporting the patient, so concentration and patient-centred care is essential.

Epidural anaesthesia

Similar to the spinal procedure above, epidurals are inserted in the back, but into the epidural space. The epidural space contains only the spinal roots and is a much larger physical space, so a larger volume of local anaesthetic can be given and more control achieved. Epidurals can be used for post-procedure analgesia for bowel surgery, caesarean section and a range of pelvic/abdominal procedures.

The positioning of the patient is similar to that used in spinal anaesthesia, with the same staff numbers involved. The main difference is the equipment used, in particular the needle. The Tuohy needle (Figure 9.7) has its distal opening on the side of the needle rather than on the end. This facilitates the positioning of the epidural catheter, which is left in situ when the needle is withdrawn. The needle is also graduated in 1 cm sections so that the needle depth can be monitored and recorded.

The technique proceeds as for spinal anaesthesia initially. The in-dwelling catheter and 0.2 μm filter are flushed and left prepared. With the patient positioned to open the vertebrae, the anaesthetist, in gown and gloves, pushes the needle through the skin of the back. A loss of resistance (LOR) syringe, filled with saline, is attached to the back of the needle. The needle is slowly advanced a few millimetres at a time, with the LOR plunger being pressed gently at the end of each movement. If the distal end of the needle is up against tissue bulk, the saline cannot escape so resistance is felt in the syringe. As the needle tip breaks into the epidural space, the saline in the syringe, when pressed, will flow easily and into the space. This indicates a successful procedure.

The syringe is then removed and a thin catheter fed down the lumen of the needle. The patient may experience some discomfort as the catheter brushes against the nerve roots on the way to its final location. This is usually transient. The distal tip of the catheter can be directed by rotating the needle, with its side aperture, to locate the catheter in the desired position. Local anaesthetic is injected down the catheter once a filter has been connected. The volume of local anaesthetic is greater than that used for spinal anaesthesia and the effect is not so profound. The degree of block is dose-dependent and a complete block can be achieved if desired, for example to allow surgical delivery of a baby, with the mother awake and pain-free.

Once the catheter is in place, it is imperative that it is not moved and to ensure this a locking dressing is applied, followed by secure taping of the catheter to the patient's back. The site of injection must be monitored to ensure it remains infection free and to check that there is no haemorrhage. Care must be taken while moving and positioning the patient.

Peripheral nerve blocks

As well as the techniques described above, the anaesthetist has a wide range of options available for alternative or augmented analgesia, including the blocking of regional nerves (e.g. sciatic, femoral or brachial plexus). This technique requires the nerve proximal to the site of surgery to be located, or an anatomically appropriate location selected, away from important structures and organs. The needle used is covered by a thin insulating layer, with just the tip exposed. This allows a low-voltage current to activate the tip so that when it comes into contact with the nerve it causes stimulation and the corresponding muscle contracts, indicating which nerve has been found.

The nerve is approximated following careful positioning and then stimulated by the electrical impulse produced by a peripheral nerve stimulator (PNS) device.

The technique commences with checking the equipment, battery power and function, collecting the appropriate drugs and checking expiry dates. The patient has the procedure explained to them and they are assisted to position themselves appropriately. The negative electrode wire is connected to the needle and the positive attached to an ECG electrode and affixed to the patient, near to the injection site. The anaesthetist flushes the needle with local anaesthetic and then withdraws the syringe. This allows for a free flow of blood in case a vessel is inadvertently punctured en route to the nerve. The needle is used to puncture the skin and advanced towards the nerve. Once close to the nerve, the PNS is turned on and set to 1 mA at 2 Hz. When the identified nerve responds by contracting strongly, the current is reduced to as low as possible, while still maintaining visual stimulation. Then 1 mL of local anaesthetic is injected through the needle, after aspiration to ensure that it is not in a blood vessel. Muscle twitch should be eliminated.

The rest of the prescribed dose is then administered in short volumes with aspiration between, and the needle is removed. The entry site is checked to ensure that it is not bleeding. The local anaesthetic will need to develop for approximately 20 minutes.

The skin pain receptors are stimulated prior to the commencement of surgery to ensure that an adequate block has been achieved. Topping up may be required during the procedure and is usually administered by the surgeon directly into the tissues.

Ultrasound-guided transabdominal plane blocks

Transabdominal plane (TAP) blocks involve the placement of epidural catheters using a Tuohy needle, guided by an ultrasound scanner, into the neurovascular plane between the internal oblique muscles and transverse abdominal muscles. The block is usually carried out after the administration of a general anaesthetic. The purpose of the technique is to block the sensory and motor nerves of the abdominal wall, which is especially useful for bowel, gynaecological and pelvic floor surgery, including those carried out with endoscopes.

The equipment and techniques must be learnt prior to involvement and will form part of the CPD for new practitioners.

References

AAGBI (Association of Anaesthetists of Great Britain and Ireland) (2003) *Syringe Labelling in Critical Care Areas*. London: AAGBI.

AAGBI (2004) *Checking Anaesthetic Equipment 3*. London: AAGBI, pp. 1–2.

AAGBI (2007) *Recommendations for Standards of Monitoring During Anaesthesia and Recovery*, 4th edn. London: AAGBI.

AAGBI (2010) *The Anaesthesia Team 3*. London: AAGBI. http://www.aagbi.org/sites/default/files/anaesthesia_team_2010_0. pdf (accessed March 2012).

Al-Shaikh B and Stacey S (2007) *Essentials of Anaesthetic Equipment*, 3rd edn. China: Churchill Livingstone.

Association for Perioperative Practice (2011) *Standards and Recommendations for Safe Perioperative Practice*, 3rd edn. Harrogate: AfPP.

Carlisle J (2006) In Allman KG and Wilson I (eds) *Oxford Handbook of Anaesthesia*. Oxford: Oxford University Press, p. 4.

College of Operating Department Practice (2009) *Scope of Practice*. London: CODP, London, p. 4.

Gopee N and Galloway J (2009) *Leadership and Management in Healthcare*. London: Sage, p. 20.

Hughes S and Mardell A (2009) *Oxford Handbook of Perioperative Practice*. Oxford: Oxford University Press.

MHRA (Medicines and Healthcare Regulatory Agency) (2002) *Medical Devices Regulations SI 2002/618*. www.mhra.gov.uk/ Howweregulate/Devices/index.htm available from www.legislation.gov.uk/uksi/2002/618/contents/made (accessed 15 December 2011).

National Patient Safety Agency (2009) *WHO Surgical Safety Checklist, NHS*. http://www.nrls.npsa.nhs.uk/resources/ clinical-specialty/surgery/ (accessed 15 December 2011).

NHS Estates (2005) *Health Building Note 26: Facilities for Surgical Procedures*, Vol. 1. London: Stationery Office.

NHS Institute for Innovation and Improvement (2009) *The Productive Operating Theatre – Team Working*. London: NHS Institute for Innovation and Improvement, p. 103.

Oakley M and Van Limburgh M (2005) Care of the patient undergoing anaesthesia. In Woodhead K and Wicker P (eds) *A Textbook of Perioperative Care*. London: Elsevier Churchill Livingstone, pp. 147–160.

Pattnaik SK and Bodra R (2000) Ability of cuff to confirm the correct intratracheal position of the endotracheal tube in the intensive care unit. *European Journal of Anaesthesiology* 17: 587–590.

Radford M, County B and Oakley M (2004) *Advancing Perioperative Practice*. Cheltenham: Nelson Thornes.

Rees GJ and Gray TC (1950) Methyl-*n*-propyl ether. *British Journal of Anaesthesia* 22: 83.

Russell J (2005) *Introduction to Psychology for Health Carers*. Cheltenham: Nelson Thornes, p. 3.

Thompson R (2009) *Introduction to Anaesthetics*, Technic Journal, CODP, London.

Wicker P and O'Neil J, (2006) *Caring for the Perioperative Patient*. Oxford: Blackwell Publishing.

Williams T and Smith B, (2008) *Operating Department Practice A–Z*. Cambridge: Cambridge University Press, p. 12.

Wolverson A (2008) Chapter 4. In Brooks A, Mahoney PF and Rowlands B (eds) *ABC of Tubes, Drains, Lines and Frames*. Chichester: BMJ Books, Wiley-Blackwell, p. 19.

Younger J (2000) Changing roles, changing titles in the perioperative environment. In Hind M and Wicker P (eds) *Principles of Perioperative Practice*. London: Churchill Livingstone, p. 148.

CHAPTER 10
Medicines Management
Joanne Dickson

Introduction

This chapter explores the principles of medicines management in the perioperative environment. It covers issues related to the law, as well as those relevant to professional practice. Most patients in the acute environment will be given medicines, and safety in their use is particularly relevant in the perioperative environment. The chapter will focus primarily on the administration of medicines, although aspects related to prescribing, where relevant, will be discussed.

The Law Governing Medicines

The process of administering medicines has developed due to both legal and professional regulation. In the UK, the Medicines Act was first passed in 1968, and has had various additions in the form of amended directions since then. It governs many aspects of medicines use, and categorises medicines into three main types:

- GSL (General sales list) – medicines that may be sold directly to a consumer without a prescription or intervention from a healthcare professional
- P (Pharmacy medicines) – can be sold without prescription under the supervision of a registered pharmacist, in a registered premises
- POM (Prescription only medicines) – available from a pharmacist using a prescription from an authorised prescriber.

Prescriptions may be generated using either of two methods: a patient-specific direction or a patient group direction.

A *patient-specific direction* is the traditional written instruction, from a doctor, dentist, nurse or pharmacist independent prescriber, for medicines to be supplied or administered to a named patient. The majority of medicines are still supplied or administered using this process (Department of Health 2006). Examples of patient-specific directions are the inpatient drug chart used in most NHS hospitals, or in the theatre environment, an anaesthetic chart determined to be suitable by the organisation using it.

Manual of Perioperative Care: An Essential Guide, First Edition. Edited by Kate Woodhead and Lesley Fudge.
© 2012 John Wiley & Sons, Ltd. Published 2012 by John Wiley & Sons, Ltd.

A *patient group direction* (PGD) is a written instruction for the supply or administration of a licensed medicine (or medicines) in an identified clinical situation, where the patient may not be individually identified before presenting for treatment (Department of Health 2006). A PGD is drawn up locally by a group of health professionals and must meet certain legal criteria and approved by the organisation in which it is to be used. PGDs can only be used by the following registered healthcare professionals, acting as named individuals: nurses, midwives, health visitors, paramedics, optometrists, chiropodists and podiatrists, radiographers, orthoptists, physiotherapists, pharmacists, dieticians, occupational therapists, prosthetists and orthotists, and speech and language therapists. Of note is the fact that registered operating department practitioners (ODPs) are not named on this list. Some organisations will have a local agreement which allows the use of PGDs by ODPs, although in practice they are not routinely used in the theatre environment.

Medicines may also be prescribed by qualified non-medical prescribers. Over the last 15 years, the role has developed significantly in order that patients can receive medicines in a more timely fashion. This development also ensures that the skills of appropriate healthcare professionals are better utilised, and that multi-disciplinary teams can develop processes to improve the patient pathway. This extension of responsibility now allows qualified and registered (with the Nursing and Midwifery Council (NMC)) nurse prescribers to prescribe any medicine to a patient with any medical condition, including **some** controlled drugs, if it is within their sphere of competence (Department of Health 2006). Pharmacist and optometrist prescribers may also now prescribe independently, but not controlled drugs, and other professional groups (physiotherapists, podiatrists and radiographers) may be trained to prescribe using a supplementary prescribing route.

Any suitably trained member of staff can legally administer medicines that have been prescribed by an authorised prescriber for an individual patient. This principle applies to registered and non-registered staff at all levels. However, non-registered staff cannot administer medicines using a PGD, and cannot train to prescribe medicines. Most NHS organisations have policies in place that limit the administration of medicines by non-registered practitioners to an identified list of medicines used in given situations. An example of this would be the administration of a 0.9% sodium chloride flush following insertion of a peripheral cannula.

Medicines used in the UK are granted a licence for use by the Medicines and Healthcare products Regulatory Agency (MHRA). The licence is granted for use of the medicine for defined indications, and is given following the pharmaceutical company providing proof of its safety and efficacy. Any medicine used for an indication outside of that for which it is licensed is used 'off licence'. This must be at the direction of an appropriate prescriber, and patients should be informed of medicines used in these circumstances.

Professional Practice and Medicines

All healthcare regulators and most healthcare organisations will set standards for the prescribing and administration of medicines. The NMC *Standards for Medicines Management* (Nursing and Midwifery Council 2008) contains guidance relevant to all healthcare professionals administering medicines.

Patient identification is an essential step in ensuring safety. The patient wristband is most often used as the method of identification in theatres, and should be used to confirm identity before medicines are given.

Prior to administration of medicines, allergies or hypersensitivities must be confirmed and documented. Usually this will be on the patient's medications prescription.

Organisational policy will determine who can document allergies, but in most cases this will include any registered professional who is competent to do so. In documenting an allergy, it is important to also determine the reaction type and severity. Some allergies will affect others, for example an allergy to benzylpenicillin will mean that a patient should be documented as allergic to all penicillins. Individuals who are allergic to penicillins may also be hypersensitive to other antimicrobials, and a pharmacist will usually be involved to determine appropriate medication choices in this group of patients. In some cases it may be determined by a prescriber that medicines should be prescribed and given even though the patient has a documented sensitivity. In these instances, the person administering the medicine is responsible for confirming the credentials of the prescriber, and ensuring they are aware of any documented allergy before administration.

The practitioner responsible for the administration of a medicine must not rely solely on the information contained within the prescription. Mistakes in prescribing can occur, and the person administering must understand the indication for the medicine, as well as potential side-effects and usual doses. It is important to consider these factors in context with the patient's past medical history as well as his or her current diagnosis. This information is particularly important for certain medicines, for example digoxin where the patient's pulse rate must be known or preparations of intravenous fluids containing potassium, where the blood levels must be known.

When preparing the medicine for administration, a non-touch technique should be used, and an appropriate method of administration chosen. This may involve choosing liquid or dispersible preparations. If medicines are to be given in liquid form by mouth, an oral syringe designed specifically for this purpose must be used (NPSA 2007). In practice, these are usually purple in colour to distinguish them from those used for intravenous administration, and they must have connectors which prevent them from being inadvertently fitted onto an intravenous device. Medicine preparations must also be checked for their suitability for use, particularly that they are being given prior to the expiry date set by the manufacturer.

Paper-based systems for medicines prescription can be problematic in terms of their legibility. Many hospitals are moving towards electronic methods for prescription, administration, pharmacy validation and supply and also for discharge prescriptions and information to colleagues based in primary care. Distinct benefits will be seen in the legibility, timeliness, accuracy of prescriptions and patient safety through use of decision support, but it is essential that all users are given opportunity to be trained on their use, as well as understanding the local governance arrangements.

When you have administered a dose of a medicine, you must clearly document the date and time of administration, ensuring the name, dose and route are also clear. All of this information can be paper-based or electronic. There must also be a signature recorded for each medicine, and in the case of a controlled drug the signature of a second registered practitioner. Some organisations also mandate a second signature on other occasions, for example when the medicine is given via the intravenous route.

Where medicines are not administered for any reason, this must also be documented. The NPSA (2010) have highlighted the problem of missed and delayed doses of medicines, reporting incidences of patient harm. It is essential that medicines due for administration are obtained and administered promptly, especially where timeliness is essential such as antimicrobials, anticoagulants and medicines for treatment of Parkinson's disease. Of particular importance in the perioperative environment is that all administrations are documented clearly in order that colleagues subsequently caring for the patient have all the information they need. For example, they can only safely determine a time for a second dose of paracetamol if they have clear information about when the previous dose was given.

Section 3

Medicines Storage

Different clinical areas will have different guidance on storage of medicines, which are likely to be documented as part of the overarching medicines policy. All cupboards and cabinets must conform to the appropriate national standards, usually BS 2881:1989, Specification for cupboards for the storage of medicines in healthcare premises.

There should be guidance in place about the locking of cabinets and cupboards. This will generally state that in normal circumstances all medicines cupboards must be kept locked when not in use, and the key held by a registered practitioner, usually a nurse, midwife or ODP. Some theatre areas will have guidance in place which allows cupboards to remain open during a theatre list, as long as there is an individual responsible for monitoring the removal of medicines during this time.

Medicines must be stored in the container in which they are supplied. Medicines should not be transferred from one container to another, nor should they be taken out of their containers and left loose. Some medicines need to be stored at a certain temperature, including some which must be stored in a fridge. If a medicine needs to be stored at low temperature, this will be highlighted on its packaging. The fridge must be specifically designated for storage of medicines, and should not contain other items. The fridge must have a thermometer, and it is essential that someone is designated to be responsible for monitoring and recording the fridge temperature .

Controlled Drugs

The registered nurse or midwife in charge of an operating theatre or theatre suite is responsible for the safe and appropriate management of controlled drugs. Even if the theatre or theatre suite is managed by an ODP, the most senior registered nurse or midwife present is responsible for controlled drugs under the present regulations (Department of Health 2007). The registered practitioner in charge will usually delegate control of access (i.e. key-holding) to the controlled drugs cupboard to another, such as a registered nurse or an ODP. Similar considerations apply to requisitioning and checking of controlled drugs. There are designated responsibilities for professional groups who are involved in the management of controlled drugs in theatres;

(a) The registered nurse, midwife or ODP for:
  (i) ordering, receiving, checking, recording and storing stock;
  (ii) recording the amount issued to medical staff;
  (iii) returning unused ampoules to stock;
  (iv) amending balances accordingly.
(b) Medical staff for:
  (i) signing for the controlled drugs received in the operating theatre controlled drugs register;
  (ii) properly recording in the patient's records the amount of drugs administered;
  (iii) returning any unopened ampoules;
  (iv) safe disposal of any unused controlled drugs that remain in an open ampoule or syringe.
(c) The pharmacist for:
  (i) supply of controlled drugs to each stock location;
  (ii) regular audit of local policies;
  (iii) checking controlled drug stocks and registers at least once every three months (AAGBI 2006).

It is essential that practitioners make themselves aware of the local guidance agreed. It is likely to give specific information about the regularity of stock balance checks, documentation of administration, transport of controlled drugs and the controlled drugs registers in use within that organisation.

Legislation around wastage of controlled drugs requires that unused part doses should be disposed of promptly, and this must be witnessed by a second registered healthcare professional. The controlled drug to be disposed of must be rendered irretrievable by placing it in a sharps bin designated and marked as pharmaceutical waste. Some healthcare organisations choose to further 'denature' controlled drugs with the use of substances in the form of granules or pads, which solidify liquid controlled drug waste.

Controlled drugs are subject to additional standards for their storage (Misuse of Drugs [Safe Custody] Regulations 1973). They must be stored in a locked metal cupboard, and the keys must be held by a registered practitioner determined as being appropriate by their employing organisation.

Pharmacology

The complexity of medicines management means that it is essential that all healthcare professionals have a good understanding of the way that medicines work. A good knowledge of pharmacology is necessary to ensure that medicines are prescribed and administered correctly, and that patient safety is maintained.

Pharmacokinetics is the study of medication activity as it moves through the body. The four phases of pharmacokinetics are absorption, distribution, metabolism and excretion.

- *Absorption*: Medicines exert their effect on the body by being absorbed at the site of administration and then being distributed throughout the body. The site of administration has an effect on absorption. Other factors that affect absorption include the preparation of the medicine (e.g. modified release preparations are absorbed more slowly than immediate release), and the lipid solubility of the medicine.
- *Distribution*: The rate of distribution of a medicine is affected by the organ which is involved in processing it, as well as blood flow at the site of absorption. For example, well-perfused organs such as the brain and the liver will have an increased rate compared to others such as fat and bone. Distribution of a medication is determined by its solubility. The brain is an organ with high lipid content; therefore, a lipid-soluble medication will rapidly travel from the blood to the brain. An example of this is a lipid-soluble anaesthetic, which can quickly move from the blood to the brain and rapidly produce the desired effect.
- *Metabolism*: The process of transformation of the medicine from its original form to a water-soluble form ready for excretion. The liver is the most common site for medication metabolism. When medications are metabolised they are changed into either inactive metabolites that are excreted or active metabolites capable of their own pharmacologic action. This process can be affected by genetic factors, which cause some individuals to metabolise medications more rapidly or more slowly than others.
- *Excretion*: Medication excretion refers to the rate of and method through which the body eliminates the medication. This may be before it is excreted from the body, primarily through the kidneys. Other routes of elimination include the biliary tract, sweat, saliva and the respiratory system.

Section 3

Pharmacodynamics is the effect of the drug on the body. It refers to the way in which it works to produce the desired effect. A drug may be used for its properties as an agonist or antagonist. A good example of an antagonist reaction is the use of naloxone to counteract the effect of opioid medicines. Naloxone works by blocking and preventing the activation of receptors for morphine.

The amount of a medicine needed to provide the desired response in an individual can vary. The margin for safe use of a medicine is known as the therapeutic index. It is the measure of a medication's therapeutic effect and its adverse effects. A high therapeutic index indicates that the medication is relatively safe. The therapeutic index is calculated by using the effective dose for 50% of patients versus the dose that would be toxic in 50% of patients. Digoxin is an example of a medication with a low therapeutic index, which indicates that there is a greater risk of toxicity with digoxin.

Considerations when Administering Medicines

When reviewing a prescription prior to administering medicines, the practitioner must consider the individual to whom it will be given. The age of the patient is important. The two groups generally identified as needing special consideration are children and the elderly. The weight of a patient may be important for patients of all ages with certain medicines, for example some low molecular weight heparins (LMWH). In paediatric practice the weight of the child is important in calculating the dose of all medicines and with some, practitioners can become complacent due to their familiarity with a particular medicine, but their unfamiliarity with how it is affected by weight. Recent incidents where adolescents were given inappropriate doses of intravenous paracetamol, based on their age rather than their weight, have demonstrated that practitioners must ensure that they are familiar with all aspects of a medicine when involved in its administration.

The UK has an increasing elderly population, who are likely to be taking medicines for chronic conditions when being prepared for surgical procedures. Patients undergoing surgical procedures to repair fractures are often found to have suffered balance problems or recorded reduced blood pressure due to this 'polypharmacy'. With age, a reduction in the size of the liver and the reduced efficiency of the kidneys will also mean that medicines may vary widely in their effects.

Liver disease itself is another factor affecting medicines. Individual patients will be affected very differently, despite similar conditions. It is therefore essential that blood results are monitored carefully in the perioperative period in order to determine early effects which are likely to impact on the metabolism of medicines.

The kidneys are the organ most often responsible for the elimination of medicines from the body, and therefore patients with renal impairment also need special consideration. As with patients with liver disease, patients with kidney problems will need to be monitored carefully. This may often involve communication between the surgical and renal team in order to make sure the patient is safely anaesthetised. Many medicines need to be given in smaller doses or less often to patients with renal impairment, in order that their kidneys are able to complete the required excretion.

Medicines Administration

Medicines can be administered using a variety of different methods, however in the theatre environment there are likely to be a smaller number of routes of administration that are commonly used.

Oral administration is the most commonly used for awake patients, and so will be used for preoperative medication, and on occasion in the postoperative recovery environment. It relies on a patient being alert enough to swallow, and also usually being able to tolerate oral fluids. It is not used where rapid effects of medicines are needed, for example in an emergency situation. Related methods may be used in perioperative practice, for example the sublingual (under the tongue) or buccal (by absorption into the buccal membrane in the mouth) routes. Sublingual administration is most commonly used for glyceryl trinitrate (GTN) in the cardiac chest pain of angina. Medicines via the sublingual or buccal routes must not be swallowed, and the patient must have the ability to understand this if they are to be used effectively.

Medicines may also be administered using feeding tubes, in place because a patient requires nutritional supplementation. Such tubes may be placed either via the nose into the stomach (nasogastric) or directly into the stomach (gastrostomy) or jejunum (jejunostomy). If these tubes are in use, issues around interaction between feed substances and also use of liquid preparations need to be considered. Crushing of tablets for administration via a tube should only be considered following discussion with a pharmacist, as some medicines when crushed can cause damage to the tube, or may be harmful in their crushed form to the patient or to the person preparing.

The rectal route of administration, where medicines are absorbed via the rectal mucosa, is often used perioperatively and may be appropriate where a patient is unable to swallow. This route is commonly used for the administration of paracetamol in patients unable to swallow, and would usually be seen as the second-line choice (after oral) prior to considering an intravenous administration of this drug. Absorption via the rectal route is generally slower, and more unpredictable, and is therefore not used in emergency situations.

Parenteral administration

The most commonly used route intraoperatively is the *intravenous* route. Medicines are delivered directly into the bloodstream via a vein, usually through a peripherally or centrally inserted line. These lines must be inserted and accessed using non-touch aseptic technique (ANTT), to reduce the risk of bacteraemia.

The intravenous route is used for medicines which lose their potency during transit through the digestive system. It is also used where a rapid effect, or high concentrations of the medicine are required. Intravenous administration should only be performed by practitioners who have been specifically trained to do this. Often, intravenous administration of medicines is part of the role of the anaesthetist in the theatre environment. However, in certain perioperative environments it is appropriate for registered nurses and ODPs to be trained to use this route. Allergic or anaphylactic reactions are much more common following intravenous administration and the knowledge and skills about what to do when this happens must be an integral part of any training package.

Medicines can be given intravenously using the bolus technique, where the drug is either mixed with a suitable dilutent, or may be given without dilution. The full bolus dose will usually, for safety reasons, be given over a period of at least 3–5 minutes. There are a limited number of medicines, for example adenosine, which need to be given as a rapid bolus followed by an appropriate flush of the intravenous device. Bolus administration is used where a peak plasma concentration of the drug is needed immediately. Drugs can also be given as intravenous infusions. This technique is used where a medication is intended to be given over a longer period, at a constant or variable rate. A continuous infusion is used where a consistent or controlled therapeutic response is required. It may also be used to permit greater dilution than is usually possible with an intermittent infusion, and in order to avoid toxicity.

Analgesic medicines in the form of *patient-controlled analgesia systems* (PCAS) are another method of giving small boluses of analgesia (often opioid-based) in controlled doses where the patient is able to determine when a subsequent dose is needed. They press a button on a hand held device, and a small dose will be given as long as the patient is within the limits of dose which have been set by the healthcare professional.

When administering injectable medicines it may be necessary to perform calculations in order to determine the appropriate dose to be administered. Incorrect calculations can lead to serious complications, and even death. The incorrect placement of a decimal point can lead to 10 or 100 times doses being given. All practitioners performing calculations must have the correct numeracy skills, and some organisations will insist these are tested prior to or during a term of employment. You will always need to ensure that on occasions where you are checking your calculation with a second registered healthcare professional (as guided within the NMC standards for medicines management), that each of you performs the calculation independently, and does not rely on one person to be correct.

Other injectable routes may also be used in the perioperative period, including *subcutaneous injection* (into the subcutaneous tissue of the skin). LMWH preparations, commonly used for prophylaxis for venous thromboembolism (VTE) are administered via this route, delivering a slower rate of absorption into the bloodstream.

Intramuscular injections are used where the increased blood supply of muscle tissue (over fatty tissue of subcutaneous injection) is needed. This route needs to be used with caution, as physical landmarks need to be known and followed in order to prevent inadvertent injection of the nerve fibres which are near to the muscle tissue.

Transdermal administration is increasingly common. Manufacturers have developed patches filled with drugs which are absorbed slowly through the skin at a controlled rate. Patches may be used for long-term pain control or for smoking cessation. It is important to consider the possible placement of transdermal patches in the perioperative environment. Patients may forget to inform healthcare professionals that they use patches when asked about their routine medicines. They will often be left in situ during operative procedures, and addition of further medicines will need to be considered with the background dose via the patch in mind.

Topical administration of medicines means the drug is administered directly to the tissue, for example the ear, eye or skin. Local anaesthetic creams which may be used prior to the placement of intravenous devices would be applied topically.

Inhalation is used routinely in theatre, where the lungs are used as the method of absorption of medication. Many anaesthetic drugs are given via this route, and this will be discussed further in other chapters.

Epidural administration is used in perioperative practice for the administration of local anaesthetics and analgesia for pain control. This route must only be used by suitable qualified practitioners, and in UK practice this is likely to be an anaesthetist. The epidural route may be used for single bolus doses, or epidural catheters are often placed for ongoing drug delivery. Perioperative practitioners involved in the care of epidural infusions will need to ensure local guidelines and policies (usually developed by specialist pain teams) are followed.

Arterial lines are commonly placed during major operative procedures. They are not routinely used for the administration of medication in theatres, although they are used for direct injection of vasodilators and thrombolytic agents during arterial recanalisation. In addition, various chemotherapeutic treatments are more effective by the arterial route and may be administered through intermittent catheterisation or by placement of subcutaneous ports. The presence of an arterial line is an important factor to consider when monitoring patients in theatre, and administering drugs via other routes. Lines must be easily identifiable, as administration via the incorrect route can lead to significant patient harm. Reported examples include local anaesthetic drugs given intravenously, rather than epidurally (leading to patient death) and drugs for oral administration (e.g. Oramorph) given intravenously, leading to extravasation injury.

Sources of Information on Medicines

In order to ensure practice with medicines is safe and clinically effective, practitioners should be aware of up-to-date and reliable sources of information. In the clinical area this may be in the form of clinical guidelines and policies, which are often developed by a group of experienced peers, who will use regional, national and international sources of evidence.

There are also sources of information readily available in the clinical area, including the British National Formulary (BNF) which is a reference book that contains a wide spectrum of information and advice on prescribing and pharmacology of medicines. Copies can be found in most healthcare organisations, and the electronic version is easily accessible. There are other similar reference sources (including MIMS and Food and Drugs Board data) which may also be available.

The National Institute for Heath and Clinical Excellence makes recommendations to the NHS on new and existing medicines, treatments and procedures and about treating and caring for people with specific diseases and conditions.

The National Patient Safety Agency (NPSA) is the body responsible for monitoring patient safety. They encourage healthcare organisations and those working within them to report patient safety incidents. They collate these reports in order to inform and educate about potential risks.

The Nursing and Midwifery Council (NMC) (2008) published *Standards for Medicines Management*. As well as regulating all registered nurses, it reports its primary role as being to protect the public, and it is as part of this patient safety function that it publishes guidance on medicines management.

The National Prescribing Centre (NPC) supports the NHS and those working for it to improve safety, quality and value for money in the use of medicines for the benefit of patients and the public. It publishes resources and guidance relevant to prescribers, both medical and non-medical, and other healthcare professionals.

In order to remain up to date, you will also need to review current practice developments published in healthcare books and journals, conference papers and promotional material generated by pharmaceutical companies. In all of these instances it is important that you are able to appraise the information contained within them for its relevance and possibly its generalisability. This will inform your decision-making, alongside guidance produced locally and the experience and knowledge of colleagues from your own and other professional disciplines.

Conclusion

This chapter has introduced you to important aspects of medicines management which need to be considered throughout your career in the perioperative environment. It has highlighted legal and professional aspects of care, and related them to their impact on patient safety. It is expected that you will continue to build on this knowledge and develop your practice in this area throughout your career.

Section 3

References

AAGBI (Association of Anaesthetists of Great Britain and Ireland) (2006) *Controlled Drugs in Perioperative Care*. London: AAGBI.

Department of Health (2006) *Medicines Matters*. London: Department of Health.

Department of Health (2007) *Safer Management of Controlled Drugs: A guide to good practice in secondary care*. London: Department of Health.

NPSA (National Patient Safety Agency) (2007) *Promoting Safer Measurement and Administration of Liquid Medicines via Oral and Other Enteral Routes*. NPSA/2007/19: Patient Safety Alert 19. http://www.nrls.npsa.nhs.uk/resources/?entryid45=59808 (accessed March 2012).

NPSA (2010) *Reducing Harm from Omitted and Delayed Medicines in Hospital*. NPSA/2010/RRR009: Rapid Response Report 009. http://www.nrls.npsa.nhs.uk/resources/?EntryId45=66720 (accessed March 2012).

Nursing and Midwifery Council (2008) *Standards for Medicines Management*. London: NMC.

Further Readings

Kelly J and Wright D (2009) Administering medicines to adult patients with dysphagia. Nursing Standard 23: 29, 61–68.

Lawson E and Hennefer D (2010) *Medicines Management in Adult Nursing*. Exeter: Learning Matters.

National Patient Safety Agency (NPSA) (2007) *Promoting Safer Use of Injectable medicines*. NPSA/2007/20: Patient Safety Alert 20. http://www.nrls.npsa.nhs.uk/resources/?EntryId45=59812.

Royal Marsden Hospital (2008) *The Royal Marsden Manual of Clinical Nursing Procedures*, 7th edn. London: Wiley Blackwell.

Royal College of Nursing (RCN) (2005) *Standards for Infusion Therapy*. London: Royal College of Nursing.

Useful Websites

Medicines and Healthcare products Regulatory Agency (MHRA) www.mhra.gov.uk

British National Formulary (BNF) http://bnf.org/bnf/

National Electronic Library for Medicines http://www.nelm.nhs.uk/en/

National Prescribing Centre www.npc.co.uk

Nursing and Midwifery Council www.nmc-uk.org

Health Professions Council http://www.hpc-uk.org/

CHAPTER 11

Fluid Replacement and Blood Transfusion

Fiona Martin

Crystalloid and Colloid Fluid

We give perioperative intravenous (IV) fluids because:

- patients often receive insufficient fluid before their operation
- patients lose fluid during the operation (e.g. bleeding, evaporation from wounds, urine)
- fluids are needed to deliver drugs (e.g. antibiotics)
- patients need the ions or compounds contained in the fluids to maintain homeostasis (e.g. K^+, glucose)
- IV fluids may reduce postoperative nausea and vomiting (Maharaj et al. 2005).

Intravenous fluids are often described as crystalloid or colloid. Crystalloids are mainly water with specific mineral salts and water-soluble molecules added (e.g. K^+, Na^+, lactate). Colloids contain larger insoluble molecules which are thought to slow its leakage into the peripheral tissues as interstitial fluid. The choice of crystalloid versus colloid fluid has been subject of much research. The World Health Organization (WHO) recommends that blood loss can be replaced with equal amounts of colloid but three times as much crystalloid may be needed (WHO Blood Transfusion Safety 2002). A Cochrane Review of the use of crystalloids and colloids in the critically ill (Perel and Roberts 2011) found no evidence that colloids reduce mortality.

Table 11.1 shows the contents of commonly used crystalloid and colloid fluids and the ion levels in venous blood for comparison.

Assessment of Volume Status

It is difficult to be precise about how much fluid a patient needs, but a judgement can be made using the following pieces of information and also by observing trends in their clinical observations with time. The British Consensus Guidelines on Intravenous Fluid

Table 11.1 Constituents of commonly used crystalloid and colloid fluids with plasma blood levels for comparison.

	Na⁺ (mmol/L)	Cl⁻	K⁺	Ca²⁺	Lactate	Glucose	Other	pH	Osmolality (mOsm/kg)
Plasma concentration	135–145	95–105	3.5–5.0	2.1–2.5 (total)	0.5–2	3.6–5.8 mMol/L (approx.0.6–1 g/L)	–	7.35–7.45	285–295
Reference ranges vary slightly in each hospital									
0.9% (normal) Saline	154	154	–	–	–	–	–	5.5	308
5% Glucose	–	–	–	–	–	50 g/L	–	4.2	278
10% Glucose	–	–	–	–	–	100 g/L	–	3.5–6.5	555
Hartmann's solution (very similar to US Ringer's lactate)	131	111	5	4	29	–	–	6.5	279
Gelatin (Gelofusine®)	154	125					Gelatin 40 g/L MW 30 kDa	7.4	308
Starch (Voluven®)	154	154	–	–	–	–	Hydroxyethyl starch 6 g/L MW 130 kDa	4.0–4.5	308

Therapy for Adult Surgical Patients (Powell-Tuck *et al.* 2008) contain evidence-based recommendations on assessment of fluid status and fluid prescribing in surgical patients.

- *History*: Has the patient been nil by mouth for long? Have they been suffering from diarrhoea and vomiting. Do they feel thirsty? Do they have a fever?
- *Charts*: Input/output charts comparing oral/IV intake with urine output and nasogastric/stoma losses can help to guide decisions about fluid prescription. However, urine output can be misleading after surgery, diarrhoea and vomiting is hard to quantify and charts are often incomplete. Patient weight is a good guide to hydration. Patients needing haemodialysis are weighed at each dialysis session.
- *Clinical signs of dehydration*: These are dry skin, sunken eyes, reduced skin turgor, rapid respiratory rate, tachycardia, poor urine output and a sunken anterior fontanelle in a baby. Critically ill patients often lose intravascular fluid to their tissues as oedema, which can mask some of these signs.
- *Intraoperative fluid loss*: Open abdominal surgery causes fluid losses of around 5 mL/kg per hour from evaporation. Blood loss can be hard to quantify (e.g. during transurethral resection of the prostate).

Methods of Administration and Warming

Intravenous fluids are administered via a sterile giving set to an IV cannula. Simple fluid-giving sets are suitable for slow to moderate flows of fluid and can be used with biometric pumps to ensure that the correct rate and volume of fluid is given. When faster flows are needed, wide bore sets are used. These often contain a screen filter (particle limit 170–200 µm) to prevent infusion of clumps of cells when infusing blood products.

Cold intravenous fluids cause hypothermia which impairs wound healing, blood clotting and increases metabolic demands, so fluids should be warmed whenever anything other than small volumes are being administered (NICE 2008). Fluid warmers work by heating IV fluid to body temperature by directly heating it or by running it by warm plates or warm water. Most systems have an additional chamber to collect air bubbles produced by the heated blood.

As IV fluid cannot currently carry oxygen, large blood losses must be replaced with transfused blood. As a guide, blood transfusion should be considered when 20% of the patient's circulating volume has been lost, taking into account the patient's haemoglobin level before and after the loss.

Blood volume is approximately:

- 70 mL/kg in adults (ideal body weight)
- 80 mL/kg in children
- 85–90 mL/kg in neonates (Cherian and Emmanuel 2002).

Special Considerations

Paediatrics

Fluid volumes need to be precise when dealing with children because of the small volumes involved. Children's maintenance fluid in millilitres per hour is estimated by the formula: 4 mL/kg for the first 10 kg + 2 mL/kg for the next 10 kg + 1 mL/kg for the remainder of their weight (e.g. a 15 kg 3-year-old would receive $(4 \times 10) + (2 \times 5)$ mL/h = 50 mL/h.

Section 3

This fluid has a small volume so must be given precisely by a syringe pump, a volumetric pump or by using a volume-controlled burette which is filled with only the amount intended to be given.

Neurosurgery

The blood supply to the brain depends on the brain itself being at a lower pressure than the blood pressure. If the brain has swollen, the skull cannot expand so the pressure in the brain goes up. Mannitol (a 6-carbon sugar) is used as an osmotic diuretic to cause the pressure in the brain to decrease. Some units use hypertonic saline for the same purpose.

Dextrose-only solutions are not used for patients with head injuries or having neurosurgery because they increase cerebral oedema.

Blood Transfusion

Whole blood consists of red blood cells which carry oxygen, white blood cells which fight infection, platelets which are a key component the blood clotting system and plasma which contains further clotting factors and albumin. Donated whole blood is split into red cells, plasma and platelets. Red cells can be stored for 35 days. Plasma is frozen (fresh frozen plasma, 'FFP') or further processed to make cryoprecipitate which contains clotting factors and fibrinogen. Platelets can only be kept for 5 days.

Donated blood is screened for some viruses but still presents a risk to the recipient as the donor may have been in the incubation phase of a disease, or may have a disease which is not tested for. For this reason, and because of the expense, lack of availability and other complications such as transfusion related lung injury, great effort is made to avoid blood transfusion.

Blood groups and crossmatching

There are four ABO blood groups. These are genetically determined by the antigens in the blood (Table 11.2).

A patient cannot receive donated blood with antigens they do not possess or they will have a transfusion reaction which can lead to hypotension, renal failure and death (Table 11.3).

Table 11.2   The ABO blood groups with their red cell antigens and antibodies in plasma.

Blood group	A antigen	B antigen	Anti-A antibody	Anti-B antibody
O	No	No	Yes	Yes
A	Yes	No	No	Yes
B	No	Yes	Yes	No
AB	Yes	Yes	No	No

Table 11.3   Compatibility of ABO blood donors and recipients.

Blood group	O recipient	A recipient	B recipient	AB recipient
O donor	√	√	√	√
A donor	No	√	No	√
B donor	No	No	√	√
AB donor	No	No	No	√

Group O blood can be given to anyone (O is the 'universal donor'). An AB patient can receive any donated blood (AB is the 'universal recipient').

There are over 50 further antigens in the blood which can cause a transfusion reaction. If donated blood contains an antigen absent in the patient's blood, the patient makes an antibody to it. The next time the patient receives blood containing this antigen, these antibodies attack the blood and cause a transfusion reaction.

Rhesus D

Ninety per cent of people have the Rhesus D antigen (Rh D positive). A Rhesus negative woman may carry a Rhesus positive baby. If there is mixing of fetal and maternal circulation (e.g. during delivery), the mother will produce antibodies which will affect any subsequent babies who are Rhesus D positive and give them severe anaemia. Women of childbearing age of unknown blood group should always receive Rhesus D negative blood in an emergency, and Rhesus D negative women receive injections of Anti D antibody to destroy any Rhesus D positive cells which may have leaked into their circulation during delivery or trauma (RCOG 2011).

When donated blood is selected for a recipient, the laboratory staff match the groups and antigens as closely as possible by testing the sample to see if it reacts with donated units of blood. If the laboratory has a recent blood sample demonstrating the patient has no antibodies then an electronic crossmatch may be possible which only takes a few minutes. Otherwise, a full crossmatch takes around an hour. If the situation is urgent, the laboratory can abbreviate the crossmatch to provide group-specific blood in about 15 minutes. If the situation is immediately life-threatening, the patient can be given emergency O negative ('universal donor') blood which is normally kept in the fridge in the emergency department, the operating theatres and the labour ward.

Other blood products

After donation, whole blood is split into plasma (which is often frozen), platelets and packed red cells. Packed red cells are usually suspended in a solution of saline, adenine, glucose and mannitol (SAGM) to keep them alive. As a rough guide, one unit of packed cells increases a patient's haemoglobin by 1 g/dL. It has no clotting factors, so when more than two to four units are used, the patient will need to receive FFP and possibly platelets. Recent battlefield surgery experience indicates that using packed cells, FFP and platelets in a ratio of 1 : 1 : 1 may decrease mortality in major trauma but further evidence is needed before extrapolating this to civilian practice (Borgman *et al.* 2007).

Full crossmatching is not necessary for FFP transfusion but it should be group compatible. Donor plasma contains antibodies to any antigen not present in the person's blood group (Table 11.2). Therefore, for FFP group AB (no antibodies) is the universal donor and O (no antigens for the antibodies to react to) is the universal recipient (Table 11.4).

Table 11.4   ABO compatibility of fresh frozen plasma donors and recipients.

Blood group	O recipient	A recipient	B recipient	AB recipient
O donor	√	No	No	No
A donor	√	√	No	No
B donor	√	No	√	No
AB donor	√	√	√	√

Immunocompromised patients are given irradiated blood products, otherwise the T lymphocyte cells in the donated blood can attack the patients' lymphoid tissue and prevent them from making any blood cells. This is called transfusion graft-versus-host disease and is often fatal.

Reasons and Criteria for Transfusion

The decision to transfuse a patient is based on haemoglobin level, general state of health, the amount of blood lost and ongoing losses. The Cochrane Review on transfusion thresholds (Hill *et al.* 2010) recommends that transfusion can be withheld until the Hb is 7.0 g/dL unless there is ongoing bleeding. Those with significant heart disease may need a higher haemoglobin of around 10.0 g/dL (Hébert *et al.* 1999). The decision to transfuse may be based on formal laboratory tests, or a bedside haemoglobin fingerprick test (e.g. Hemocue®).

Blood Product Checking and Administration

The National Patient Safety Agency issued a Safer Practice Notice (NPSA 2006) stating that everyone involved in blood product ordering, sample taking, collection of products and product infusion should have specific training and assessment of competency to minimise the risks of error. The sample must be labelled with the patient's full name, date of birth and hospital or NHS number in the presence of the patient with reference to their name bands. Donated blood must also be checked in the same way and appropriate measurements of the patient's vital signs made before, during and after transfusion.

Jehovah's Witnesses

Jehovah's Witnesses refuse transfusions of blood and blood products on religious grounds even if it results in their death. Depending on individual beliefs, some Jehovah's Witnesses may accept cell salvage, cardiac bypass or acute normovolaemic haemodilution if they consider that the blood remains in a constant circulation with their body. Many Jehovah's Witnesses carry an advance directive to document their exact wishes with regard to specific blood products and salvage systems. They may change their mind at any time, but their wishes cannot be overridden by a clinician except in rare circumstances such as the patient being a child and the hospital being in possession of a court order.

Techniques to Reduce Need for Transfusion

Preoperative

- Iron supplementation can be used for patients with iron deficiency anaemia (common in pregnancy).
- Erythropoeitin, a renal hormone injection which increases bone marrow red cell production, may be administered.

Intraoperative

In the intraoperative period any of the following may be applied as appropriate:

- surgical techniques
- meticulous haemostasis (electrocautery, microwave, ultrasound, argon beam, radiosurgery, laser surgery, cryosurgery, tissue sealants)

- tourniquets
- patient positioning
- arterial embolisation (also a radiological technique).

Anaesthetic techniques

Anaesthetic techniques that may be applied to reduce the need for transfusion include:

- maintenance of normal body temperature to preserve the blood clotting mechanisms
- hypotensive anaesthesia, in which blood loss is reduced by reducing the patient's blood pressure (carries a risk of stroke, heart or kidney damage)
- drugs, such as tranexamic acid, aprotinin (both stop clot breakdown), recombinant Factor VIIa
- minimisation of blood loss from frequent sampling (especially important on intensive care units)
- cell salvage (see below)
- acute normovolaemic haemodilution, in which blood is removed from the patient at the start of surgery, replaced with crystalloid or colloid and then retransfused after blood loss has finished. Many Jehovah's Witnesses will accept this if the blood which is removed remains connected to the cannula.

Autologous transfusion

Autologous transfusion is a method of returning blood cells to the patient by collecting them and processing them to remove impurities before retransfusion. This can occur intraoperatively using a cell salvage machine or postoperatively by using an adapted wound drain system.

Intraoperative cell salvage

Cell salvage starts with a suction tubing system supplied with anticoagulant fluid (heparin or citrate based) so that blood lost during surgery can travel to the cell salvage machine without clotting. The anticoagulated blood passes through a filter into a reservoir where it is washed in normal saline and spun to remove platelets, white blood cells and anticoagulant. Centrifuged blood is collected in a bag which may then be infused into the patient.

Cell salvage is considered where expected blood loss is 20% of the patient's circulating volume or for patients who have a bleeding tendency or difficult blood to cross-match. Its use is increasing, especially in obstetrics.

Cell salvage is contraindicated where blood has been contaminated with bowel contents. In addition to this, orthopaedic cement and amniotic fluid should not enter the salvage suction system.

Operators of cell salvage equipment must be trained and assessed in its use. The UK Blood Transfusion and Tissue Transplantation Service provide a competency framework (UKBTTS 2007).

Postoperative cell salvage

This is an adapted vacuum wound drain which collects blood from a wound for retransfusion. This system is suitable for some orthopaedic operations (e.g. knee replacements). The blood must be re-infused within 6 hours.

With all forms of cell salvage, the blood retrieved must be correctly labelled and prescribed.

Section 3

References

Borgman MA, Spinella PC, Perkins JG *et al.* (2007) The ratio of blood products transfused affects mortality in patients receiving massive transfusions at a combat support hospital. *Journal of Trauma* 63(4): 805–813.

Cherian MN and Emmanuel JC (2002) Clinical use of blood. *Update in Anaesthesia* 14: 18–22. http://update.anaesthesiologists.org/2002/06/01/clinical-use-of-blood/ (accessed November 2011).

Hébert PC, Wells G, Blajchman MA *et al.* (1999) A multicenter, randomized, controlled clinical trial of transfusion requirements in critical care. *New England Journal of Medicine* 340(6): 409–417.

Hill SR, Carless PA, Henry DA *et al.* (2010) Transfusion thresholds and other strategies for guiding allogeneic red blood cell transfusion. *Cochrane Database of Systematic Reviews*, Issue 10: CD002042.

NICE (National Institute for Health and Clinical Excellence) (2008) *The Management of Inadvertent Hypothermia in Adults.* CG65. London: National Institute for Health and Clinical Excellence. London. http://www.nice.org.uk/CG65 (accessed December 2011).

NPSA (National Patient Safety Agency) (2006) *Right Patient, Right Blood: Advice for safer blood transfusions. NPSA/2008/ SPN14.* London: National Patient Safety Agency. http://www.nrls.npsa.nhs.uk/resources/collections/right-patient-right-blood/ (accessed November 2011).

Maharaj CH, Kallam SR, Malik A, Hassett P, Grady D and Laffey JG (2005) Preoperative intravenous fluid therapy decreases postoperative nausea and pain in high risk patients. *Anesthesia and Analgesia* 100: 675–682.

Perel P and Roberts I (2011) Colloids versus crystalloids for fluid resuscitation in critically ill patients. *Cochrane Database of Systematic Reviews* Issue 3: CD000567.

Powell-Tuck J, Gosling P, Lobo DN *et al.* (2008) *British Consensus Guidelines on Intravenous Fluid Therapy for Adult Surgical Patients GIFTASUP.* London: The Intensive Care Society. http://www.ics.ac.uk/intensive_care_professional/standards_and_guidelines/british_consensus_guidelines_on_intravenous_fluid_therapy_for_adult_surgical_patients__giftasup__2008 (accessed November 2011).

RCOG (Royal College of Obstetricians and Gynaecologists) (2011) *The Use of Anti-D Immunoglobulin for Rhesus D Prophylaxis. Green top Guideline No. 22.* London: RCOG. 1998, Revised 2002 and 2011. http://www.rcog.org.uk/womens-health/clinical-guidance/use-anti-d-immunoglobulin-rh-prophylaxis-green-top-22 (accessed November 2011).

UKBTTS (UK Blood Transfusion and Tissue Transplantation Services) (2007) *Intra-operative Cell Salvage Competency Assessment Workbook*, version 2. http://www.transfusionguidelines.org.uk/docs/pdfs/htm_edition-4_all-pages.pdf (accessed November 2011).

WHO Blood Transfusion Safety (2002) *WHO Handbook: The Clinical Use of Blood.* Geneva: WHO. http://www.who.int/bloodsafety/clinical_use/en/Handbook_EN.pdf (accessed November 2011).

CHAPTER 12

Intraoperative Care

Paul Rawling

This chapter aims to enable the reader to consider the overarching principles of intraoperative care without negating the fact that this is a very large and very complex area for discussion. As practitioners we are in a privileged position of caring for patients when they are at potentially their most vulnerable. We are educated from an early stage of training to understand that we are the patient's advocate and have a voice that patients do not have when they are in a general anaesthetic drug-induced coma or are so anxious that perhaps they are less capable of logical consideration of issues involving their immediate care. The message to take from this chapter is that the intraoperative practitioner is the patient's guardian. You are the person who will keep the patient safe.

Patient Safety

Safety of the patient during the operative procedure is the primary concern of every member of the surgical team in the operating theatre (Rothrock 2011). Widely accepted in healthcare is the philosophy 'First, do no harm' and this is the mantra for everyone to meet in intraoperative care. Overall, the intraoperative practitioner is working to help restore the patient's health. A by-product of the patient's surgery and intervention will be a degree of physical harm. This harm is caused via the deliberate surgical damage to the tissues being operated upon.

The Evidence Centre (2010, p. 1) states that 'The NHS strives to make all surgery safe and effective but sometimes incidents occur.' This is where the intraoperative care practitioner fits neatly into the process. The intraoperative care practitioner works methodically in a manner to minimise the risk that surgical care poses to patients while they remain in our care.

Teamwork

At a time of great change in the National Health Service (NHS), where all clinical staff are encouraged to participate in quality improvement (Darzi 2008), teamworking becomes more critical. Teams are described as a cooperative group working toward a

Manual of Perioperative Care: An Essential Guide, First Edition. Edited by Kate Woodhead and Lesley Fudge.
© 2012 John Wiley & Sons, Ltd. Published 2012 by John Wiley & Sons, Ltd.

collective goal (Corbett 2009). The team philosophy should be aimed at collaboration and cooperation. The focus on interaction and a unilateral outcome of very high-quality patient care for every patient must be the priority. Organisational priorities must include treating patients on operating lists. The lists must be completed effectively and efficiently which will provide the trust with monetary income to enable the continuation of this care for the community and also to invest in development of further services.

Teamwork is a critical area to consider within intraoperative care. Everything we do in perioperative care is related to another area and without the team the patient would be at much greater risk of harm. The number of different professional groups that work within intraoperative care dictates that cooperation and collaboration must occur or the risk of critical events increases. Corbett (2009) reminds us very clearly that as practitioners we do not work in isolation. Patient care would be significantly affected if we did and the quality of care would be reduced.

Within every multi-disciplinary arena, effective functioning of a team will depend on the reduction and elimination of obstacles (Gillespie *et al.* 2008). In operating departments there are medical staff, nursing staff, operating department practitioners and support workers who are also an important group of staff upon whom much practice depends. Each group will effectively have a separate agenda, in part shaped by the organisation's expectation and the individual role descriptors provided. Breakdowns in team working have been described as a major cause of adverse events and errors (Rothrock 2011) within perioperative care. This is relatively easy to see and a reason why many departments now prefer settled teams even if that only includes core staff. Working in teams has also been considered positive for work morale and a sense of mutual trust and cooperation, which again was described as enhancing safety (Alfredsdottir and Bjornsdottir 2007).

The key message here is collaboration, cooperation, trust and appreciation that individual disciplines bring a variety of knowledge and skills which all help to produce high-quality safe intraoperative care.

Communication

Within operating departments communication is crucial to the effective, safe and efficient provision of quality care (Wicker and O'Neill 2006). Communication remains the basis for all interaction including verbalising and listening and allows rapport to be developed between practitioners, patients and the multi-disciplinary team. Communication not only involves the verbal exchange of information but can also be in written form. Consideration to body language and the overall perception that the receiver of the information gains is important as rapport is built on two-way interaction.

Communication must enable the intraoperative practitioner to provide holistic, individualised patient care throughout the patient's perioperative journey. The theatre environment is very changeable. As such, accurate communication is crucial within perioperative practice. Communication between practitioners, medical staff and patients is essential (Woodhead and Wicker 2005, Spry 2009) and must not be considered simply verbal. Completion of documentation with accuracy is equally important. A number of examples in intraoperative care are preoperative patient checking, instrument checks, documentation of histology specimens, reporting and documenting the swab, needle and instrument counts and handover reports to postoperative recovery practitioners.

Wicker (2011) suggests that the challenge of improving communication in the context of patient safety and the World Health Organization Checklist is essentially within the control of the theatre staff, who are the people who will begin the process with introductions in theatre during the often referred to 'time out'. The key message is that inappropriate or inaccurate communication could potentially lead to catastrophe (Gillespie *et al.* 2008). Interaction between disciplines and individuals can be clouded by previous experience and may lead to potential breakdown in the efficiency and coherence of the team. The other extreme is that good communication will lead to greater satisfaction as the quality of patient care will improve, staff will feel more comfortable within the multi-disciplinary team and as such perform at a higher and more cohesive level.

Care and Dignity

Patient dignity is always a consideration in intraoperative care (Smith 2005, Spry 2009). The majority of people would feel embarrassed if they had their clothes removed and were exposed in an environment filled with strangers. This is an issue often forgotten in the intraoperative phase of the perioperative journey. In the author's experience perioperative practitioners act in a professional manner and do avoid exposing patients to the environment on the majority of occasions, but lapses occur in all areas of practice. Baillie and Ilott (2010) remind us that patient perception of quality of care is often based on an expectation that they will be treated with dignity. Underpinning this issue is the NHS Constitution (Department of Health 2009) and the associated values of the NHS which include respect and dignity as the first of the six core values.

Allowing the patient to remain covered is essential. This can be difficult to achieve if the surgical site is required to be marked and is in an intimate area (Baillie and Ilott 2010). This could, however, be performed in private on the ward if the surgeon or surgical specialist carries out a preoperative visit. When the patient is anaesthetised and lying in theatre on a cold operating table surface they are at risk from inadvertent perioperative hypothermia (NICE 2008). This can have serious implications for both the patient and the hospital. Anecdote tells us that patients are seen arriving in theatre departments around the nation wearing flimsy theatre gowns open at the back with patient dignity compromised and the author cannot help but feel embarrassed for the patient.

The patient has to feel confident in the perioperative practitioners caring for their needs and this clearly applies to dignity, with concern that the staff ensure the patient is covered as far as possible during the entire intervention. Some patients allow all control to pass to the healthcare practitioners as soon as the perioperative journey begins. Baillie and Ilott (2010) express that patient dignity may be compromised in a manner that affects the patient's own self-perception of dignity. Privacy is a related issue that is perhaps difficult to provide in the operating department for patients but it is the practitioner's role to ensure that respect and dignity are maintained and not compromised.

Role of the Circulating Practitioner

The circulating practitioner role can be viewed as a supporting role. However, without this support, the running of the theatre list and patient care would be of a poorer quality. The role involves the preparation for surgery, support during the intraoperative period, and postoperative care for the patient, providing dressings and assisting with transportation of the patient to postoperative recovery (Phillips 2007). The roles and responsibilities of the circulating practitioner are numerous but perhaps the most important is the link between the scrub practitioner and the rest of the team.

The circulating role is a complex process and also requires a good level of communication. Spry (2009, p. 7) considers that the circulating role can be defined as 'managing and implementing activities outside the sterile field'. The author agrees and

Section 3

suggests that this aspect of perceived control of the situation is important. In an area that contains a multitude of staff from a variety of disciplines, control from an outside viewpoint is important to ensure the overarching aim of quality care and a successful surgical outcome for the patient is achieved.

The practitioner working in the circulating role will have shared responsibility for preparation and stocking of the theatre, ensuring instrument sets are available and the environment is clean and tidy and is ready for use (Wicker and O'Neill 2006). An outline of the circulating role was described by Wicker and O'Neill (2006, p. 143) to include 'Preparing surgical gowns and gloves', opening the outer layers of instrument sets, 'helping with patient positioning', 'ensuring the patients dignity is maintained' throughout, providing the 'required skin preparation fluids' and sutures as per the surgeons preference, 'collecting and storing specimens', communicating effectively on a variety of levels both verbally and in writing, assisting with 'transporting the patient to the Postoperative Recovery area' following surgery and ensuring the theatre is clean, tidy and prepared to receive the next patient on the operating list.

The key message here is cooperation, communication, support and organisation. These are the inherent skills required by practitioners working in this role.

Role of the Scrub Practitioner

The role of the scrub practitioner is again aimed at safe surgical care for the patient. This includes providing skilled support to the surgeon. Checking of patient details for correct patient, correct operation, correct site, skin preparation fluids, surgical instruments, safe sharps management, dressings, drains and occasionally drugs including local anaesthetics for wound infiltration. This, like any other role requires skill, knowledge and dexterity and the ability to speak on behalf of the patient as their advocate. The World Health Organisation (WHO) *Safe Surgery Saves Lives* document (World Health Organization 2008) explains clearly the need for the process of ensuring that the right patient receives the right surgery. This is achieved through the implementation of the WHO checklist and 'time out' introductions prior to commencement of surgery. It is normally the scrub practitioner who initiates this check prior to the patient being prepared for surgery.

The scrub practitioner should remain with the patient postoperatively until the patient has left the operating theatre for the postoperative recovery room. This level of support is critical as this is a period of increased vulnerability for the patient. The scrub practitioner's contact with the patient continues, as he or she is required to provide a detailed handover to the recovery practitioner.

The scrub practitioner's role clearly requires an in-depth appreciation of surgery, instruments, anatomy and an ability to anticipate the need of both surgeon and patient. This can be considered to be a highly technical role (Spry 2009). Many surgical operations require a large number of instrument sets and a range of both simple and complex instruments, some of which may be powered, need to be assembled or both. It could be considered that the actual scrubbing up and setting of an instrument trolley is the least technical part of this role when the other aspects of the role are considered. The role includes planning, delivery of care, organisation and an ability to communicate and delegate on a variety of levels to ensure the smooth outcome of a patient receiving high-quality care in a timely and safe manner. This is achieved often by the perioperative staff working in distinct teams where skill and knowledge can be shared, evidence-based practice embraced, and skills honed in a more limited number of specialities. Within the scrub role it becomes increasingly difficult to be expert in all specialities. The scrub role principles remain the same, but instruments, logistics, types of patients, anatomy and surgeon preferences will change.

Developing Role of Advanced Scrub Practitioner

The Perioperative Care Collaborative (2007) discussed the need for practitioners to undertake the role of advanced scrub practitioner (ASP) when there has been a lack of surgical trainees available to assist the surgeons in theatre. The ASP role should only be undertaken by a registered perioperative practitioner who is trained to provide competent and skilled assistance under the direct supervision of the operating surgeon while not performing any form of surgical intervention. Local first assistant programmes remain available in some hospitals. Formalised training is available through some universities.

The ASP should be an additional member of the intraoperative team and not be expected to practice in a dual role of ASP and scrub practitioner (Perioperative Care Collaborative 2007). This suggestion from the PCC should be supported with a local trust policy which will safeguard the practitioner and the patient. Competencies and skills will be attached to the underpinning knowledge (Timpany and Mcalevey 2010) and be supported by the Trust. From experience, the author has seen the positive impact that this role has on the intraoperative care environment, enabling the patient to receive the level of care they deserve. On the other hand, the dual role could potentially increase the risk of errors during surgical procedures.

Surgical intervention is normally not sanctioned for this role, including cutting tissue, direct diathermy application to tissue, application and cutting of sutures and applying clamps or ligatures. Brame (2011) reminds us that some experienced staff have been undertaking roles of this nature for many years without recognition or protection from the hospital. Professional accountability dictates that practitioners only work within these roles if they are trained and deemed as competent and feel that they themselves are competent and able to perform these roles. The clear definition of set parameters is vital. This allows practitioners in training to work toward these tasks and for trained ASPs to know, with a degree of certainty they are not working out-with their remit (Bernthal 1999) and would in fact be covered with vicarious liability from the hospital. Personal limits are important for every practitioner and must be accepted honestly.

Developing Role of Surgical Care Practitioner

Surgical care practitioners (SCP) carry out roles traditionally undertaken by medical staff (Nicholas 2010). Because of European Working Time Directive (EWTD) rules, there are fewer medical staff available to carry out these tasks. This group of staff although relatively new are in a difficult position. SCPs are mainly (but not all) recruited from existing registered nurses or operating department practitioners in the theatre staff, but then are as SCPs effectively working within a specific surgical team (Quick *et al.* 2010). A number of these practitioners have personal caseloads and carry out minor surgery with supervision from a consultant surgeon. The SCP normally works within a single speciality. Honesty is required and patients must be made fully aware that they are being treated by a non-medically qualified practitioner. As suggested earlier, trust is a vital part of professional practice and no more so than in intraoperative care.

The training and education for SCPs is rightly aligned with the training and competence that would be achieved by medical staff carrying out the same procedures (Quick *et al.* 2010).

This speciality is growing and there remains a non-standard application of tasks and roles. Essentially, the practitioners are able to perform delegated duties in theatres, manage patients postoperatively, adjust treatment plans, discharge and follow-up

Section 3

patients. Training for such roles normally involves postgraduate study at Masters degree level using the agreed Royal College of Surgeons Curriculum. The SCP role does include prepping and draping patients, surgical intervention like cutting and applying sutures, tissues, applying indirect diathermy, camera holding for minimally invasive surgery, securing drains, female catheterisation and application of suction, under the supervision of a surgeon (Department of Health 2006).

References

Alfredsdottir H and Bjornsdottir K (2007) Nursing and patient safety in the operating room. *Journal of Advanced Nursing* 61(1): 29–37.

Baillie L and Ilott L (2010) Promoting the dignity of patients in perioperative practice. *Journal of Perioperative Practice* 20(8): 278–282.

Bernthal E (1999) The nurse as first assistant to the surgeon: Is this a perioperative nursing role. *British Journal of Theatre Nursing* 9(2): 74–77.

Brame K (2011) The advanced scrub practitioner role: a student's reflection. *Journal of Perioperative Practice* 21(4): 118–122.

Corbett S (2009) Teamwork: How does this relate to the operating room practitioner? *Journal of Perioperative Practice* 19(9): 278–281.

Darzi A (2008) *High Quality Care for All. NHS Next Stage Review final report.* http://www.dh.gov.uk/en/Publicationsandstatistics/Publications/PublicationsPolicyAndGuidance/DH_085825 (accessed 10 December 2011).

Department of Health (2006) *The Curriculum Framework for the Surgical Care Practitioner.* http://www.dh.gov.uk/en/Publicationsandstatistics/Publications/PublicationsPolicyAndGuidance/DH_4133018 (accessed 11 December 2011).

Department of Health (2009) *NHS Constitution.* http://www.dh.gov.uk/en/Publicationsandstatistics/Publications/PublicationsPolicyAndGuidance/DH_113613 (accessed 10 December 2011).

Evidence Centre (2010) *Prioritising Patient Safety; Implementing the Surgical Safety Checklist.* www.patientsafetyfirst.nhs.uk/ashx/Asset (accessed 11 December 2011).

Gillespie B M, Chaboyer W and Lizzio A (2008) Teamwork in the OR: enhancing communication through team-building interventions. *ACORN* 21(1): Autumn 2008.

NICE (National Institute for Health and Clinical Excellence) (2008) *The Management of Inadvertent Perioperative Hypothermia in Adults.* London: NICE.

Nicholas M (2010) The surgical care practitioner: a critical analysis. *Journal of Perioperative Practice* 20(3): 94–99.

Perioperative Care Collaborative (2007) *The Role and Responsibilities of the Advanced Scrub Practitioner.* London: PCC.

Phillips N (2007) *Berry and Kohns Operating Room Technique*, 11th edn. St. Louis, MO: Mosby Elsevier.

Quick J, Williams S and Addison S (2010) Surgical care practitioners…. our experience. *Journal of Perioperative Practice* 20(9): 320–321.

Rothrock JC (2011) *Care of the Patient in Surgery.* St. Louis, MO: Elsevier Mosby.

Smith C (2005) Care of the patient undergoing surgery. In Woodhead K and Wicker P (eds) *A Textbook of Perioperative Care.* London: Elsevier Churchill Livingstone, pp. 161–180.

Spry C (2009) *Essentials of Perioperative Nursing*, 4th edn. Sudbury: Jones and Bartlett Publishers.

Timpany MD and Mcalevey J (2010) Perioperative role development. *Journal of Perioperative Practice* 20: 13–18.

Wicker P (2011) Perioperative communication: the surgical safety checklist. *Journal of Perioperative Practice* 21(7): 221.

Wicker P and O'Neill J (2006) *Caring for the Perioperative Patient.* Oxford: Blackwell Publishing.

Woodhead K and Wicker P (2005) *A Textbook of Perioperative Care.* London: Elsevier Churchill Livingstone.

World Health Organization (2008) *Safe Surgery Saves Lives.* Geneva: WHO.

CHAPTER 13

Safer Moving and Handling and Patient Positioning

Susan Pirie

This chapter will discuss the principles of moving and handling and the key surgical positions that practitioners will encounter in the perioperative environment. It will also focus on the need for risk assessment, both for the manual handling elements and the required position for the planned perioperative intervention. The reader will also be informed of complications that can arise from poor patient positioning, and the need to be familiar with the equipment used, particularly identified weight limits. Finally, guidance on the steps to take in the event of an adverse or potential adverse incident, and the potential consequences for the registered practitioner will be discussed.

Key Principles of Moving and Handling

Manual handling is a key element of practice in the perioperative environment, as patients are transferred from bed or trolley to operating tables prior to the surgical start and in reverse following completion of the intervention. Manual handling is a key element of health and safety legislation in the UK and employers and employees have legal duties to fulfil in relation to these tasks according to the Health and Safety at Work Act 1974 and Manual Handling Operations Regulations 1992. These duties place a responsibility on employers to ensure that initial training and regular updates on manual handling are provided, and, in turn, employees are required to access this training and updates in order to ensure that their knowledge and practice are current (AfPP 2009).

The main manual handling tasks in the perioperative environment are lifting (trays, surgical sundries, stores, etc.) and pushing and pulling movements in patient transfers. It is important to undertake a risk assessment for each task, and one form of assessment that can be adapted for use within the perioperative environment is the TILE method (AfPP 2007):

- *Task*: In this part of the assessment practitioners should consider if the task actually needs to be undertaken and should identify the movements that will be required
- *Individual*: Has the practitioner involved in the manual handling task received sufficient training and do they possess the ability to undertake the task?

Manual of Perioperative Care: An Essential Guide, First Edition. Edited by Kate Woodhead and Lesley Fudge.
© 2012 John Wiley & Sons, Ltd. Published 2012 by John Wiley & Sons, Ltd.

- *Load*: This element of the assessment considers factors such as the weight involved in the manoeuvre and the stability of the practitioner involved.
- *Environment*: This part of the assessment involves practitioners considering the number of staff that are required for the task. In addition, factors such as space considerations and additional equipment should also be assessed.

Once the risk assessment has been completed it is important to consider the principles for safe lifting and pushing and pulling, and these are as follows:

Lifting

- Consider what is involved before lifting and plan accordingly.
- Ensure that the load is kept close to the waist and the body for as long as possible during the manoeuvre.
- Ensure that positioning is stable with one leg slightly ahead of the other and be prepared to change position as the lift progresses. If the load is at floor level, then feet should be placed alongside the load.
- It is important to have a good hold on the load and to hold it as close to the body as possible.
- When starting a lift, the best posture to minimise the risk of injury is to have the back slightly bent forward and the hips and knees partially flexed.
- It is important not to flex the back any further during the lift.
- It is imperative to avoid twisting movements during the lift and/or to lean to one side. Shoulders should be facing forward and in line with the hips. If it is necessary to change direction during the lift, then it is important to move the feet into the required direction, with the rest of the body following through, in order to avoid injury.
- By keeping the head up and looking forward and not down, a practitioner will minimise their risk of injury.
- Ensure that all movements in the lift are smooth as jerky or rough movements can affect the stability of the load.
- Do not attempt to lift anything more than is easily manageable, as although it is possible to lift more than the comfortable lift, to do so will decrease the safety of the lift.
- If precise positioning is required, then it is important that the load is put down and then adjusted into the required position.

Pushing and pulling

In general situations the following principles should be considered:

- In order to make the move easier, practitioners should ensure that their feet are well away from the load.
- It is estimated that in order to move a load over a flat service, an effort of at least 2% of the total load weight is required.
- If the load in question has to be moved over an uneven surface, then the effort ratio in relation to the weight of the load can increase to 10%.
- In the event that a load needs to be pushed down or pulled up a slope then the force required to move the load may exceed the recommended weight limits for both men and women. If such an action is required, then it is essential that two or more people complete the move in order to minimise the risk of injury.
- Handling devices such as trolleys, Patslides, etc. should have handles at waist height (Health and Safety Executive 2006).

Risk Assessment of Patients in Relation to the Surgical Position

Another important process relevant to patient positioning is that of risk assessment. Undertaking a risk assessment prior to positioning a patient for surgery is an essential element of safe perioperative practice and a high standard of patient care.

Risk management, of which risk assessment is an integral part, has been defined as follows: 'Involves highlighting an activity and assessing the risks in comparison to need and then making changes and/or substitutions' (Smith and Williams 2004).

Risk assessment is part of clinical governance procedures and a requirement of health and safety legislation. The Clinical Governance Framework places a corporate responsibility on the healthcare organisation, but individual practitioners are not exempt from undertaking risk assessments. An employer will expect practitioners to undertake risk assessments in their own area of practice and it is also considered to be a professional responsibility. Both the Nursing and Midwifery Council (NMC) and the Health Professions Council (HPC) require their registrants to maintain their knowledge and skills and to work within the limits of their competence (HPC 2008, NMC 2008). In addition, the NMC specifically requires its registrants to manage risk (NMC 2008). Risk assessment is an integral part of health and safety legislation.

The risk assessment related to patient positioning should consider factors relating to the individual patient as well as factors relevant to the intraoperative phase of patient care. Some of these factors are listed in Table 13.1.

A key element of undertaking risk assessments is the ability to identify a hazard and then to assess the risk associated with the hazard. A hazard is defined as something which has the potential to cause harm and a risk is defined as the probability or potential for the hazard to cause actual harm as well as an assessment of the severity of harm that may occur (Champion 2000).

Table 13.1 Factors to be considered in risk assessment relating to patient positioning.

Patient considerations	Intraoperative considerations
Age, height and weight	Anaesthetic access to the patient when positioned for surgery
Body mass index	The length of time that it is anticipated that the patient will be in the surgical position
Skin condition	The surgical position that is required
Presence of studs and other jewellery that cannot be removed	
Nutritional status	
Allergies	
Pre-existing medical conditions	
Physical or other mobility issues	
Pre-existing prosthesis or implanted devices such as pacemakers	
Pre-existing external factors such as urinary catheters, drains from previous surgery	

From Association of Perioperative Room Nurses (2008).

Section 3

Table 13.2   Simple matrix for a risk scoring system.

Likelihood	Risk rate	Severity of harm	Risk rate
Low	1	Minimal harm	1
Medium	2	Moderate harm	2
High	3	Major/catastrophic harm	3

It is important that perioperative practitioners are involved in undertaking the risk assessments as they are the people most likely to be familiar with the equipment and processes that are being assessed. It is often the case that the risk assessment process is thought to be complicated, but it actually comprises five distinct and separate steps as follows:

1. Plan the assessment
2. Look for hazards
3. Evaluate the risks
4. Prepare an action plan for controlling the risks
5. Review and revise the assessments (Champion 2000).

Planning the assessment enables a practitioner to clearly identify the activity or task under scrutiny, which in turn can assist the practitioner in identifying the hazards associated with the activity or task. It is important to note the significance of each hazard, as well as evaluating the risk associated with the hazard. A recognised risk scoring system such as high, medium or low will facilitate a prediction of the likelihood of harm and the severity of harm that will occur, thus creating a risk score (Champion 2000, Health and Safety Executive 1997). This can be measured in a simple matrix as shown in Table 13.2.

The level of risk can be assessed by a simple multiplication of the risk rates of the likelihood of harm and the severity of harm, which can then allow a warning system of red, amber and green to be used to assess the risk level as high, medium or low. For example, a risk score of 6–9 would be classed as red and require immediate action to reduce the risk, an amber risk would range between 3 and 6 and require action within an agreed timescale whereas a score of 1–3 would be identified as green and monitored to ensure that it remains at this level.

Having established the risk assessment and management principles to be applied to patient positioning, it is now pertinent to consider the range of patient positions available. The purpose of a specific surgical position is to ensure that the maximum view of the operative field is obtained whilst maintaining the comfort and safety of the patient at all times (Adeeji *et al.* 2010). A further compromise in the choice of patient position can be related to the type of anaesthetic used and the access that the anaesthetist will require during the procedure. The range of key surgical positions is described in the following section.

Key Surgical Positions

The key surgical positions are lateral, lithotomy, prone, supine, Trendelenburg and reverse Trendelenburg, with supine being the most commonly used position for perioperative procedures (Smith 2005).

Lateral

In this position, the patient is placed on their side and is supported by the use of a table accessory positioned against the patient's abdomen, with a further support against their lower back. The upper arm is supported in a gutter support. Care must be taken to ensure that the lower limbs are protected from undue pressure by placing a suitable pillow or other pressure-relieving device between the legs to reduce pressure on bony prominences, as well as the use of gel pads to protect against pressure on the lower heel (Smith 2005). This position is often used in thoracic surgery, some renal surgery and also in hip surgery.

Lithotomy

In this position the patient is initially placed in a supine position and then the legs are raised and the feet supported in stirrups or other leg supports, thus allowing the lower end of the table to be removed in order to facilitate access for gynaecological, urological and some lower bowel surgical procedures. It is important that the patient's legs are moved simultaneously into position on the leg supports, which are at the same height, in order to reduce the risk of flexion beyond 90°. If the patient is to be positioned in lithotomy poles, then their legs should be positioned on the outside of the poles in order to prevent pressure on the peroneal nerve. The patient's buttocks must be aligned with the break in the table, and in a position that will support the sacrum, once the base of the table has been removed. The patient's arms should be supported on arm boards with less than a 90° angle in order to prevent injury (AfPP 2007, Association of Perioperative Room Nurses 2008).

Prone

The prone position is used for some neurosurgical, spinal and vascular procedures. The patient will initially be in the supine position, prior to being rolled into a face down position. It is essential that sufficient people are present in order to position the patient safely, including ensuring that the patient's cervical alignment is maintained and that the patient is positioned on a headrest which allows access to the airway. It should be noted that one person should be in command of the instructions to move the patient, and that this person is most likely to be the anaesthetist, as he or she has responsibility for the patient's airway. The headrest should provide adequate protection to the forehead, eyes and chin. The patient's arms should be positioned by their sides or, if this is not possible, then on arm boards, with an abduction of less than 90°, and with the elbows flexed and palms facing downwards. Placing the patient's arms above their head can cause injury to the brachial plexus (AfPP 2007, Association of Perioperative Room Nurses 2008). One person, preferably the anaesthetist, is in control of the moving and turning of patients.

Supine

In this position, the patient lies flat and it is important that their spine is kept in alignment, and that the patient's head and upper body are in alignment with their hips and that their legs are parallel. Heel supports should be provided to reduce pressure and the arms should be placed on suitably aligned arm boards. Pregnant women may require a 20° tilt to the left in order to prevent pressure on the inferior vena cava (AfPP 2007, Association of Perioperative Room Nurses 2008, Pirie 2010).

Trendelenburg

The Trendelenburg position is often used for pelvic surgery where the patient is positioned in a supine position initially and then the operating table is tilted to a head down position which does not exceed a 20° tilt. It is essential that a non-slip mattress is

Section 3

used in order to prevent the patient from moving either during positioning or during the procedure itself (AfPP 2007, Pirie 2010).

Reverse Trendelenburg

This position, as the name suggests, is where the patient is positioned in the supine position prior to being tilted into a head up position. This position is used for head and neck surgery such as thyroid surgery as well as for some shoulder and abdominal surgery, such as cholecystectomy (AfPP 2007, Pirie 2010).

It is important to note that there are some variations to the above positions which are also recognised perioperative positions. These are described below.

Dorsal recumbent position

This is similar to the supine position, but at least one arm will be positioned at the side of the patient, with the other arm extended on an arm board to facilitate venous access. The arm that is placed at the side of the body should not be subjected to undue pressure. The elbows should also be protected to prevent injury. This position can be used in abdominal surgery (AfPP 2007).

Lloyd–Davies position

This is essentially an adaptation of the lithotomy position which is used for genitourinary surgery and lower bowel surgery where access to the abdominal and perineal areas is needed. Care should be taken to ensure that the patient's hands are padded and secured safely at their sides in this position, and that their calves are supported adequately (AfPP 2007).

Jack-knife/knee chest position

This is an adaptation of the prone position and is used for rectal surgery and some spinal surgery. In this position, pillows should be placed to provide support to the body, and thus protect the abdomen, pelvis, spine and neck from unnecessary pressure. The patient's head should be fully supported and turned to one side, while maintaining adequate airway access for the anaesthetist. The patient's position should be maintained during the procedure with the use of appropriate table supports (AfPP 2007, Pirie 2010).

Complications Arising from Poor Patient Positioning and How to Minimise the Risks

Complications that can arise from poor patient positioning are identified as skin damage as a result of pressure, nerve damage, deep vein thrombosis and compartment syndrome (Adeeji *et al.* 2010, Beckett 2010).

Skin damage

It is recognised that there are a range of extrinsic and intrinsic factors associated with skin damage in the perioperative phase of a patient's journey. Extrinsic factors such as friction and shear during the transfer to and from the operating table, and/or pressure sustained during the operative procedure have been identified. Intrinsic factors such as age, hypotension, poor oxygen perfusion, poor nutrition and reduced mobility have all been recognised as factors that can compromise skin integrity (Parker 2004).

Therefore, it is important that a patient's skin is examined prior to positioning for surgery and that any untoward blemishes or marks are recorded. In order to minimise the risk of skin damage during patient transfer, transfer equipment such as Patslides and slide sheets should be used with sufficient staff for safe transfer and patient positioning. Such actions will minimise the risk of skin damage from friction or shearing forces.

Pressure damage may also occur in the intraoperative phase, although such damage may not be immediately obvious. Pressure damage occurs as a consequence of either the occlusion of a major blood vessel or as a result of a reduction in capillary perfusion. Tissue damage can occur as a result of the compression of the skin, bone and muscle against the hard surface of the operating table as gravity forces a patient's weight downwards onto the operating table. These forces can interrupt the normal processes of tissue perfusion, potentially creating ischaemia and tissue oedema, thus increasing the risk of tissue damage. In addition, it is known that failing to maintain normothermia can also increase the risk of pressure damage occurring (Parker 2004, Pirie 2010).

There are a wide range of products such as gel pads and other pressure-relieving devices that minimise the risk of pressure damage. It is important to ensure that all bony prominences are adequately padded and that the correct positioning aids are used as appropriate. Particular care is required when a patient is in the prone position to ensure that no damage is sustained to the occiput.

Nerve damage

Nerve damage is another factor that is associated with poor patient positioning (Adeeji *et al.* 2010, Beckett 2010). It has been demonstrated that a number of factors can contribute to the potential for nerve damage, such as compression, the surgical position itself and positioning devices such as stirrups.

Compression occurs when a nerve (e.g. the ulnar or peroneal nerves) is compressed by a bony prominence once the patient has been positioned. Similarly, nerve damage can be caused when vascular ischaemia, caused by compression, restricts the supply of blood to neural tissue. Damage to long nerves such as the brachial plexus and sciatic nerves can be caused by unnecessary stretching and traction during the time it takes to position the patient and the time that they are left in that surgical position.

Other factors that can increase the risk of nerve injury include pre-existing physiological disease processes, such as diabetes and peripheral vascular disease, among others. Other factors that can influence the risk of nerve injury are the body mass index (BMI). If a patient is overweight or underweight, this is known to increase the risk of nerve injury (Adeeji *et al.* 2010, Beckett 2010).

Deep vein thrombosis

A deep vein thrombosis (DVT) can occur as a result of prolonged inactivity which in turn can cause blood stasis, thus increasing the risk of a clot forming in a deep vein. A DVT is also closely associated with the risk of pulmonary embolism, which can prove to be fatal. The risks of DVT have been recognised and are now checked by undertaking a venous thromboembolism (VTE) assessment when a patient is admitted to hospital. Patients identified as being at risk are given prophylactic treatment such as anti-embolism stockings and pharmacological measures such as low molecular weight heparin (NICE 2010). The need for a VTE assessment is also included in the Safer Surgery Checklist (National Patient Safety Agency 2009).

Compartment syndrome

Compartment syndrome is a recognised complication of some perioperative interventions, notably trauma, and is defined as 'a condition where the circulation and function of tissues within a closed space are compromised by an increase of pressure in that

Section 3

space' (Matsen 1975). If compartment syndrome is not recognised as an acute surgical emergency, then the consequences can include amputation, multi-organ failure and ultimately death.

Compartment syndrome has been linked to abdominal, urological or gynaecological procedures, regardless of whether the positioning devices have been lithotomy poles or Lloyd–Davies supports. Pressure in the anterior compartments of the lower limbs of up to 30 mmHg when a patient has been in the lithotomy position for more than 4 hours have been identified (Malik *et al.* 2009).

The immediate management of suspected compartment syndrome necessitates the removal of dressings, plaster casts or other external pressure devices. The limb should be elevated to the level of the heart or above to reduce blood flow in the affected limb. The maintenance of normotension, and ongoing assessment of hypovolaemia, metabolic acidosis and myoglobinaemia are necessary to reduce the risk of renal failure. However, the surgical operations of fasciectomy, the treatment for compartment syndrome, should not be delayed (Malik *et al.* 2009).

Using Equipment and Weight Limits

All medical equipment is defined as a medical device and is subject to the requirements of the European legislation relating to medical devices. A medical device is defined as 'an instrument, apparatus, appliance, material or other article, whether used alone or in combination, together with any software necessary for its proper application' (Medical Device Directive 1993).

Integral to the legislation relating to medical devices is the requirement for the manufacturer to produce guidance on decontamination processes if applicable (O'Brien 2009), and for all instrumentation to have instructions for use. Failing to use medical devices for the purpose they have been designed, or in a different way to the instructions for the device, may absolve the product liability for the device from the manufacturer. In this situation, the product liability may be transferred to the organisation or the individual who is responsible for this alternative use (AfPP 2009).

As stated above, equipment should only be used for the purposes that it has been designed for, and it is important that staff are familiar with how to use the equipment. It is also helpful if staff are aware of any approved steps to take in the event of equipment failure. For example, staff should be familiar with the mechanisms for moving or unlocking electric operating tables in the event of a power failure. Product training should be implemented before new equipment is introduced into the department. It is essential that this criterion is adhered to irrespective of whether it is equipment on loan or newly purchased equipment. Staff who are operating or using equipment without full instruction will find that they are in breach of the legal duty of care, and potentially breaching their duty to their employer, as well as their professional registration if applicable (AfPP 2009).

In view of this legislation and guidance, it is imperative that practitioners are aware of the limitations of the products that they use in connection with their duties within the perioperative environment. It is acknowledged that there has been an increase in obesity in the general population and that there has been a subsequent increase in obese or morbidly obese patients, which in turn has led to the development of specific bariatric equipment in order to provide safe care to these patients. It is therefore imperative that perioperative practitioners are aware of the weight limits of the equipment that they use and that they are informed in advance of patients whose weight may indicate a problem, so that all relevant equipment can be checked to ensure that it is suitable for the patient.

When Something Goes Wrong with Patient Positioning

As discussed earlier in this chapter, there are occasions when a patient can come to harm as a direct result of the surgical position that has been required for their perioperative intervention. Also it should be noted that there may be factors other than patient positioning that can cause a patient harm. Irrespective of the harm caused, or the potential harm that can occur, it is important that such incidents are reported. While it is likely that these reports may be verbal in the first instance to a more senior member of the multi-disciplinary team, it is important that they are reported. Staff should be familiar with the adverse incident reporting mechanisms within their organisation and should also be aware of the need for incidents or potential incidents to be reported to external bodies. In addition, the incident or potential incident should be recorded in the patient's notes, on the safer surgical checklist, theatre register and other relevant contemporaneous documentation. In the event of equipment failure, it may be that the actual or potential incident should be reported to the Medicines and Health Care Regulatory Agency (MHRA). It may also be relevant to report the incident to a patient safety organisation such as the National Patient Safety Agency, who facilitate a specific reporting system. Staff should be familiar with how such incidents are reported within their organisation, and should follow up on any subsequent investigation, regardless of whether it is an internal or external investigation.

Professionally registered practitioner such as nurses and operating department practitioners are required to abide by, and practice within, their professional codes and standard of practice. Both the Health Professions Council (HPC) and the Nursing and Midwifery Council (NMC) require practitioners to be responsible for patient safety, and to report their concerns if they feel that this is compromised or potentially compromised by their actions or lack of action (HPC 2008, NMC 2008).

Staff at all levels, whether registered or not, should feel confident to raise any concerns they may have that could impact on actual or potential patient safety, in either an informal or formal process. However, it is irrelevant how concerns are raised, the important factor is that staff feel empowered to raise them in the environment in which they work. Failing to raise such concerns can have far-reaching consequences.

References

Adeeji R, Oragul E and Khan Wand Maruthainar N (2010). The importance of correct patient positioning in theatres and implications of mal-positioning. *Journal of Perioperative Practice* 20(4): 143–147.

AfPP (Association for Perioperative Practice) (2007) *Standards and Recommendations for Safe Perioperative Practice.* Harrogate: AfPP.

AfPP (2009) *Safeguards for Invasive Procedures: The Management of Risks.* Harrogate AfPP.

Association of Perioperative Room Nurses (2008) *Perioperative Standards and Recommended Practices.* Denver: AORN.

Beckett AE (2010) Are we doing enough to prevent patient injury caused by positioning for surgery? *Journal of Perioperative Practice* 20(1): 26–29.

Champion J (2000) Risk assessment a five-step process. *British Journal of Perioperative Nursing* 10(7): 350–353.

Health and Safety Executive (1997) *Successful Health and Safety Management*, 2nd edn. http://www.hse.gov.uk/pubns/priced/hsg65.pdf (accessed 27 February 2011).

Health and Safety Executive (2006) *Getting to Grips with Manual Handling.* http://www.hse.gov.uk/pubns/indg143.pdf (accessed 27 February 2011).

HPC (Health Professions Council) (2008) *Standards for Conduct, Performance and Ethics.* London: HPC.

Malik AA, Khan W S A, Chaudry A, Ihsan M and Cullen N P (2009) Acute compartment syndrome – a life and limb threatening surgical emergency. *Journal of Perioperative Practice* 19(5): 137–141.

Matsen FA (1975) Compartmental syndrome. *A unified concept. Clinical Orthopaedic and Related Research* 113: 8–14.

Medical Device Directive (1993) *Council Directive 93/42/EEC of 14 June 1993 Concerning Medical Devices.*

Section 3

National Patient Safety Agency (2009) *WHO Surgical Safety Checklist*. London: NPSA. http://www.nrls.npsa.nhs.uk/resources/clinical-specialty/surgery/?entryid45=59860 (accessed 4 December 2011).

NICE (National Institute for Health and Clinical Excellence) (2010) *Venous Thromboembolism: Reducing the risk*. London: NICE. http://www.nice.org.uk/CG92 (accessed 4 December 2011).

NMC (Nursing and Midwifery Council) (2008) *The Code: Standards of conduct, performance and ethics for nurses and midwives*. London: NMC.

O'Brien V (2009) Controlling the process: legislation and guidance regulating the decontamination of medical devices. *Journal of Perioperative Practice* 19(12): 428–432.

Parker A (2004) Principles of surgical practice. In Radford M, County B and Oakley M (eds) *Advancing Perioperative Practice*. Cheltenham: Nelson Thornes.

Pirie S (2010) Patient care in the perioperative environment. *Journal of Perioperative Practice* 20(7): 244–247.

Smith B and Williams T (2004) *Operating Department Practice A–Z*. London: Greenwich Medical Media.

Smith C (2005) Care of the patient undergoing surgery. In Woodhead K and Wicker P (eds) *A Textbook of Perioperative Care*. Edinburgh: Churchill Livingstone.

Further Readings

Bale E and Berrecloth R (2010) The obese patient: anaesthetic issues. *Journal of Perioperative Practice* 20(8): 294–299.

Health and Safety Executive (2006) *Five Steps to Risk Assessment*. http://www.hse.gov.uk/pubns/indg163.pdf (accessed 4 December 2011).

Marklow A (2006) Body positioning and its effect on oxygenation – a literature review. *Nursing in Critical Care* 11(1): 16–22.

Richardson C (2004) Use of leg positioning holders. *British Journal of Perioperative Nursing* 14(3): 127–130.

Wilde S (2004) Compartment syndrome the silent danger related to patient positioning and surgery. *British Journal of Perioperative Nursing* 14(12): 546–552.

CHAPTER 14

Pressure Area Care and Tissue Viability

Zena Moore

Introduction

Pressure ulcers have been known to exist since ancient Egyptian times, and probably for as long as humans have been in existence (Robertson *et al*. 1990). They are largely a preventable problem, yet despite the advances in technology, preventative aids and increased financial expenditure, remain a common and debilitating concern (EPUAP 2002). Pressure ulcers are painful, impacting negatively on all domains of the activities of daily living (Gorecki *et al*. 2009). They commonly occur in those who cannot reposition themselves to relieve pressure on their bony prominences (Robertson *et al*. 1990), such as the very old, the malnourished, those with acute illness and those undergoing surgery (Robertson *et al*. 1990). Thus, it is suggested that the majority of pressure ulcers occur during an episode of hospitalisation of an individual in an acute care setting (EPUAP 2002). This has significant implications for the health service, as length of stay is protracted for those with pressure ulcers when compared to their matched counterparts (Graves *et al*. 2005). Furthermore, direct resource costs are also increased, all of which serve to impact negatively on achieving diagnostic related goals (Bennett *et al*. 2004).

Definition of a Pressure Ulcer

The European Pressure Ulcer Advisory panel and the National Pressure Ulcer Advisory Panel (EPUAP/NPUAP 2009) suggest that a pressure ulcer 'is localized injury to the skin and/or underlying tissue usually over a bony prominence, as a result of pressure, or pressure in combination with shear. A number of contributing or confounding factors are also associated with pressure ulcers; the significance of these factors is yet to be elucidated.' Understanding the exact definition of a pressure ulcer is important as it provides a clear description of the key aetiological factors that cause pressure ulcers (i.e. pressure or pressure in combination with shear).

Manual of Perioperative Care: An Essential Guide, First Edition. Edited by Kate Woodhead and Lesley Fudge.
© 2012 John Wiley & Sons, Ltd. Published 2012 by John Wiley & Sons, Ltd.

Prevalence and Incidence

From the international literature, pressure ulcer prevalence figures vary from 6.8% to 53.2% (Davis and Caseby 2001, Bours *et al.* 2002, Tannen *et al.* 2006, Capon *et al.* 2007, Keelaghan *et al.* 2008, Paquay *et al.* 2008). As with prevalence data, incidence figures differ across countries and across clinical settings. The literature reports figures of between 9.7% and 38.1% (Martin *et al.* 1995, Bergstrom *et al.* 1996, Goodridge *et al.* 1998, Ooi *et al.* 1999, Davis and Caseby 2001, Horn *et al.* 2004, Defloor *et al.* 2005, Vanderwee *et al.* 2007). Among surgical patients, specifically, pressure ulcer prevalence rates of 8.5% and 33% (Versluysen 1986, Karadag and Gümüskaya 2006), and incidence rates of between 14.1% and 54.8% (Schoonhoven *et al.* 2002a, Lindgren *et al.* 2005, Aronovitch 2007) have been reported. The majority of ulcers are noted on the heel and the sacrum, and are mainly stage 1 and 2 pressure ulcer damage. Furthermore, it is suggested that 23% of all nosocomial pressure ulcers develop in the operating department (Aronovitch 1999).

Pressure Ulcer Classification

Blanching erythema

After a period of pressure on superficial tissues, there will be a corresponding deprivation of oxygen to that area (Mayrovitz *et al.* 1999). To compensate for the loss of oxygenation after removal of pressure, there is a rapid increase in blood flow to the affected part. This is called reactive hyperaemia and is one of the body's compensatory mechanisms (Bliss 1998). The aim of this process is to restore normal blood flow and to prevent tissue death. Reactive hyperaemia is evident to the naked eye as a reddened patch over the affected skin (Bliss 1998). Blanching hyperaemia, when the reddened area blanches (turns white) on gentle compression of the skin (Collier 1999), indicates that no permanent damage has occurred; however, it is pathologically different to normal skin (Witkowski and Parish 1982).

Non-blanching erythema

The classification of early pressure ulcer damage, non-blanching erythema, has been widely welcomed by practitioners. However, the original definition, 'tissue redness that does not blanch (turn white) when pressed' was not without problems because the definition is unsuitable for individuals with darkly pigmented skin (Henderson *et al.* 1997). To overcome the limitations of the original definition of non-blanching erythema, the EPUAP/NPUAP (2009) suggest that 'darkly pigmented skin may not have visible blanching; its color may differ from the surrounding area. The area may be painful, firm, soft, warmer or cooler as compared to adjacent tissue.'

Pressure ulcer classification systems

A variety of pressure ulcer classification tools are currently in use; perhaps the most common are the Stirling Scale (1 or 2 digit) in the UK (Reid and Morison 1994), the original NPUAP Scale in the USA (NPUAP 1989) and the original EPUAP Scale (EPUAP 1999). The Stirling Scale has five stages ranging from no damage to full-scale tissue destruction, and includes a subset of descriptors for each stage (Reid and Morison 1994). While working on the latest guidelines for prevention and management of pressure ulcers (EPUAP/NPUAP 2009), the EPUAP and NPUAP developed a common international definition and classification system for pressure ulcers. The system includes four categories/stages from non-blanchable erythema to full thickness tissue loss. For the USA, two additional categories/stages have been included: 'unstageable/unclassified', which is full thickness skin or tissue loss where the depth is unknown, and 'suspected deep tissue injury', where the depth of damage is unknown (EPUAP/NPUAP 2009). A recent systematic review concludes that there is insufficient evidence to suggest which pressure ulcer classification system to recommend for clinical practice (Kottner *et al*. 2009). Studies conducted are so heterogeneous that it is impossible to synthesise the evidence in a clear and meaningful way (Kottner *et al*. 2009).

Risk Assessment Tools

Risk has been defined as the probability of an individual developing a specific problem (i.e. a pressure ulcer) (Deeks *et al*. 2002). In a study exploring risk factors for pressure ulcer development among surgical patients, Karadag and Gümüşkaya (2006) noted that of the 84 patients who scored not at risk preoperatively (Braden Scale), 54.8% went on to develop a pressure ulcer after surgery (97.9% developed within the first 3 days postoperatively). This suggests that the risk assessment tool was not sufficiently sensitive to capture the true risk status of the group. Indeed, the risk status of the population changed from the immediate preoperative period to the immediate postoperative period. The authors identified that 85.7% of the group were at risk of pressure ulcer development postoperatively. This risk gradually reduced over the 6 days after surgery. The duration of immobility increases with the length of surgery. Indeed, prevalence rates increase from 6% to 13% as surgery time increases from 3 hours to 7 hours or more (Aronovitch 1999, Scott *et al*. 2001, Price *et al*. 2005). As such, it is clear that undergoing surgery is an important risk factor, with intraoperative and postoperative immobility being a key consideration (Schoonhoven *et al*. 2002b). It can be argued that this immobility is not sufficiently weighted in the current risk assessment tools to enable an accurate assessment of the patient's risk status (Moore and Cowman 2008). Indeed, the current risk assessment tools do not adequately reflect the risk of pressure ulcer development in the operating department (Price *et al*. 2005).

Risk Factors

In those undergoing surgery, a number of risk factors have been identified (Schoonhoven *et al*. 2002a, Lindgren *et al*. 2005, Aronovitch 2007). These factors have been catagorised into patient-related factors and surgery. Lindgren *et al*. (2005) identified female gender, American Society of Anesthesiologists (ASA) status or New York Heart Association (NYHA) status and food intake to be the strongest predictors of pressure ulcer development (odds ratio (OR) 0.27; 95% confidence interval (CI) 0.11–0.68, $P = 0.003$; OR 2.30; 95% CI 1.21–4.38, $P = 0.011$; OR 0.53; 95% CI 0.31–0.91, $P = 0.022$, respectively). Conversely, Aronovitch (2007) found no statistically significant relationship between co-morbid conditions and an increased risk of intraoperatively acquired ulcers. Indeed, of the 48% with no co-morbid conditions, 7% still went on to develop a pressure ulcer, compared to 9% of those with at least one co-morbid condition. Aronovitch (2007), noted that the greater the surgery time, the greater the prevalence of pressure ulcers, arguing that even with few co-morbidities, patients still go on to develop pressure ulcers. Similarly, Schoonhoven *et al*. (2002b) found no statistical significant relationship between patient risk factors and surgery-related risk factors and pressure ulcer development. The only risk factor which remained statistically significantly associated with perioperative pressure ulcer development was length of surgery. Indeed, for every 30 minutes of surgery over 4 hours, the risk of developing a pressure ulcer increased by 33% (95% CI 13–56%). A more recent study (Connor *et al.* 2010) supports the work of Schoonhoven *et al.* (2002b) where patient and surgery factors were not found to statistically significantly influence the occurrence of pressure ulcers. However, the relationship between anaesthesia duration and pressure ulcer development was confirmed (OR 1.005; 95% CI 1.000–1.010; $P = 0.038$).

Pressure ulcers occur due to prolonged unrelieved exposure to externally applied mechanical forces (Kosiak 1959). Those who are vulnerable to exposure to this pressure are the immobile (Bergstrom *et al.* 1996, Goodridge *et al.* 1998, Casimiro *et al.* 2002, Moore 2008). For the surgical patient, it is logical that activity and mobility are the highest predictors of risk, as it is these factors that cause an individual to be exposed to pressure (Defloor 1999). Individuals undergoing surgery have immobility induced upon them and are also not able to feel pain, the stimulus that a change in position is required (EPUAP/NPUAP 2009). Not being able to move increases the risk of pressure ulcer development due to exposure to prolonged interface pressures between the skin and the relatively hard operating table (EPUAP/NPUAP 2009). Thus, for the surgical patient, addressing pressure redistribution and reduction of shearing forces are central in providing adequate pressure ulcer prevention in the operating department (Schoonhoven *et al.* 2002b).

Conclusion

Almost 23% of nosocomial pressure ulcers occur in the operating department, with length of surgery emerging as one of the most important risk factors for patients within this clinical environment. Pressure is the prime cause of pressure ulcers and immobility is the key factor that exposes the individual to this pressure. For those undergoing surgery, immobility is imposed upon them due to anaesthesia, impairing their ability to feel pain and to reposition spontaneously. The duration of surgery compounds this problem, with prevalence rising in keeping with increasing duration of surgery. The literature outlines the challenges with risk assessment in this cohort of patients, as risk status changes from the preoperative, intraoperative and postoperative phases. Indeed, some individuals assessed as not at risk preoperatively develop pressure ulcers, suggesting the key link between the intraoperative period and pressure ulcer risk. Unfortunately, the current risk assessment tools do not accurately reflect this changing risk status, compounding the challenges in providing adequate protection for patients within the operating department. Therefore, it is contended that all those undergoing surgical procedures with protracted surgery duration are at risk of pressure ulcer development. This makes it imperative that pressure redistribution and reduction of shearing forces are included as integral components of patient safety within the operating department.

References

Aronovitch S (1999) Intraoperative acquired pressure ulcer prevalence. *Journal of Wound, Ostomy and Continence Nursing* 26: 130–136.

Aronovitch SA (2007) Intraoperatively acquired pressure ulcers: are there common risk factors? *Ostomy Wound Management* 53: 57–69.

Bennett G, Dealey C and Posnett J (2004) The cost of pressure ulcers in the UK. *Age and Ageing* 33: 230–235.

Bergstrom N, Braden B, Kemp M, Champagne M and Ruby E (1996) Multi-site study of incidence of pressure ulcers and the relationship between risk level, demographic characteristics, diagnoses, and prescription of preventive interventions. *Journal of the American Geriatric Society* 44, 22–30.

Bliss MR (1998) Hyperaemia. *Journal of Tissue Viability* 8, 4–11.

Bours G, Halfens RJG, Abu-Saad HH and Grol RTPM (2002) Prevalence, prevention and treatment of pressure ulcers: descriptive study in 89 institutions in the Netherlands. *Research in Nursing and Health* 25, 99–110.

Capon A, Pavoni N, Mastromattei A and Di Lallo D (2007) Pressure ulcer risk in long-term units: prevalence and associated factors. *Journal of Advanced Nursing* 58, 263–272.

Casimiro C, García-de-Lorenzo A and Usán L (2002) Prevalence of decubitus ulcer and associated risk factors in an institutionalized Spanish elderly population. *Nutrition* 15, 408–414.

Collier M (1999) Blanching and non-blanching hyperaemia. *Journal of Wound Care* 8, 63–64.

Connor T, Sledge J, Bryant-Wiersema L, Stamm L and Potter P (2010) Identification of pre-operative and intra-operative variables predictive of pressure ulcer development in patients undergoing urologic surgical procedures. *Urologic Nursing* 30, 289–295.

Davis CM and Caseby NG (2001) Prevalence and incidence studies of pressure ulcers in two long-term care facilities in Canada. *Ostomy and Wound Management* 47, 28–34.

Deeks J, Higgins J, Riis J and Silagy C (2002) Module 11: Summary statistics for dichotomous outcomes data. In Alderson P and Green S (eds) *Cochrane Collaboration Open Learning Material for Reviewers*. Chichester: John Wiley and Sons, pp. 87–102.

Defloor T (1999) The risk of pressure sore: a conceptual scheme. *Journal of Clinical Nursing* 8, 206–216.

Defloor T, De Bacquer D and Grypdonck MH (2005) The effect of various combinations of turning and pressure reducing devices on the incidence of pressure ulcers. *International Journal of Nursing Studies* 42, 37–46.

EPUAP (European Pressure Ulcer Advisory Panel) (1999) Guidelines on treatment of pressure ulcers. *EPUAP Review* 2, 31–33.

EPUAP (2002) Summary report on the prevalence of pressure ulcers. *EPUAP Review* 4, 49–57.

EPUAP/NPUAP (European Pressure Ulcer Advisory Panel and National Pressure Ulcer Advisory Panel) (2009) *Prevention and Treatment of Pressure Ulcers: Quick Reference Guide*. Washington DC: National Pressure Ulcer Advisory Panel.

Goodridge DM, Sloan JA, LeDoyen YM, McKenzie JA, Knight WE and Gayari M (1998) Risk-assessment scores, prevention strategies, and the incidence of pressure ulcers among the elderly in four Canadian health-care facilities. *Canadian Journal of Nursing Research* 30: 23–44.

Gorecki C, Brown JM, Nelson EA *et al.* and on behalf of the European Quality of Life Pressure Ulcer Project group (2009) Impact of pressure ulcers on quality of life in older patients: a systematic review. *Journal of the American Geriatrics Society* 57: 1175–1183.

Graves N, Birrell F and Whitby M (2005) Effect of pressure ulcers on length of hospital stay. *Infection Control Hospital Epidemiology* 26: 293–297.

Henderson CT, Ayello EA, Sussman C *et al.* (1997) Draft definition of stage 1 pressure ulcers: inclusion of persons with darkly pigmented skin. *Advances in Wound Care* 10: 16–19.

Horn SD, Bender SA, Ferguson ML *et al.* (2004) The National Pressure Ulcer Long-Term Care Study: pressure ulcer development in long-term care residents. *Journal of the American Geriatric Society* 52: 359–367.

Karadag M and Gümüskaya N (2006) The incidence of pressure ulcers in surgical patients: a sample hospital in Turkey. *Journal of Clinical Nursing* 15: 413–421.

Keelaghan E, Margolis D, Zhan M and Baumgarten M (2008) Prevalence of pressure ulcers on hospital admission among nursing home residents transferred to the hospital. *Wound Repair Regeneration* 16: 331–336.

Kosiak M (1959) Etiology and pathology of ischaemic ulcers. *Archives of Physical Medicine and Rehabilitation* 40: 62–69.

Kottner J, Raeder K, Halfens R and Dassen T (2009) A systematic review of interrater reliability of pressure ulcer classification systems. *Journal of Clinical Nursing* 18: 315–336.

Lindgren M, Unosson M, Krantz A-M and Ek A-C (2005) Pressure ulcer risk factors in patients undergoing surgery. *Journal of Advanced Nursing* 50: 605–612.

Martin BJ, Devine BL and MacDonald JB (1995) Incidence of pressure sores in geriatric long-term hospital care. *Journal of Tissue Viability* 5: 83–87.

Mayrovitz HN, Macdonald J and Smith JR (1999) Blood perfusion hyperemia in response to graded loading of human heels assessed by laser-doppler imaging. *Clinical Physiology* 19: 351–359.

Moore Z (2008) Risk factors in the development of pressure ulcers. *Acta Med Croatica* 62: 9–15.

Moore ZEH and Cowman S (2008) Risk assessment tools for the prevention of pressure ulcers. *Cochrane Database of Systematic Reviews* 16: CD006471.

NPUAP (National Pressure Ulcer Advisory Panel) (1989) Pressure ulcers prevalence, cost and risk assessment: consensus development conference statement. *Decubitus* 2: 241.

Ooi WL, Morris JN, Brandeis GH, Hossain M and Lipsitz LA (1999) Nursing home characteristics and the development of pressure sores and disruptive behaviour. *Age and Ageing* 28: 45–52.

Paquay L, Wouters R, Defloor T, Buntinx F, Debaillie R and Geys L (2008) Adherence to pressure ulcer prevention guidelines in home care: a survey of current practice. *Journal of Clinical Nursing* 17: 627–636.

Price M, Whitney J, King C and Doughty D (2005) Development of a risk assessment tool for intraoperative pressure ulcers. *Journal of Wound Ostomy and Continence Nursing* 32: 19–30.

Reid J and Morison M (1994) Classification of pressure sore severity. *Nursing Times* 90: 46–50.

Robertson J, Swain I and Gaywood I (1990) The importance of pressure sores in total health care. In Bader DL (ed.) *Pressure Sores, Clinical Practice and Scientific Approach*. London: Macmillan Press, pp. 3–13.

Schoonhoven L, Defloor T and Grypdonck HHF (2002a) Incidence of pressure ulcers due to surgery. *Journal of Clinical Nursing* 11: 479–487.

Schoonhoven L, Defloor T, van der Tweel I, Buskens E and Grypdonck M (2002b) Risk indicators for pressure ulcers during surgery. *Applied Nursing Research* 16: 163–173.

Scott EM, Leaper DJ, Clark M and Kelly PJ (2001) Effects of warming therapy on pressure ulcers-a randomized trial. *AORN Journal* 73: 921–927, 929–933, 936–928.

Tannen A, Bours G, Halfens R and Dassen T (2006) A comparison of pressure ulcer prevalence rates in nursing homes in the Netherlands and Germany, adjusted for population characteristics. *Research in Nursing and Health* 29: 588–596.

Vanderwee K, Grypdonck MHF, De Bacquer D and Defloor T (2007) Effectiveness of turning with unequal time intervals on the incidence of pressure ulcer lesions. *Journal of Advanced Nursing* 57: 59–68.

Versluysen M (1986) How elderly patients with femoral fracture develop pressure sores in hospital. *British Medical Journal* 292: 1311–1313.

Witkowski JA and Parish L (1982) Histopathology of the decubitus ulcer. *Journal of the American Academy of Dermatology* 6: 1014–1021.

CHAPTER 15

Thermoregulation

Eileen Scott

This chapter aims to discuss thermoregulatory mechanisms, the effects on them of anaesthesia, and the adverse consequences of hypothermia. Most of what is required for everyday practice is included, however, for more detailed information, see the 'Further Reading', particularly the NICE *Clinical Guideline on Perioperative Hypothermia* and some selected papers relating to my own research.

It is important to know at the outset that, from an anaesthetic perspective, there are two forms of hypothermia: inadvertent and induced. The latter is a deliberate and controlled anaesthetic technique used for specific types of surgery. Induced hypothermia, through the use of cardiac bypass systems and chilled infusions, is an anaesthetic technique used to slow metabolic rate and therefore reduce oxygen demands during, for example, cardiac surgery. In some, highly controlled, situations mild hypothermia can have a beneficial effect in accelerating neurological recovery after cerebral ischaemia and brain injury and extreme hypothermia is known to have a protective mechanism against ischaemia and hypoxia. This specialised temperature control is beyond the scope of this chapter.

Temperature Regulation

All humans need to maintain a nearly constant internal temperature, which is optimal at 37 °C. The normal process of thermoregulation has three components: afferent thermal sensing, central regulation, and efferent responses. Autonomic thermoregulatory control is determined by heat and cold receptors. These are widely distributed in the body, including the skin surface, and send signals via the central nervous system, to the hypothalamus which is the primary thermoregulatory centre. The most efficient response is vasomotor activity, and although sweating and active vasodilation are the responses to heat, it is vasoconstriction which is the first defence against cold.

Anaesthesia

The induction of anaesthesia can cause changes in normal responses. Normally a deviation of only 0.2 °C from the optimal 37 °C will trigger responses, but in the anaesthetised patient this threshold is widened to a value approximately 20 times the normal range. Although abnormally high temperatures, defined as malignant hyperthermia, can be triggered by anaesthetic agents, especially by suxamethonium combined with halothane, this is a rare and life-threatening event. Thyroid crisis, a rare complication following thyroidectomy for Graves' disease, can also result in abnormally high temperatures. However, a more common side-effect of anaesthesia is hypothermia, which results from a combination of impaired thermoregulation, exposure to the cold environment of the theatre and skin preparation methods. Anaesthetic drugs inhibit thermoregulation in a dose-dependent manner and the vasoconstriction and shivering responses to cold are inhibited about three times as much as is the sweating response to heat.

Hypothermia

Hypothermia is usually defined as a temperature less than 36 °C and is classified as mild if not less than 32 °C. Inadvertent hypothermia is a recognised complication of anaesthesia when normal thermoregulation is inhibited. All surgical patients are at risk of intraoperative hypothermia and it has been estimated that 70% of all patients might suffer from its effects during the immediate postoperative period, although this figure could be as high as 85%. Hypothermia may not be immediately resolved and patients may still be affected up to 4 hours after surgery. There is evidence to suggest that a high proportion of patients (over 20%) were returned to the ward with temperatures of less than 35 °C. This situation should not arise today in view of a raising awareness of the problems of hypothermia and resulting changing practices, including the implementation of NICE guidelines.

Temperature changes caused by anaesthesia

Temperature changes caused by anaesthesia are in three stages. Induction of anaesthesia causes vasodilation, which allows movement of heat from the centre with no net loss of body heat. This postinduction core-to-peripheral redistribution of body heat is followed by heat loss through radiation, convection, conduction and evaporation, which gradually decreases core temperature until the 'plateau phase' is reached. However, this plateau, which is a result of thermoregulatory vasoconstriction segregating metabolic heat to the core thermal compartment, may not be reached until after 3–4 hours of anaesthesia. Despite possible stabilisation of core temperature during this final stage, the net heat loss from the periphery may still continue. If the halt in temperature decline has been achieved because of vasoconstriction, which decreases cutaneous heat loss and acts to hold meta-bolic heat in the body core, this type of core-temperature plateau is potentially dangerous from a clinical point of view. This is because the total body heat content continues decreasing even though the core temperature remains constant, thus the shivering response is not triggered. In some situations, preoperative warming may be beneficial and also delayed intraoperative warming (determined by patient core temperature) can still be effective; however it may be impractical to begin warming once a procedure has started.

Intraoperative procedures

The greatest temperature drops may occur within the first 40–60 minutes of anaesthesia and may also relate to patient exposure during skin preparation and positioning.

Significant reductions in core temperature have also been noted at the end of orthopaedic procedures after tourniquet deflation. Hypothermia may be affected by ambient temperatures and by longer periods of surgery. It is more likely to occur in surgical procedures where large surface areas of the body are exposed, in situations when the peritoneal cavity is opened, and perhaps when large amounts of unwarmed irrigation fluids are used.

Regional and general anaesthesia

Although hypothermia is associated with both regional and general anaesthesia, it may be less likely to occur if regional techniques are employed, perhaps because the hypothalamic thermoregulation remains intact. However, vasodilation still occurs and there is still an impairment of shivering in the area of the block. It may be because of this usual absence of shivering that routine temperature monitoring is less likely to be carried out, resulting in hypothermia sometimes remaining undetected in these patients. If a combination of regional (epidural) and general anaesthesia is used, the risk of hypothermia may be increased because of the combined effects on the thermoregulatory mechanisms.

Inequalities of risk

Intraoperative reductions in temperature may be more severe in patients with a low content of body fat, perhaps if preoperative haemoglobin levels are low and if anxiolytics have been given preoperatively. Although it is thought that the precision of thermoregulatory control is not affected by gender, some researchers have suggested that women may be at greater risk. However, it may be that the women (as sometimes tends to be the case) were older than the men. There is certainly widespread opinion that thermoregulatory control is inhibited with advancing age, perhaps because of limited cardiovascular reserve. The greater effect in the elderly was not dependent on type of surgery and reductions in core temperatures have been found in minor, and relatively short, procedures.

The demographic changes which have resulted in more elderly patients undergoing sometimes extensive surgery may have increased the scale of the problem of intraoperative hypothermia. While each individual risk factor is important, it is patients with multiple risk factors, most likely also to be elderly, who are more likely to become hypothermic.

Consequences of hypothermia

Known and suspected adverse effects of hypothermia are diverse and meta-analysis has demonstrated not only the extent of the risk of adverse outcomes but also the implications for cost effectiveness. Hypothermia is associated with variations in serum potassium levels, postoperative instability, an increased risk of myocardial ischaemia in the first 24 hours following surgery and increased mortality. Hypothermia can have an impact on arterial blood pressure, is associated with cardiovascular complications, is thought to affect protein metabolism and, through vasoconstriction, to decrease subcutaneous oxygen tension. These effects on skin oxygen tension have also been shown to increase the incidence of surgical wound infection and to increase the risks of pressure ulcers. It has also been suggested that if hypothermia develops, this leads to a longer overall hospital stay. Furthermore, the incidence of perioperative morbid cardiac events was higher in hypothermic patients, who were known to be at high risk of coronary disease, and who had abdominal, thoracic or vascular surgical procedures.

Section 3

Hypothermia impairs coagulation through inhibiting the series of enzymatic reactions of the coagulation cascade which controls the haemostatic system. It is therefore a contributory factor to abnormal bleeding and the development of coagulopathy after shock, trauma or massive transfusion; coagulopathy itself is associated with high morbidity and mortality rates.

There may also be a delayed metabolism of anaesthetic drugs and this, combined with attempts to treat hypothermia during the initial postoperative period, lead to longer stays in recovery. Patients who remain hypothermic during immediate recovery often experience episodes of shivering. Shivering has different causes but, whether it stems from hypothermia, or from a clonic type of tremor caused by a differential 'awakening' of the central nervous system from anaesthesia, its afferent stimulus is cold skin. This involuntary emergency response to a sensed heat loss is an unpleasant, and sometimes distressing, experience which can increase oxygen demands by 400–500% above basal requirements. This sudden and extreme test of cardiorespiratory reserve has been likened to the strain on the cardiovascular system of an Olympic event, difficult for young people, but perhaps fatal for the elderly. Therefore, although the immediate postoperative effects of hypothermia may be modest in relatively young, healthy patients, shivering is potentially dangerous for anyone with limited cardiorespiratory reserves. Neither does an absence of shivering necessarily mean that the patient is normothermic and adequate monitoring is essential.

Temperature measurements

Traditionally, oral, rectal and axillary routes have been used for routine temperature monitoring. Core temperature is, however, more reliably measured in the pulmonary artery, tympanic membrane, distal oesophagus or nasopharynx. The most accurate measure is via the pulmonary artery, although such invasive techniques are only used in critical care areas. New technology has resulted in electronic thermometers which measure the core temperature non-invasively, and with a high degree of accuracy, for example using tympanic thermometers. Tympanic readings represent a close correlation to core temperatures because of the proximity of the carotid arteries which vascularise both the tympanic membrane and the hypothalamus. Assuming this accurate representation, in comparison, rectal and bladder readings may overestimate core temperatures while oral measures may underestimate them. Electronic axillary readings have also been shown to be a poor indicator of core temperature.

As with all thermometers, it is essential that measurement techniques are accurate, that probes are placed correctly and those differences between sites are taken into account. The day-to-day use of tympanic thermometers is part of the skill-base of all anaesthetic and recovery practitioners. Also, with current Department of Health regulations it is important that training in the use of medical devices is carried out. The choice of device is related to hospital procurement policies; the important thing is that whatever is used intraoperatively should also be used in the recovery ward/PACU and the general surgical wards. Otherwise trends cannot be accurately recorded.

Warming therapies

As with thermometers, there is a range of products on the market. Research evidence has demonstrated safety and efficacy but the clinical effectiveness of each may not have been fully assessed. There are new products becoming available all the time and cost is always an issue but should not be an overriding concern. As with thermometers you will be constrained by procurement policies. It is essential that perioperative staff ensure that their voice is heard relating to practicalities and effectiveness when such decisions are made.

BOX 15.1

Key priorities for implementation of perioperative care (adapted from 'CG 65 Inadvertent perioperative hypothermia: the management of inadvertent perioperative hypothermia in adults. London: NICE. Available from www.nice.org.uk/ Reproduced with permission. NICE 2008a)

Patients (and their families and carers) should be informed that:

- staying warm before surgery will lower the risk of postoperative complications
- the hospital environment may be colder than their own home
- they should bring additional clothing, such as a dressing gown, a vest, warm clothing and slippers, to help them keep comfortably warm
- they should tell staff if they feel cold at any time during their hospital stay.

When using any device to measure patient temperature, healthcare professionals should:

- be aware of, and carry out, any adjustments that need to be made in order to obtain an estimate of core temperature from that recorded at the site of measurement
- be aware of any such adjustments that are made automatically by the device used.

Preoperative phase

Each patient should be assessed for their risk of inadvertent perioperative hypothermia and potential adverse consequences before transfer to the theatre suite. Patients should be managed as higher risk if any two of the following apply:

- American Society of Anesthesiologists (ASA) grade II–V (the higher the grade, the greater the risk)
- preoperative temperature below 36.0 °C (and preoperative warming is not possible because of clinical urgency)
- undergoing combined general and regional anaesthesia
- undergoing major or intermediate surgery
- at risk of cardiovascular complications.

If the patient's temperature is below 36.0 °C:

- forced air warming should be started preoperatively on the ward or in the emergency department (unless there is a need to expedite surgery because of clinical urgency, for example bleeding or critical limb ischaemia)
- forced air warming should be maintained throughout the intraoperative phase.

Intraoperative phase

- The patient's temperature should be measured and documented before induction of anaesthesia and then every 30 minutes until the end of surgery.
- Induction of anaesthesia should not begin unless the patient's temperature is 36.0 °C or above (unless there is a need to expedite surgery because of clinical urgency, for example bleeding or critical limb ischaemia).
- Intravenous fluids (500 mL or more) and blood products should be warmed to 37 °C using a fluid-warming device.
- Patients who are at higher risk of inadvertent perioperative hypothermia and who are having anaesthesia for less than 30 minutes should be warmed intraoperatively from induction of anaesthesia using a forced air warming device.
- All patients who are having anaesthesia for longer than 30 minutes should be warmed intraoperatively from induction of anaesthesia using a forced air warming device.

Postoperative phase

- The patient's temperature should be measured and documented on admission to the recovery room and then at 15-minute intervals.
- Ward transfer should not be arranged unless the patient's temperature is 36.0 °C or above.
- If the patient's temperature is below 36.0 °C, they should be actively warmed using forced air warming until they are discharged from the recovery room or until they are comfortably warm.

Further Readings

Alexander R, Alfonsi P, Campos J *et al.* (2007) Survey on intraoperative temperature management in Europe. *European Journal of Anaesthesia* 24: 668–675.

Melling A, Ali B, Scott EM and Leaper DJ (2001) The effects of preoperative warming on the incidence of wound infection after clean surgery: a randomized controlled trial *The Lancet* 358: 876–880.

NICE (National Institute for Health and Clinical Excellence) (2008a) *Inadvertent Perioperative Hypothermia: The management of inadvertent perioperative hypothermia, Clinical Guideline 65.* London: NICE. http://www.nice.org.uk/Search. do?keywords=perioperative+hypothermia&newSearch=true&searchType=Guidance (accessed 7 September 2011).

NICE (2008b) *Surgical Site Infection: Prevention and treatment of surgical site infection, Clinical Guideline 74.* London: NICE. http://www.nice.org.uk/Search.do?keywords=surgical+site+infections&searchsubmit=GO&searchSite=on&searchType=All&newSearch=1 (accessed 7 September 2011).

Scott EM (2000) Hospital acquired pressure sores in surgical patients. Unpublished PhD thesis, University of Teesside, Middlesbrough.

Scott EM and Buckland R (2006) Intra-operative warming for the prevention of post- operative complications: a systematic review. *AORN Journal* 83(5): 1090–1113.

Scott EM, Leaper DJ, Clark M and Kelly PJ (2001) Effects of warming therapy on pressure ulcers – a randomized trial. *AORN Journal* 73(5): 921–938.

Sessler DI (1997) Current concepts: mild perioperative hypothermia *The New England Journal of Medicine* 336(24): 1730–1737.

Sessler DI (2000) Perioperative heat balance. *Anesthesiology* 92(2): 578–596.

Young CC and Sladen RN (1996) Temperature monitoring. *International Anesthesia Clinics* 34(3): 149–174.

Section 3

CHAPTER 16

Venous Thrombosis Prophylaxis

Sue Bacon

This chapter will describe the background to prevention of venous thromboembolism (VTE), how a deep vein thrombosis (DVT) forms and what the risk factors are. It will also describe how to assess a patient's risk of VTE and provide some knowledge of methods of thromboprophylaxis. It will also provide knowledge of the signs and symptoms of DVT as some patients attending the preassessment clinic may have already developed a DVT if they have become increasingly immobile preoperatively.

Background to Venous Thromboembolism

For many years (since the 1960s) the risk of patients dying from thrombosis has been well documented. Kakker was a pioneer in this field of medicine. He demonstrated that DVT was common in both medical and surgical inpatients and that the use of subcutaneous heparin reduced the incidence of DVT (Kakker *et al.* 1970). It is amazing that it has taken so many years for the prevention of venous thromboembolism (VTE) to have finally reached the top of the health agenda in England. It has been a top priority in the USA (Shojania *et al.* 2001).

There has been an apparent increase in the incidence of VTE in America with a prediction that the rate will increase from 0.95/1000 to 1.82/1000 by 2050 (Deitelzweig *et al.* 2011).

In 2005 in the UK, the Commons Health Select Committee produced a report on VTE prevention (Department of Health 2005) which made many recommendations, all of which were agreed by the Department of Health.

The 2005 report estimated that there were 25 000 people in the UK alone who were dying each year from VTE, a disease that is largely preventable. The management and treatment of VTE and post-thrombotic syndrome (PTS) was reported as costing the NHS £640 million a year. PTS is an unpleasant condition which may develop as a consequence of DVT.

The National Institute for Health and Clinical Excellence (NICE) was commissioned to give guidance on VTE prevention in surgical hospitalised patients and this guidance was published in 2007.

Manual of Perioperative Care: An Essential Guide, First Edition. Edited by Kate Woodhead and Lesley Fudge.
© 2012 John Wiley & Sons, Ltd. Published 2012 by John Wiley & Sons, Ltd.

An independent working group looked at the remaining group of patients; those admitted with medical conditions and who were also at risk of developing a VTE and recommendations were made (Department of Health 2007).

Since 2007 there have been many forward steps in the prevention of VTE, culminating in further NICE guidance (CG92) in 2010 for all patients admitted to hospital (NICE 2010b).

The All Party Parliamentary Thrombosis Group (APPTG) ensured that VTE prevention was pushed to the top of the agenda and since 2007 has undertaken an audit of all acute hospital trusts in the UK. In 2010 this audit showed that only 41% of all acute trusts were assessing patient's risk of VTE on admission (All Party Parliamentary Thrombosis Group 2010). In 2011 the Department of Health introduced a Commissioning for Quality and Improvement (CQUINS) target, mandating that 90% of patients admitted to hospital must be risk assessed within 24 hours of admission. The CQUIN payment framework ensures that a proportion of a hospitals income is conditional on improving quality thus, unless the target is achieved, there will be a reduction in income. Mandating risk assessment was welcomed, as, while it was clear that patients must be assessed for their risk of VTE, assessment was not at the top of the agenda and thus often pushed aside. When the National Patient Safety Agency (NPSA) took an audit of warfarin therapy to reduce harm to patients there was rapid compliance.

In April 2011 the Department of Health also indicated that their risk assessment criteria must be used; this was frustrating for a number of hospitals that had developed their own methodology but an incentive for those hospitals struggling to agree a format.

The NHS is now strongly focused on VTE prevention and it is part of the NHS outcomes framework, to 'reduce the incidence of avoidable harm' (Department of Health 2010).

The NICE quality standard for VTE prevention will also help to make thrombo-prophylaxis the norm in all our hospitals and will no doubt help to frame future commissioning, focusing on reducing VTE events (NICE 2010a).

VTE prevention is now part of medical training and the Royal College of Nursing (RCN) is recommending inclusion in nurse education. There are many online resources for education, including VTE exemplar centres such as Kings Thrombosis and the RCN websites.

How does a Deep Vein Thrombosis Develop?

Knowledge of how a thrombus can develop is helpful in understanding the rationale behind VTE prevention. In 1856, it was recognised by Virchow that there were three contributory factors in developing a thrombosis:

- venous stasis (pooling of the blood – for example, increased immobility)
- vessel damage (following injury to the vein – for example during surgery)
- hypercoagulopathy (a tendency for the blood to 'stick together' such as occurs when dehydrated, the patient has a clotting disorder, or the patient is taking drugs that may affect the clotting – for example the oral contraceptive pill).

These three factors became known as Virchow's triad (Figure 16.1).

Risk Factors

According to NICE (2010b), the main risk factors for VTE are:

- active cancer or cancer treatment
- age over 60 years

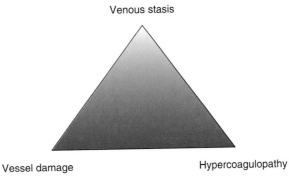

Figure 16.1 Virchow's triad.

- critical care admission
- dehydration
- known thrombophilia
- obesity (BMI > 30 kg/m^2)
- one or more medical co-morbidities (for example acute infectious disease, heart failure)
- personal or first-degree relative with a history of VTE
- use of hormone replacement therapy
- varicose veins with phlebitis
- women who are pregnant or have given birth in the previous six weeks.

While considering the patient's individual risk of thrombosis it is important to also consider the patient's individual risk of bleeding:

- active bleeding
- acquired bleeding disorder
- concurrent use of anticoagulants
- lumbar puncture/spinal anaesthesia within 4 hours
- lumbar puncture/spinal anaesthesia planned in the next 12 hours
- acute stroke
- low platelet level (<75 × 10^9/L)
- uncontrolled hypertension (230/120 mmHg or higher)
- inherited bleeding disorders – haemophilia/von Willebrand's disease.

How to Assess a Patient's Risk of Venous Thromboembolism

Risk assessment is the first step in VTE prevention and is used to accurately identify those patients at risk of developing a VTE.

Each patient has individual risk factors for thrombosis and bleeding (as listed above) and these need to be assessed carefully.

All hospitals now have a risk assessment form based on the Department of Health form which should be completed, dated and signed within 24 hours. This is to comply with the CQUINS target, but is essential for the wellbeing of the patient, regardless of targets.

When the risk factors are related to an individual patient, one can understand why some patients are more 'at risk' than others. For example, an elderly patient undergoing a hip replacement who has had a previous VTE event is at a higher risk of VTE than a young patient having day-case surgery, with no previous history of VTE (young, no perceived immobility, no major vessel damage and no expected dehydration or thrombophilia).

Section 3

It is at preassessment that the patient is fully informed of the impending surgery and the associated risks. At this time the patient should be given documentation to take home and read about preventing VTE.

Methods of Thromboprophylaxis

Once an assessment of the thrombosis and bleeding risk is made, a decision for type of thromboprophylaxis is required. This decision may also be influenced by the reason for the hospital admission, and these risks are identified on the assessment form as 'admission-related' risks; for example, a patient may have a high risk of thrombosis due to a previous event, have a thrombophilia and family history of thrombosis, (thus carrying a high risk of VTE) but the procedure for which they have been admitted carries a high risk of bleeding (neurosurgery) and this may alter the decision on the type of thromboprophylaxis.

All patients, regardless of their risk of thrombosis or bleeding, require some form of non-interventional thromboprophylaxis, often just referred to as 'reducing the risk of VTE' or 'general advice to patients' and 'best practice'. In the author's opinion, this method of thromboprophylaxis is often undervalued and underused, probably as it is almost impossible to evaluate, but it is essential for all patients. It involves:

- *Patient education*: Many patients will not be aware of the words 'deep vein thrombosis' or 'pulmonary embolism' but have heard of blood clots, so it is important to ascertain the patients understanding of the condition prior to further discussion. All patients should be informed of their individual risk and how they can reduce the risk.
- *Early mobilisation*: All patients should be encouraged to move as soon as is practically possible and it is very important that all healthcare professionals are proactive in encouraging this. Ideally the level of mobility achieved each day should be documented and increased immobility addressed. Those patients who are immobile should be taught simple leg exercises and, if they are unable to perform these, the healthcare professionals can perform simple passive exercises while attending to the patient hygiene. Advice from a physiotherapist may be required.
- *Hydration*: This also plays an important part (Virchow's triad) and dehydration should be avoided at all costs. A study by Kelly found that dehydration played an independent role in the incidence of VTE in acute stoke patients (Kelly *et al.* 2004). Healthcare professionals must ensure that patients have water within reach, and that patients should be reminded to drink.

Interventional thromboprophylaxis is either mechanical or pharmacological. The choice of thromboprophylaxis should be based on local policies, the clinical condition of the patient, the surgical procedure and also patient preference (NICE 2010b).

Mechanical Thromboprophylaxis

Mechanical devices are used to prevent blood pooling in the legs and to encourage venous return. There are three main methods of mechanical thromboprophylaxis: anti-embolism stockings, intermittent pneumatic compression and foot pumps.

Anti-embolism stockings

These stockings provide graduated compression; they have a higher compression at the ankle than the calf, and should comply with the compression of 14–15 mmHg at the calf (NICE 2010b). There has been much discussion regarding the recommended length of stocking as to whether knee or thigh length should be used. NICE guideline CG46 (now obsolete) recommended the use of thigh length but recent NICE guidance (CG92, NICE 2010b) recommends simply thigh or knee length. From the authors' experience, below knee socks seems most appropriate – patients are more compliant, the stockings do not roll down or cause a tourniquet effect behind the knee when the knee is bent and they are easier to apply for both patient and healthcare professionals and they are more cost-effective.

It may be appropriate at this stage to distinguish between graduated elastic compression socks (GECS) and anti-embolic stockings (AES). The former tend to have a higher compression and usually used to treat patients with poor venous return. These are worn during the day and removed at night. GECS may include lower compression but AES have only lower compression and are worn 24/7 and changed daily. There is often confusion between the two.

Surgical patients who are deemed at risk of VTE should have AES fitted, unless they have contraindications, mainly peripheral vascular disease, excessive oedema of the legs and skin conditions which may be exacerbated by the application of stockings (see NICE guidance C92, for full list of contraindications). Some patients may have a leg deformity that precludes successful fitting. It is important to also use one's own clinical judgement in deciding whether to fit AES or not, and advice should be sort if in doubt.

Careful measuring and fitting of the AES is important, and all healthcare professionals involved in fitting AES must have appropriate training. Each manufacturer has guidance for measuring and fitting their product and further guidance can be sought from them. Incorrect fitting can cause harm to the patient. A patient with an epidural may not realise that the top of the sock is too tight for example, which can lead to necrosis.

The AES should be changed daily and the foot and ankle observed for signs of pressure sores. In the CLOT study, looking at the effectiveness of AES in preventing VTE in acute stroke patients, it was found that some patients developed pressure sores and from this trial it was recommended that AES are not fitted in medical patients (Dennis *et al.* 2009). It is important that patients are told about the care and management of wearing AES so that they can ensure that they are removed daily. Patients also need to be informed about how to apply the AES and not to pull them up high and then turn down the top if they are too long as this produces a tourniquet effect and could cause rather than prevent a DVT. Should the calf measurements be different, further advice should be sought as this could indicate the presence of a DVT. Failure to mention this anomaly could endanger the patient's life as it is dangerous to carry out surgical procedures or fit mechanical devices with an undiagnosed DVT.

Intermittent pneumatic compression

These devices are fitted to the patient's legs in the form of inflatable leggings or boots and an air pump provides intermittent pulsing pressure to the chambers of the leggings. The exact method of inflation is different for each manufacturer but the principle is the same, encouraging venous return and also stimulating fibrinolysis, the breaking down of clots (Morris and Woodcock 2004).

Foot pumps

Foot pumps are fitted to the patient's feet and an air pump alternately inflates a cushion in the venous plantar area of the foot and simulates the action of walking, thus increasing venous return.

Section 3

These devices – intermittent pneumatic compression and foot pumps – are most often used for patients who are deemed at risk of VTE but have a contraindication for pharmacological thromboprophylaxis, for example following neurosurgery and daily evaluation of the requirement for the intermittent pneumatic compression should be documented.

There are two further important points with regard to the use of intermittent pneumatic compression and foot pumps:

- They must not be fitted to patients who have a suspected DVT.
- They should not be placed back on the patient when they have been removed for a number of hours (time determined locally and as per manufacturers advice) as, if the patient has been immobile, there is potential for a DVT to have developed and thus fitting the devices could cause an embolus to move to the lungs.

Pharmacological Thromboprophylaxis

The decision for which drug to be used is based upon local policies and individual patient risk factors, as well as the clinical condition of the patient, for example renal failure and also patient preferences, for example the patient may prefer an oral drug to a daily injection.

Anticoagulants work of different parts of the 'clotting cascade,' and in order to understand the action of these drugs it is worth gaining an understanding of this (Bacon 2011). Anticoagulants include:

- *low-molecular-weight heparin* (LMWH, Factor X inhibitor, subcutaneous injection), which is the drug of choice, with enoxaparin, tinzaparin and dalteparin being the most commonly used (Caution needs to be taken in patients with renal failure (defined as eGFR <30 mL/min), depending on the choice of LMWH.)
- *fondaparinux* (synthetic pentasaccharide Factor Xa inhibitor, subcutaneous injection)
- *unfractionated heparin* (s/c injection) may be used in patients with renal failure.

New oral agents on the horizon include dabigatran etixalate (Pradaxa), a direct thrombin inhibitor, and rivaroxaban (Xarelto) Factor X inhibitor, currently licensed for prevention of VTE following hip and knee replacements.

Warfarin is NOT recommended for VTE prevention, but patients who are previously anticoagulated with warfarin may be restarted post operatively, using LMWH to 'bridge' until the INR is therapeutic.

Aspirin is also NOT recommended for VTE prophylaxis (it is an antiplatelet agent and thus not as effective in preventing venous clots).

Pharmacological prophylaxis should be commenced as soon as haemostasis has been established and the risk of bleeding reduced – hence the requirement for daily assessment of the patient.

Signs and Symptoms of Deep Vein Thrombosis

It is worth having some basic knowledge of signs and symptoms of DVT as it is possible that patients attending the preassessment clinic may have already developed a DVT. Signs/symptoms include:

- pain/aching
- swelling
- oedema

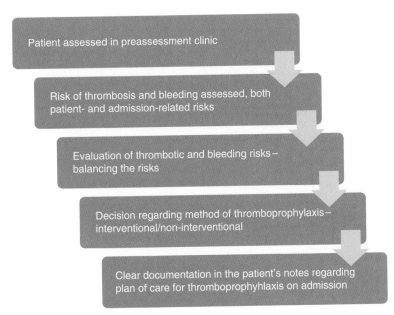

Figure 16.2 Pathway for venous thromboembolism risk assessment.

- warmth
- whole leg swelling.

Should the patient complain of any of the above, they should be referred for further assessment.

The pathway for the VTE risk assessment is illustrated in Figure 16.2.

Summary

You should now have the confidence to assess a patient's risk of thrombosis and give advice regarding the plan of care they can expect on admission.

References

All Party Parliamentary Thrombosis Group (2010) *Fourth Annual Audit of Acute NHS Hospital Trusts 2010.* www.kingsthrombosiscentre.org.uk (accessed 14 December 2011).

Bacon S (2011) The management of VTE: a practical guide for nurse prescribers. *Nurse Prescribing* 9(4): 172–179.

Deitelzweig SB, Johnson BH, Lin J and Schulman KL (2011) Prevalence of clinical venous thromboembolism in the USA: Current trends and future projections. *American Journal of Hematology* 86(2): 217–220.

Dennis M, Sandercock PA, Reid J *et al.* (2009) Effectiveness of thigh-length graduated compression stockings to reduce the risk of deep vein thrombosis after stroke (CLOTS trial 1): a multicentre, randomised controlled trial. *Lancet* 373(9679): 1958–1965.

Department of Health (2005) *The Prevention of Venous Thromboembolism in Hospitalized Patients.* Second Report of Session 2004–5. House of Commons Health Committee. London: Stationery Office.

Department of Health (2007) *Report of the Independent Expert Working Group on the Prevention of Venous Thromboembolism in Hospitalized Patients.* April 2007. London: Stationery Office.

Department of Health (2010) *The NHS Outcomes Framework 2011/12.* http://www.dh.gov.uk/prod_consum_dh/groups/dh_digitalassets/@dh/@en/@ps/documents/digitalasset/dh_123138.pdf (accessed March 2012).

Kelly J, Hunt BJ, Lewis RR *et al.* (2004) Dehydration and venous thromboembolism after acute stroke. *International Journal of Medicine* 97(5): 293–296.

Section 3

Kakker VV, Howe CT, Nicholaides AN, Renney JT and Clarke MB (1970) Deep vein thrombosis of the leg. Is there a high risk group? *American Journal of Surgery* 120(4): 527–530.

Morris RJ and Woodcock JP (2004) Evidence-based compression; prevention of stasis and deep vein thrombosis. *Annals of Surgery* 239: 162–171.

NICE (National Institute for Health and Clinical Excellence) (2010a) *Venous Thromboembolism Prevention Quality Standard*. London: NICE. http://www.nice.org.uk/aboutnice/qualitystandards/vteprevention/vtequalitystandard.jsp (accessed March 2012).

NICE (2010b) *Venous Thromboembolism – Reducing the Risk*. CG92. London: NICE.

Shojania KG, Duncan BW, McDonald KM, Wachter RM and Markowitz AJ (2001) Making healthcare safer: A critical analysis of patient safety practices. *Evidence Report/Technology Assessment (Summary)* (43)i–x: 1–688.

Further Readings

Thrombosis Adviser. www.thrombosisadvisor.com (accessed 5 December 2011).

The Thrombosis Charity: Lifeblood. www.thrombosis-charity.org.uk (accessed 5 December 2011).

CHAPTER 17

Care of Surgical Instruments

Jane Smith

Introduction

Since the very early days of surgery it has been recognised that a surgeon's ability is not only reliant on a good technique but also on the fine manipulation of the tools required in order to elicit the desired outcome for the patient. Hippocrates alluded to this, asserting that 'What concerns surgery are the patient, operator, assistants and instruments; the light' (Debakey 1991, Zimmerman and Veith 1993). This insight from 'the father of western medicine' supports the notion that the art of surgery is a partnership, and thorough consideration must be dedicated to each aspect of it; this will incorporate the acquisition and care of the surgical instrument.

The term 'surgical instrument' includes everything on a spectrum from simple scalpel to highly specialised technologically advanced medical equipment; these are often referred to as medical devices.

> Several different international classification systems for medical devices continue to exist however, the World Health Organization, with its partners, is working towards achieving harmonisation in medical device nomenclature, which will have a significant impact on patient safety. (World Health Organization 2003)

Surgical Instrument Procurement

Patient safety and outcome is paramount and therefore the integrity of the instruments and their procurement must be subject to a rigorous process. Before an instrument or set of instruments is chosen, careful consideration has to be given to its quality to prevent inadvertent harm to the patient, which could be attributed to the instrument. This will include deciding whether the instrument could become scratched or dented, and whether it is manufactured from a durable substance that will withstand numerous decontamination cycles or is assembled from several parts that could become detached in a patient cavity or misplaced.

Manual of Perioperative Care: An Essential Guide, First Edition. Edited by Kate Woodhead and Lesley Fudge.
© 2012 John Wiley & Sons, Ltd. Published 2012 by John Wiley & Sons, Ltd.

Each organisation will have its own procurement process and this will determine how instruments are purchased and managed effectively. All organisations, however, should use a prepurchase research procedure which has contribution and input from the infection prevention and control team, sterile services and other specialisms that govern aspects of patient safety, to ensure that any instruments or equipment under consideration for purchase can be accommodated within existing cleaning and sterilisation standards and controls.

Information should also be sought, as part of this procedure, from the instrument manufacturers as they should provide the required reprocessing information in accordance with the requirements of the Institute of Decontamination Sciences (Beesley and Pirie 2005, Institute of Decontamination Sciences 2011). Regardless of which process is in operation, it is important that prior to purchasing any new instrumentation, dialogue has occurred between the manufacturers, sterile services, infection control and the theatre personnel. The Institute also stipulate that it is up to the purchaser to ensure that the recommended reprocessing guidelines such as the sterilisation method and cycle (including temperature and recommended exposure time) can be followed on site and that these comply with current decontamination guidelines. If they do not, the product should not be purchased as failure to have these conversations could prove costly (Medicines and Healthcare products Regulatory Agency 2006).

> The Health and Social Act 2008, updated 31st December 2010, has determined through its Code of Practice, overall requirements for healthcare providers in relation to infection prevention and control practices; it also details the overall requirements for decontamination of medical devices. (Institute of Decontamination Sciences 2011)

Regardless of whether single components or sets of instruments are being purchased, training for both the sterile services staff and theatre personnel should be an integral part of the agreement package from the manufacturer supplying the instrumentation (Medicine and Healthcare products Regulatory Agency 2006).

Prior to the purchase and introduction of any new instrumentation, research into responsibilities and procedure for maintenance and repair needs to be undertaken. If it is possible for repairs to be carried out in-house, authorisation must be obtained from the manufacturers to do this, especially within any agreed warranty period.

Training

The training delivered by the manufacturer to the sterile services personnel should incorporate the correct methods of decontamination and sterilisation in accordance with the Institute of Decontamination Sciences guidelines. It is recommended that this will include the number of components that make up each instrument by disassembling and rebuilding each one.

The training provided by the manufacturer for the theatre staff should include the names of the instruments and their specific use. In addition, the training should cover the surgical technique. This could be delivered to the theatre team, including the specific surgeons, who are likely to be using the instruments. For new theatre personnel it is recommended that individual personal competencies are in place to cover the use and function of the instruments (Beesley and Pirie 2005).

The process for learning surgical procedures will vary depending on the organisational structure within the theatre team. Consideration should be given to the different individuals' learning styles within the team and the teaching of instruments and surgical techniques adapted accordingly (e.g. the use of acronyms or photographs). It is at this point in the practitioner's development that emphasis is given to ensure that instruments are only used for the purpose for which they were surgically intended. There will no doubt be a time when a scrub practitioner will be asked for a certain instrument to be used for a different function and this should be prohibited. Instruments such as artery forceps should not be used to secure drapes as this could strain the mechanism and render them useless. Within the training package, reference should be made to the correct way in which instruments are handed to the surgeon as there is a right and wrong way of doing this (Beesley and Pirie 2005). Empowering a new trainee is key to ensuring safe systems of work are adopted and maintained.

Inclusion in Surgical Counts

Ensuring quality assurance of an instrument, prior to the commencement of each procedure, is vital. These checks should include that all parts of the instrument are present, functional and sharp if appropriate. The practitioner performing the check should make sure that all clamps close properly and in the case of instruments that have a ratchet that this is effective and easy to use; and that the tips can approximate and that moving joints move freely (Pirie 2010).

Visual inspections should be carried out to ensure that there is no rusting, pitting or scratches to either the outside or inside of any instrument with or without a lumen.

These assurances and inspections, although primarily the remit of sterile services, should be standardised practice prior to any use on patients.

One message that needs to be emphasised is that when the scrub practitioner is ready to commence the operation, he or she must always be aware of where all the instruments are placed as ultimately they are responsible. In some places of work they stipulate that no one touches the sterile field to remove any instrument with the exception of the scrub practitioner.

Some instruments may have more than one component. Within the concept of accountability it is important that the scrub practitioner is familiar with all the parts of each instrument and can account for them all during an instrument check. This is not to suggest that each instrument be taken apart for the purpose of the instrument checks but the scrub practitioner should know, prior to each check that she or he can account for each piece that was on the tray at the start of each case and the same number is present and accounted for at the end of each check (Beesley and Pirie 2005). Another reason for the scrub practitioner to be aware of all the parts within a particular instrument is that if it happens to fail during a procedure the instrument may need to be reassembled.

It is important that all theatre personnel adhere to a recognised procedure for identifying instruments that need repairing especially during a surgical case. A faulty instrument should remain in the theatre environment until that surgical case is completed as it has been part of the instrument count. Anything contrary to this must have been discussed and written into local policy (Beesley and Pirie 2005).

Safety Aspects to be Considered

Any instrument that has a lumen should be checked prior to usage to ensure that it is clean and free from any debris which could compromise the quality of the product.

Instruments that have T junctions, namely endoscopes, tend to have a recognised blind spot that can be difficult to decontaminate effectively and the scrub practitioner needs to be mindful of this.

Section 3

Telescopes or indeed any product that has a lens should be checked by the scrub practitioner prior to the surgical case commencing. To do this they should look through the instrument and make sure there are no visible cracks or dark spots which could indicate a fault in the lens. As soon as is possible, the light source should be coupled to the scope to ensure the scope system is fully operational, to provide a safety mechanism.

Within an instrument set there may be some items that could be considered as sharp (e.g. scissors). For quality purposes there has to be an agreement between sterile services and the management of theatres as to how the scissors are to be sharpened and maintained (Radford *et al.* 2004, Pirie 2010).

With other instruments that tend to be sharp, such as Kilner's retractors, sterile services may choose to use a variety of means to protect the sharp end of the instrument. This is usually to protect the user from a sharps injury and to prevent damage to the fabric or material of the packaging. Consideration must be given to accounting for these items that are used primarily as protection, as anything additional on the tray has the potential to become a foreign body in the patient, causing inadvertent harm.

Power tools are many and varied in type, and local arrangements should be in place to ensure that sterility at the point of use is maintained, whatever means is in use. Power tools may be battery, electric or use compressed air and each will require a different approach, for example any unsterile power hose should be enclosed within a sterile sleeve of some description.

Particular care and attention should be paid to the leads that are used, regardless of whether they are sterile or non-sterile, to ensure that the quality of the lead is maintained. Damage can occur to both the outer casing and also to the internal fibres. Damage can easily occur to the casing without it being obvious. It is therefore advisable that a system is in place to ensure someone is responsible for checking the integrity of the outer casings of leads whether sterile or non-sterile (Association for Perioperative Practice, AfPP 2007).

The majority of leads that are used within the perioperative environment are light leads. This is a lead that contains a number of fibre light filaments that is used to provide a light source. Failure to routinely check if all the fibres are intact could result in a substandard source of light. The checking procedure and personnel responsible for implementing it should be determined and agreed between the theatre personnel, sterile services and the medical engineering service within the hospital. Other factors related to the efficacy of the leads are the connectors and the adaptors. The practitioner should make sure that all these are in place prior to each case commencing. In addition, it is vital that the female and male connectors are established and a method of identifying which connector is needed for each lead. For example if an unsterile lead is required for a sterile bronchoscope then the theatre practitioner must know which connector is required prior to the patient arriving in theatre to prevent any delays or possible harm to the patient.

The way that the unsterile leads are stored is crucial in the prevention of damage; they should be looped rather than coiled. This method eliminates the possibility of resistance or tension being placed on the lead. There should be no kinks or knots in the lead. Good looping also saves a lot of time when the lead is required. The same principle should also apply when a sterile lead is being stored. Keeping your unsterile leads, connectors and adaptors clean is also very important.

The same principles apply to caring for cables. However, cables such as electrosurgical equipment (e.g. diathermy cables) should also be checked for insulation integrity and circuit continuity. The integrity of the outer casing could be compromised; a minor crack may have gone undetected. Cracks in the casing pose a risk of electrical current leakage if used within a cavity, which could cause inadvertent harm to the patient, therefore it is crucial that 'All the necessary safety precautions and checks should be followed as advised in the instruction manual. The equipment should be inspected and safety features tested before every use' (Wicker 2000, AfPP 2007, O'Riley 2010). The checking of cables and leads usually takes place in the sterile services department although it is always recommended that the end user also completes a check.

Accountability

UK statute law does not dictate what particular system or method is utilised for safe surgical instrument checking within each perioperative environment. Under the accountability of ensuring a 'duty of care' it is important that there is a recognised procedure for providing assurance that each instrument can be accounted for before, during and after a clinical invasive procedure and thereby negating the risk of a foreign body being retained in a patient (Plowes 2000, AfPP 2011) The AfPP endorses for accountability purposes that a swab, needle and instrument count be used for every clinical invasive procedure to prevent foreign body retention and subsequent harm to the patient. The checking of all spare instruments and loan instruments should be included and form part of the instrument check. The whole checking process should be mandated and be evident in local policy for governance purposes (AfPP 2011).

Handling of Surgical Instruments

The smooth transition of instruments from scrub practitioner to surgeon is of paramount importance. The way that this happens should enable the surgeon to continue with surgery, there should not be any delays while the surgeon adjusts their fingers. For this to happen without any mishap, the handling of the instruments should form part of the training. Each type of instrument requires a slightly different approach by the scrub practitioner and the instrument should be handed to the surgeon in such a manner that he or she knows the instrument has left the hands of the practitioner and is now in the hands of the surgeon and he or she should be able to continue suturing, clamping, etc. (Beesley and Pirie 2005).

For any instrument that has a ratchet, it is important that everyone involved with both the sterilisation process and any handling by the theatre personnel respect the function of the ratchet and therefore take the appropriate care of these instruments. This means that the ratchet should be relaxed when sterile and packaged, which should prevent the instrument becoming sprained. Likewise, at no time should this instrument be kept tightly closed as this could cause the instrument to become sprained, causing it to fail when it is required to secure a bleeding vessel.

The Neutral Zone

It is recommended, for the safe transfer of sharp instruments, that the scrub practitioner uses a receiver to transfer a sharp instrument to the surgeon and also to receive the sharp instrument back by using this same method which should minimise the risk of needle stick injury (Beesley and Pirie 2005). This is known as the neutral zone.

Tracking and Tracing

All instruments used for invasive procedures can be a vehicle for the transmission of infection (Medicines and Healthcare products Regulatory Agency 2006). Principles of safe practice must be adopted by the surgical team and the sterile services department to reduce or eliminate this risk and every instrument should be treated as a potential threat.

A tracking system is a system of recording and monitoring instruments that have been used during a procedure and if required is a recognised methodology for an investigation should the need arise. The Institute of Decontamination Sciences asserts that any organisation that uses medical devices on patients who are at risk from transmissible spongiform encephalopathies (TSE) and should develop a specific decontamination policy on TSE exposure (Institute of Decontamination Sciences 2011). The requirements for traceability can be reduced by using disposable devices, where appropriate, during surgery on any patient suspected of being at risk of prion disease.

Single-use instrumentation is intended to be used on an individual patient during a single procedure and then discarded. It is not intended to be reprocessed and used on another patient. The labelling identifies the device as disposable and not intended to be reprocessed.

The purchasing of single-use instrumentation and also the use of procedure packs have increased dramatically over the years and this has had an impact on reusable instrumentation. Certainly, with instruments such as drill bits, drills, taps, etc. the likelihood is that these are now purchased as single-use items. The reasons for this include the reduced theoretical risk of transferring prion disease, less likelihood of cross-infection and overall perceived cost effectiveness.

References

AfPP (Association for Perioperative Practice) (2007) *Standards and Recommendations for Safe Perioperative Practice.* Harrogate: AfPP.

AfPP (2011) *Standards and Recommendations for Safe Perioperative Practice.* Harrogate: AfPP.

Beesley J and Pirie S (eds) (2005) *NATN Standards and Recommendations for Safe Perioperative Practice.* Harrogate: National Association of Theatre Nurses.

Debakey M (1991) A surgical perspective. *Annals of Surgery* 213(6): 499–531.

Institute of Decontamination Sciences (2011) *Teaching and Training Manual.* Bathgate: IDSc.

Medicines and Healthcare products Regulatory Agency (2006) *MHRA Device Bulletin: Managing Medical Devices: Guidance for healthcare and social services organisations.* DB2006 (05), November, p. 3.37.

O'Riley M (2010) Electrosurgery in perioperative practice. *Journal of Perioperative Practice* 20(9): 332.

Pirie S (2010) Introduction to Instruments. *Journal of Perioperative Practice* 20(1): 23–25.

Plowes D (2000) *Back to Basics.* Harrogate: National Association for Theatre Nurses.

Radford M, County B and Oakley M (2004) *Advancing Perioperative Practice.* Cheltenham: Nelson Thornes.

Wicker P (2000) Back to basics – electrosurgery in perioperative practice. *Journal of Perioperative Practice* 10(4): 223.

World Health Organization (2003) *Medical Devices Regulations: Global overview and guiding principles.* Geneva: WHO.

Zimmerman L and Veith I (1993) *Great Ideas in the History of Surgery.* San Francisco: Norman Publishing.

CHAPTER 18

Swab and Instrument Count

Diane Gilmour

The swab and instrument count is essential and plays a vital role in enhancing the surgical patient's safety. The unintended retention of a swab or instrument is a serious, largely preventable event which should not have occurred, and is classified as a 'never event' (Department of Health 2011). The inadvertent retention of a swab or instrument may cause serious patient harm and often requires further medical treatment. In 2009 the Pennsylvania Patient Safety Advisory detailed the results of a retrospective audit of operation records which identified an incidence of 1 in 5500 operations resulting in a retained foreign object at a potential cost to the hospital of US$166 000 (£249 000) including legal costs and on-going surgical care per patient (Pennsylvania Patient Safety Authority 2009). This does not include the financial, physical and psychological cost to the patient in prolonged treatment, possible further surgery, time off work, etc.

Pennsylvania Patient Safety Advisory also detailed the number of reports received in 2008 involving an incorrect swab and instrument count. Forty-seven per cent of reports involved incorrect needle counts, 33% incorrect instrument counts and 20% incorrect swab counts.

Greenberg *et al.* (2008) concluded that one in eight surgical cases involves an intraoperative discrepancy with the swab and instrument count, a discrepancy being defined as a count that does not agree with the previous count. They observed that 51% of discrepancies were due to misplaced items found on the floor, in the rubbish or on the drapes. Such results show that not every discrepancy resulted in harm to that patient, and were resolved as practitioners carried out manual counts in accordance with local policy. Therefore it is essential to consistently perform surgical counts according to national standards and local policy.

Within the Codes of Conduct registered practitioners as professionals will be personally accountable for their conduct, their actions and omissions in practice (Nursing and Midwifery Council 2007, Health Professions Council 2008).

The Department of Health (2011) identified that a 'never event' may indicate that within an organisation the correct systems and processes are not in place. This is substantiated by Rowlands and Steeves (2010) who concluded in their study that processes or frameworks that reduce the probability of an untoward incident such as a retained swab or instrument occurring improve patient safety practices. However, it is imperative that such events are

Manual of Perioperative Care: An Essential Guide, First Edition. Edited by Kate Woodhead and Lesley Fudge.
© 2012 John Wiley & Sons, Ltd. Published 2012 by John Wiley & Sons, Ltd.

reported so that lessons can be learnt to prevent such incidences being repeated and causing harm to other patients (Department of Health 2011).

This chapter will outline the process for undertaking a swab and instrument count, provide rationale for these actions and identify the roles and responsibilities of the different members of the surgical team. Throughout the chapter the Association for Perioperative Practice (AfPP) and Association of Perioperative Registered Nurses (AORN) standards and recommendations for practice are used.

Aim of the Swab and Instrument Count

The aim of the swab and instrument count is to ensure that all accountable items – those at risk of being retained in the patient and are used during the operative procedure – are removed from the patient in order to reduce the risk of harm and injury to that patient should an accountable item be retained. Department of Health (2011) criteria for a 'never event' include that which is a known source of risk, that there is guidance available and if that is implemented the event is largely preventable. However, on occasions a swab or instrument may be retained intentionally.

The retention of a swab or instrument is a preventable occurrence and diligence, careful counting and effective communication within the surgical team will significantly reduce such incidences.

Legislation does not mandate how the swab and instrument count should be performed but perioperative standards exist worldwide to guide practitioners in the development and formulation of local policies and guidance.

AfPP and AORN recognise within their published guidance that surgical procedures are performed within a variety of settings such as radiology, day surgery, outpatients and primary care and that such guidance should be adapted to meet local needs but are applicable wherever operative or other invasive procedures are performed and swabs or instruments could be retained (AORN 2010, AfPP 2011). Accountable items include:

- all reusable instruments including screws or detachable parts
- all single-use instruments including screws or detachable parts
- blades
- bulldogs
- cotton wool balls
- diathermy tip cleaners
- Lahey swabs (peanuts, pledgets)
- Liga reels
- local infiltration needles
- nylon tapes
- ophthalmic micro sponges
- patties
- shods
- slings/sloops
- suture needles
- Tibbs/cannula
- X-ray detectable swabs.

Roles and Responsibilities

The scrub practitioner is accountable for knowing where all the swabs and instruments, and any additional equipment used are, during the surgical procedure. The scrub practitioner usually initiates the swab and instrument count and this must be done together with and audible to, the circulating practitioner.

Each swab and instrument count must be performed by two members of staff, one of whom must be a registered practitioner (operating department practitioner or nurse) and who may be acting as scrubbed or circulating practitioner. The second person may be a support worker or student who has been assessed and documented as competent to be involved with the swab and instrument count (AORN 2010, AfPP 2011).

If a support worker is fulfilling the scrub role they are directly supervised by a registered practitioner, then the swab and instrument count must be conducted with that person (Perioperative Care Collaborative 2007).

If a scrub practitioner is not required, then the registered practitioner as circulator should perform the swab and instrument count with the operating surgeon.

If the scrub practitioner is relieved during the procedure, together with their replacement they should conduct a swab and instrument count, and record in all appropriate documentation.

The operating surgical team must allow time for the swab and instrument count to be completed without pressure.

Key Principles

- A local swab and instrument policy must be published, shared and included within new staff induction programme. If the policy is amended or altered at any time then all staff must be made aware of these changes and sign a document to state that they have read and understood these changes.
- A swab and instrument count should be performed before the procedure (as a baseline reference for subsequent counts), before closure of a cavity (to identify any retained items prior to closure of the cavity), before wound closure begins, at skin closure or end of the procedure (to identify all items counted and added in during the procedure are present), and at the time if the scrub practitioner is relieved.
- As a minimum there should be two counts performed, one before the procedure starts and one as the procedure ends.
- Each operating room should have a visual system for recording of the swab and instrument count. Ideally this should be a dry-wipe board fixed to the wall, visible to all for reference during the procedure when required.
- The local policy must detail how practitioners add swabs, needles and other miscellaneous items to the board, and how items that are discarded during the procedure are accounted (see Table 18.1).
- A swab and instrument count should be performed in the same sequence; swabs, sharps, miscellaneous items and instruments. The count should move from the immediate surgical site to the mayo stand if used to the scrub practitioner's trolley and then to discarded items. This prevents any item separated into two locations being forgotten.
- All surgical swabs, irrespective of shape or size must have an X-ray detectable marker fixed within the swab.
- Non X-ray detectable swabs used for wound dressings must be withheld from the sterile field until the wound is closed and the procedure finished.
- X-ray detectable swabs should not be cut up, used for wound dressings or postoperative packaging unless intentionally agreed by the surgeon and the reason documented in the patient's notes, care plan and in the operating register.

Table 18.1   Example of a swab and instrument count board.

Date	23/01/2012
Patient's name	Mr John Smith
Procedure	Right hemicolectomy
Small swabs	5 + 5 + 5
Medium swabs	5 + 5
Large packs	5
Blades	2
Suture needles	5 + 1 + 1
Hypodermic needles	2
Diathermy tip cleaner	1
Liga reels	2
Packs within abdomen	3

- Any items added to the sterile field during the procedure must be counted in and documented appropriately, such as on the wipe board or instrument list, and available for subsequent swab and instrument counts.
- If an accounted item is accidentally dropped off the sterile field the circulating practitioner must alert the scrub practitioner immediately and place the item, adopting standard precautions when handling the item, in a place visible to the scrub practitioner so that it can be included within the swab and instrument count.
- Once a swab and instrument count has commenced there should be no interruptions and the count completed without distractions. If the count is interrupted then it should recommence from the last recorded item.
- All items used during the procedure, including clinical waste and laundry, must remain within the operating theatre until the final swab and instrument count has been completed.
- On completion of the final swab and instrument count the scrub practitioner must inform the surgeon verbally that the count is correct. The surgeon must respond to this statement as verification to prevent any misunderstanding.

The Swab Count – Checking Procedure

- All swabs and packs, including cotton wool balls, are counted and must be in bundles of five and of uniform size and weight. Any packet that does not contain five must be removed from the count and operating theatre immediately and discarded. The batch number and lot number is noted and swabs with the same numbers also removed from stock. The manufacturer is also informed.
- Swabs are recorded on the visual record in bundles of five.
- During the swab count the integrity, particularly of the tapes on larger swabs as well as the X-ray detectable strip, must be checked.
- X-ray detectable swabs used during catheterisation should remain in the operating theatre and be included within the swab and instrument count.
- In the event of a life-threatening emergency when a swab and instrument count may not have been performed then all packaging is kept for verification and at the earliest opportunity a count performed. This is then documented in the patient's notes and care plan.

- When checking swabs at the beginning of the procedure for use and when discarding or during subsequent counts each swab must be separated, opened and shown to the circulating practitioner to ensure that it is one swab and contains no other items.
- Local policy will include how swabs are managed intraoperatively. In major and complex cases swabs may be discarded during the procedure. This may be as individuals, or as multiples of five into a suitable contained disposal system. Various applications exist but within each department the one adopted within the policy must be followed for consistency and continuity to avoid discrepancy. The policy should incorporate standard precaution infection control measures.
- When counting swabs during the surgical procedure a logical sequence will reduce the risk of error. For example large swabs progressing to smaller ones, then sharps and finally instruments.
- If a swab is introduced a cavity such as vagina or abdomen intraoperatively and its intention is to remain there this must be recorded on the visual record such as 'swab in wound' and crossed through once the item has been removed. If a swab is used as a pack within the abdomen then this should be attached to an artery clip or similar instrument as verification to all the surgical team that a pack is inside the cavity.

The Instrument Count – Checking Procedure

- All staff involved with the swab and instrument count must be able to recognise and identify the instruments being counted and used.
- All instruments on the sterile field must be inspected prior to use to ensure all parts are functioning and safe to use; for instance diathermy leads should be checked for insulation integrity. Some instruments also need assembling prior to use and all separate parts must be accounted for on the instrument sheet.
- If an instrument is found to be damaged or not working then this should be removed from use immediately and processed for repair.
- Instruments must be counted individually and correspond with the preprinted instrument sheets or the tracking of a supplementary instrument.
- If an instrument is added during the procedure the local policy for tracking and traceability and recording of the additional instrument must be followed.
- Some instruments are also included on the visual record such as bulldog clamps, shods and artery forceps and therefore form part of the count on the visual record.
- At the end of the procedure all single-use instruments must be disposed of appropriately as per the local clinical waste policy.
- Blades, sutures and hypodermic needles are recorded as single items on the visual record and when added during the procedure amended as single items or the number contained within the packet – for example, double-ended sutures.
- A logical sequence for the counting of sharps should be adopted: blades, suture needles, hypodermics for example.
- Suture packets are retained on the sterile field by the scrub practitioner as an additional check if required but practitioners need to remember that the number of suture packets may not reflect the number of needles as identified above.
- If a blade, needle or instrument breaks during the procedure the scrub practitioner must ensure that all pieces are accounted for and returned to them. The item is then removed from the sterile field, labelled and sent for decontamination before informing the relevant department, such as the manufacturer or sterile services who will action a repair or the Medical and Healthcare Products Regulatory Agency (MHRA) who may issue a safety bulletin or hazard warning.

Section 3

Table 18.2   Steps to follow when a discrepancy is noticed.

1	The scrub and circulating practitioner perform another count and the item missing identified
2	If possible, the surgical procedure should be stopped depending on the patient's condition
3	Manual inspection of the wound and surrounding area
4	Visual inspection of the area surrounding the operating table/trolley, floors, all waste bins, linen, recount of any discarded items including swabs and scrub practitioner trolley
5	If the item is found then the surgery can continue
6	If, despite a thorough search, the item is not located then a plain X-ray of the surgical site should be taken before the final closure of the wound. It is useful for the radiologist to have a similar item for comparison
7	If the item is found, local policy and 'best practice' may require that this is documented and reported as a 'near miss' so that steps can be made to address the contributing cause
8	If the missing item is microscopic and cannot be detected by X-ray, such as fine needles, then this should be documented
9	If the item is not found then this is documented on the patient's care plan, operating theatre register or electronic records, and patient's notes
10	The discrepancy and actions taken to resolve this are reported to the appropriate personnel and the organisation's formal incident-reporting procedure started including statements from all staff involved
11	The NHS organisation must then report the incident as a 'never event' to the National Patient Safety Agency, Commissioners and recorded within the monthly service quality performance report (Department of Health 2011)

- The management of sharps during the surgical procedure must follow local policy such as a neutral zone or hands-free technique, reducing the risk of a sharps injury to any of the scrubbed surgical team.
- Other miscellaneous items such as diathermy tip scratch pads, nylon tapes, and liga reels must all be included within the swab and instrument count. Small items such as these used regularly throughout the surgical procedure need to be accounted for at all times to reduce the risk of them being retained within the patient.

Managing a Discrepancy

If at any point during the surgical procedure the swab and instrument count is incorrect then the surgeon must be informed immediately and verbally acknowledge this information. Table 18.2 lists the steps that should be followed.

Documentation

The swab and instrument policy defines the aims and key principles of the process and includes what to do in the event of a discrepancy.

At the end of the operative procedure the scrub and circulating practitioners must within all the relevant documentation such as operating register, electronic records, patient care plan, surgical safety checklist, record their details, that the swab and instrument count was completed, recording any intentional retained swab or instrument or discrepancy that may have occurred and the action taken.

SIGN OUT (to be read out loud)

> Before any member of the team leaves the operating room Registered Practitioner verbally confirms with the team:
>
> • Has the name of the procedure been recorded?
> • Has it been confirmed that instruments, swabs and sharp counts are complete (or not applicable)?
> • Have the specimens been labelled (including patient name)?
> • Have any equipment problems been identified that need to be addressed?

Figure 18.1   National Patient Safety Agency Surgical Safety Checklist. From Panesar *et al.* (2009).

The 'Safe Surgery Saves Lives' Campaign launched by the World Health Organization in 2007 introduced the Surgical Safety Checklist as a framework for improving patient safety within the surgical environment (Figure 18.1). One of the key elements identified to reduce patient harm during a surgical procedure is the confirmation at 'sign out' that the swabs and instruments are correct (National Patient Safety Agency 2009).

References

AfPP (Association for Perioperative Practice) (2011) Swab, instrument and needle count. In *2011 Standards and Recommendations for Safe Perioperative Practice*. Harrogate: AfPP.

AORN (Association of Perioperative Registered Nurses) (2010) Recommended practices for sponge, sharp and instrument counts. In *2010 Perioperative Standards and Recommended Practices*. Denver, CO: AORN.

Department of Health (2011) *The 'Never Events' list 2011/12 – policy framework for use in the NHS*. London: Department of Health.

Greenberg C, Regehogen S, Lipsitz S, Diaz-Flores R and Gawande A (2008) The frequency and significance of discrepancies in the surgical count. *Annals of Surgery* 248(2): 337–341.

Health Professions Council (HPC) (2008) *Standards of Conduct, Performance and Ethics*. London: HPC.

National Patient Safety Agency (2009) *Surgical Safety Checklist*. London: NPSA.

Nursing and Midwifery Council (2007) *The Code: Standards of conduct, performance and ethics for nurses and midwives*. London: NMC.

Panesar SS, Cleary K, Sheikh A and Donaldson L (2009) Surgical safety checklist. *Patient Safety in Surgery* 3(1): 9.

Pennsylvania Patient Safety Authority (2009) Beyond the count: preventing retention of foreign objects. *Pennsylvania Patient Safety Advisory* 6(2): 39–45.

Perioperative Care Collaborative (PCC) (2007) *Position Statement: Delegation: the Support Worker in the Scrub Role*. England: PCC.

Rowlands A and Steeves S (2010) Incorrect surgical counts: a qualitative analysis. *AORN Journal* 92(4): 410–419.

CHAPTER 19

Care of Specimens

Rosanne Macqueen

Introduction

Many patients undergoing surgery have specimens taken to assist in establishing or confirming a diagnosis which then determines the most appropriate course of treatment (Hughes and Mardell 2009). Obtaining a specimen may be the only reason for performing the surgery (Hughes and Mardell 2009). Ensuring that the specimen is correctly handled, named, typed, labelled, dispatched and transported to the laboratory is the responsibility of both the scrub and circulating practitioners (Hughes and Mardell 2009), in collaboration with medical and laboratory staff (Phillips 2007, AfPP (Association for Perioperative Practice) 2011).

Incorrect handling, mislabelling and loss of specimens can result in the patient returning to theatre for the collection of additional specimens, a wrong diagnosis and/or inappropriate or delayed treatment (Hughes and Mardell 2009). Makary *et al.* (2007) reported that 4.3/1000 surgical specimens were incorrectly identified during a six-month study; 3.7/1000 of these related to theatres. In 2008, the National Patient Safety Agency (NPSA) highlighted the potential harm that could be caused through incorrect patient identification and mislabelling of specimens, and made recommendations that this be incorporated into any adaptation of the World Health Organization's (WHO) Surgical Checklist, launched in the UK in 2009 (National Patient Safety Agency 2008, 2009).

Obtaining specimens in the UK is legislated under the Human Tissue Act 2004 (Human Tissue Authority 2004) and in Scotland, the Human Tissue (Scotland) Act 2006 (Human Tissue Authority 2006). These Acts regulate the removal, storage and use of human tissue, including from the deceased, for the purposes of transplantation, research, training and education, and further stipulate that consent should always be gained before any removal, storage or use of human body tissue, which includes for the purposes of DNA analysis (except in criminal investigations). Care and handling of specimens is regulated by the Health and Safety Executive under the Health and Safety at Work Act 1974, the Management of Health and Safety at Work Regulations 1999, the Control of Substances Hazardous to Health (COSHH) Regulations 2002 (Health and Safety Executive 2000), and local policy which should be devised in collaboration with local laboratory departments (AfPP 2011).

Manual of Perioperative Care: An Essential Guide, First Edition. Edited by Kate Woodhead and Lesley Fudge.
© 2012 John Wiley & Sons, Ltd. Published 2012 by John Wiley & Sons, Ltd.

Table 19.1   Examples of specimen types.

Fluids	Tissues	Non-biological
Amniotic fluid	Bone	Retained items, e.g. swabs/instruments
Blood	Breast tissue	Foreign bodies, e.g. peanuts, glass
Bone marrow	Brushings	Explanted prosthesis, e.g. orthopaedic screws/plates
Cell washings	Calculi, e.g. gallstones	Projectiles, e.g. bullets
Cerebrospinal fluid	Donor tissue, e.g. skin	Clothing, e.g. from crime scenes
Exudate	Margins of malignant lesions	
Semen	Muscle	
Urine	Organ – solid biopsy, diseased	
	Suspicious lesions	

Types and Testing of Specimens

A sample of tissue or fluid is referred to as a biopsy (Table 19.1). By examining a biopsy histologically (tissue analysis) and cytologically (cell analysis) in a laboratory, the pathologist can determine a clinical diagnosis (Phillips 2007, Hughes and Mardell 2009). This is then verified following the removal of the whole tissue, for example, the gallbladder, referred to as the surgical specimen (Phillips 2007, Hughes and Mardell 2009). Tests performed on fluid biopsies include bacteriology, virology, cytology, cell counts and genetic studies; tests performed on tissue biopsies include histopathology, hormonal assays and tissue typing (Phillips 2007, Hughes and Mardell 2009).

Types of biopsy

Methods of taking biopsies are described in Table 19.2.

Specimen Collection

It is imperative that specimens are collected using the correct technique and equipment at the correct time and delivered to the correct laboratory without delay (Dougherty and Lister 2008). Planning for the removal of a specimen in advance can support this, for example, ensuring the pathology department is aware that a frozen section will be taken (this is the responsibility of the medical staff) (AfPP 2011).

The surgeon should identify the specimen immediately at the time it is removed (AfPP 2011). Identification includes the nature of the specimen and the site (AfPP 2011). The scrub practitioner should verify this information with the surgeon, and confirm the preparation required before relaying the same information to the circulating practitioner (AfPP 2011). This information should be 'relayed back' to ensure the information has been clearly understood (Hughes and Mardell 2009).

Preparation of the specimen is determined by the specimen type; for example, most histopathology specimens are fixed in a transport medium such as formalin (AfPP 2011). The integrity of the specimen should always be maintained, and unless sending

Table 19.2 Methods of taking biopsies.

Biopsy	Method used
Aspiration biopsy	A 22–25 gauge needle and syringe is used to enter a joint, body cavity, cyst or abscess to aspirate the fluid contents, which are then fixed in a chemical solution. Fine needle biopsies have largely reduced the need for full excisional biopsies
Bone marrow biopsy	Usually taken from the sternum or iliac crest under local anaesthesia for cytology; the biopsies are extracted using a trocar puncture or aspiration needle placed into the bone, followed by a wider bore needle to aspirate the bone marrow
Brush biopsy	Tissue samples from the respiratory and urinary tracts can be taken by using nylon or steel brushes passed through an endoscope. The brushes remove tissue by rubbing against the target structure. The cells are smeared onto glass slides and the brush tips placed in formalin
Excisional biopsy	The whole structure or mass is removed. Excisional biopsies can be taken endoscopically
Incisional biopsy	A section of the mass is removed; usually soft tissue masses in the muscle, fat or other connective tissue
Percutaneous needle biopsy	Use of a special, hollow needle introduced through the body wall, sometimes under the guidance of an image intensifier, ultrasound or CT scanner, to obtain tissue from an internal organ or solid mass
Punch biopsy	Often used for skin biopsies. A sharp, circular-shaped punch instrument is used to cut out a round 3–4 mm sample of tissue
Smear biopsy	Used for fine needle aspirations and scrapings. The sample is fixed onto a glass slide by liquid suspension or by spraying with fixative. The slide is then stained to allow for microscopic examination
Frozen section	Used to determine an immediate intraoperative diagnosis for malignancy and regional node invasion. The specimen is placed in a dry container (fixative or saline alters the freezing process used during examination) and taken straight away to the laboratory. The results are reported back immediately by the pathologist by phoning the operating theatre. A written record of these results should be made by the medical staff (AfPP 2011)
Permanent section	The specimen is made permanent by firming it in fixative, removing the water content and replacing with paraffin before embedding in wax. The specimen is then sliced and placed on glass, the process reversed and dye added to allow for diagnostic examination

Adapted from Phillips (2007).

dry, should be kept moist (Phillips 2007, AfPP 2011). Fresh and frozen specimens are not fixed in preservative (Phillips 2007), nor is it recommended that samples taken to confirm tuberculosis (TB) are fixed; these specimens should be sent dry (Thomas *et al.* 2011). Paired specimens such as tonsils, for example, which are usually both removed, should be placed in separate containers and labelled as left or right (Phillips 2007). Foreign bodies and forensic specimens should be kept dry and managed in accordance with local policy (Phillips 2007). The same process applies to orthopaedic implants, however, legal ownership of the implant should be ascertained in advance if the implant is to be destroyed (AfPP 2011). Fetal remains and retained products of conception are treated in the same way as any other removed body tissue; however, sensitivity is advised in relation to the parents' wishes (Royal College of Nursing 2007a, Human Tissue Authority 2009, AfPP 2011). Amputated limbs should be wrapped in plastic before transporting to the laboratory (Phillips 2007).

Specimen containers or pots are made from glass, plastic and in some cases waxed cardboard (Phillips 2007) and should be leak-proof and sealable (AfPP 2011). The size should be appropriate to the size of the specimen, allowing it to be fully covered. Containers filled with fixative should be labelled as hazardous in compliance with COSHH Regulations (Health and Safety Executive 2002). Sterile containers can help reduce any risk of inadvertent contamination (Dougherty and Lister 2008).

Specimens are a possible source of infection. Standard precautions should always be followed during their handling, including wearing appropriate personal protective equipment (PPE), for example, gloves, aprons and eye protection (Hughes and Mardell 2009, AfPP 2011). Gloves should be removed and hands washed after handling any specimen (Phillips 2007).

Minimal handling and ensuring that the contents do not spill should reduce the risk of damaging the specimen, and of biohazardous exposure (Phillips 2007, Hughes and Mardell 2009). If the outside of the container is contaminated it should be wiped with antiseptic solution or soap and water immediately (Phillips 2007, Department of Health 2007). Accidental exposure, for example, splash injuries, should be treated in compliance with local policy (AfPP 2011). PPE should be worn to clean up any exposure or spillage (Department of Health 2007), and be disposed of, along with the materials used to clean up the spill, into an appropriate waste receptacle for infected waste (Department of Health 2007, Royal College of Nursing 2007b). All exposures and spillages should be reported (Department of Health 2007).

Documentation of Specimens

Each specimen should be labelled accurately to ensure it corresponds with the patient and their medical records, and it should be done before the specimen is placed in the specimen container. The patient's full name, unique hospital number, date of birth, hospital, department, nature of the specimen (type and site), the date and time the specimen was removed, the fixative solution (if used) and the consultant's name should all be recorded (Phillips 2007, Hughes and Mardell 2009, AfPP 2011) and attached, usually using a preprinted identification label, to the specimen container. All of these details should be checked between the scrub and circulating practitioner (AfPP 2011). Care should be taken to avoid sticking the preprinted label to the lid of the container (AfPP 2011). Some laboratories may forbid the use of labels for particular specimen types, for example, blood cultures; therefore check local policy (AfPP 2011).

The same demographic and specimen details need to be added to the specimen request or requisition form, which accompanies the specimen to the laboratory. Also required are the contact details of the consultant, the consultant's (or designated deputy's) signature and who the report should be sent to (AfPP 2011). Clinical information is also recorded and may include clinical signs and symptoms, a provisional diagnosis, current treatment, for example, antibiotic therapy, the risk of infection, and any other significant history, for example, foreign travel (Phillips 2007, Dougherty and Lister 2008, AfPP 2011). The request form for frozen specimens should be filled out before the start of surgery (AfPP 2011).

Section 3

Transport of Specimens

There are a number of regulations which govern the transport of specimens. These are determined by the mode of transport and the category of the infectious substance as determined by the United Nations (UN) (Department of Health 2007). These in turn determine the packaging for transport (Department of Health 2007). Clinical and diagnostic specimens are classified as Category B and these types of specimens should be packaged in compliance with the UN No. 3373 P650 packaging instructions (Department of Health 2007, Health and Safety Executive 2011). For security purposes specimens should only be handled by those with designated responsibility (Department of Health 2007).

Following collection, the specimen container should be placed into a clear, plastic, sealable bag (Phillips 2007, AfPP 2011). The specimen request form must be placed in the same bag in a way that maintains patient confidentiality; specimen transport bags usually have a second pocket for the request form (Dougherty and Lister 2008, AfPP 2011). Before leaving the department the specimen and all the related details and documentation should be rechecked (AfPP 2011). AfPP (2011) recommends that all specimens related to a patient are removed from the theatre before the next patient arrives, further reducing the risk of a mix-up and of any delay to the specimen being received by the laboratory. A record of every specimen should be documented in the patient's medical notes and in the theatre register (Phillips 2007). To allow for tracking from the theatre to the laboratory, AfPP (2011) recommends that every specimen is signed for alongside a corresponding printed name as it is dispatched.

Specimens which cannot be transported to the laboratory promptly should be stored in a specially designated facility (Phillips 2007, AfPP 2011). Specimens not fixed should be stored in a designated fridge at a temperature of 4°C; this will ensure that any bacterial growth is kept to a minimum (Phillips 2007, AfPP 2011). Placing specimens in formalin into a fridge set at 4°C prevents the specimen fixing (AfPP 2011). Blood cultures which cannot be transferred immediately should be stored in an incubator set at 37°C (Phillips 2007).

References

AfPP (Association for Perioperative Practice) (2011) *Standards and Recommendations for Safe Perioperative Practice*, 3rd edn. Harrogate: AfPP, section 5, p. 227, section 8.3, pp. 319–323.

Department of Health (2007) *Transport of Infectious Substances; Best Practice Guidance for Microbiology Laboratories.* http://www.dh.gov.uk/en/Publicationsandstatistics/Publications/PublicationsPolicyAndGuidance/DH_075439 (accessed 7 August 2011).

Dougherty L and Lister A (2008) *The Royal Marsden Hospital Manual of Clinical Nursing Procedures*, 7th edn. Singapore: Wiley Blackwell, chapter 40, pp. 775–794.

Health and Safety Executive (2000) *Management of Health and Safety at Work Regulations 1999; approved code of practice and guidance.* http://www.hse.gov.uk/pubns/priced/121.pdf (accessed 7 August 2011).

Health and Safety Executive (2002) *Control of Substances Hazardous to Health Regulations.* http://www.hse.gov.uk/coshh/ (accessed 7 August 2011).

Health and Safety Executive (2011) *Infectious Substances, Clinical Waste and Diagnostic Specimens.* http://www.hse.gov.uk/cdg/pdf/infect-subs.pdf (accessed 7 August 2011).

Hughes S and Mardell A (2009) *Oxford Handbook of Perioperative Practice.* China: Oxford University Press, chapter 16, pp. 292–293.

Human Tissue Authority (2004) Human Tissue Act 2004. http://www.legislation.gov.uk/ukpga/2004/30/pdfs/ukpga_20040030_en.pdf (accessed 7 August 2011).

Human Tissue Authority (2006). Human Tissue (Scotland) Act 2006: A guide to its implications for NHSScotland. http://www.hta.gov.uk/_db/_documents/Information_about_HT_(Scotland)_Act.pdf Accessed 7 August 2011.

Section 3

Human Tissue Authority (2009) *Code of Practice 5; Disposal of Human Tissue*. http://www.hta.gov.uk/_legi (accessed 7 August 2011).

Makary MA, Epstein J, Pronovost PJ, Millman EA, Hartmann EC and Freischlag JA (2007) Surgical specimen identification errors; a new measure of quality in surgical care. *Surgery* 141(4): 450–455.

National Patient Safety Agency (2008) *Patient Identification Errors from Failure to Use of Check ID Numbers Correctly.* http://www.urls.npsa.nhs.uk (accessed 7 August 2011).

National Patient Safety Agency (2009) *Patient Safety Alert Update; WHO Surgical Safety Checklist*. 26 January. http://www.urls.npsa.nhs.uk (accessed 7 August 2011).

Phillips N (2007) *Berry and Kohn's Operating Room Technique*, 11th edn. China: Mosby Elsevier, section 5, chapter 15, p. 259, section 7, chapter 22, pp. 387–389, section 9, chapter 25, pp. 480–481.

Royal College of Nursing (2007a) *Sensitive Disposal of Fetal Remains; guidance for nurses and midwives*. Revised February. http://www.rcn.org.uk/__data/assets/pdf_file/0020/78500/001248.pdf (accessed 8 August 2011).

Royal College of Nursing (2007b) *Safe Management of Health Care Waste*. http://www.rcn.org.uk/__data/assets/pdf_file/0013/111082/003205.pdf (accessed 8 August 2011).

Thomas D, Jarvis M and Williams A (2011) No formalin please, it could be TB! *Journal of Perioperative Practice* 21(7): 249–250.

CHAPTER 20

Managing High-Risk Equipment

Chris Earl

Introduction

Management of high-risk equipment within the operating theatre department carries with it considerable responsibility and accountability. Medical devices may be used in the treatment of patients during surgery but, if used incorrectly, without sufficient training or being subject to regular maintenance, they can be the cause of unintended harm to patients.

Systems need to be in place in order that all practitioners are knowledgeable and responsible users. In the first instance a list or database of all equipment within the suite or department needs to be set up and maintained so that it is always current. Ideally, this database will hold details of purchase, regular maintenance visits and details of policies which relate to the equipments' safe use on patients. This database may be held centrally by the biomedical engineering department or the operating theatre devices lead. In addition, a training database which lists every practitioner who has been educated to use specific medical devices listed on the asset register should be in place, detailing the date of education, who provided it and any updates available.

Responsible Authorities

The UK Competent Authority for Medical Devices is the Medicines and Healthcare products Regulatory Agency (MHRA). Their useful document on the responsibilities of management relating to medical devices (MHRA 2006) identifies that there should be a board member in every organisation who is responsible for ensuring safe device management, and that the organisation has policies which address:

- decontamination
- equipment life cycle
- procurement
- records
- adverse incident reporting

Manual of Perioperative Care: An Essential Guide, First Edition. Edited by Kate Woodhead and Lesley Fudge.
© 2012 John Wiley & Sons, Ltd. Published 2012 by John Wiley & Sons, Ltd.

- actions required on the MHRA's Medical Device Alerts and manufacturers' corrective notices
- training
- technical specifications
- regulatory compliance and related issues
- rationalisation to single models, where possible
- risk management
- equipment inventory
- manufacturer's instructions
- disposal.

Appropriate device management systems should ensure that whenever medical devices are used that they are:

- fit for purpose
- used in accordance with the manufacturer's instructions
- maintained in a safe and reliable condition
- disposed of appropriately at the end of their useful life.

In addition, the medical device policy should set out clearly the mechanisms for:

- selection, acquisition, acceptance and disposal of all medical devices
- training of those who will use them
- decontamination, maintenance, repair, monitoring, traceability, record-keeping and replacement.

Each device should be given a unique identifier, a full history including the date of purchase and where and when it was put into use. There may also be specific legal requirements; whether these have been met or not (for example for laser use). Also whether the equipment has been properly installed and possibly commissioned for use (e.g. an autoclave); and the planned maintenance arrangements such as by an external contractor or internal department and the specific frequency of inspections required (e.g. an anaesthetic machine). Some devices have a recommended lifespan, which should also be included in the record. This enables appropriate planning for equipment replacement at suitable intervals.

Training

Training is an essential element of patient safety. Many medical devices in use in operating theatres are complex devices which operators must be confident to use and familiar with in order to reduce risks to patients.

Training must be given when a new device or piece of equipment is purchased and any practitioner who is going to set up or use the device must be able to manage it safely and with understanding.

New staff should be educated on local equipment as part of their induction process. Periodic refreshment may also be required as part of annual mandatory training.

Incident Reporting

All users have an additional responsibility to report to the MHRA if there are any adverse incidents involving medical devices. The process and online reporting mechanism are clearly laid out on the MHRA website (www.mhra.gov.uk). Incidents should be reported within 24 hours.

Section 3

Accountability

As theatre practitioners, we are governed by our various Codes of Conduct and guide-lines for good practice and these are quite unequivocal about our roles and responsi-bilities to patients for safe practice.

The Nursing and Midwifery Council (2008) states:

- a registrant must keep their skills and knowledge up to date
- you must have the knowledge and skills for safe and effective practice when working without direct supervision
- you must recognise and work within the limits of your competence
- you must keep your knowledge and skills up to date throughout your working life
- you must take part in appropriate learning and practice activities that maintain and develop your competence and performance.

The operating department practitioner's Code states:

- a registrant must understand the obligation to maintain fitness to practise
- understand the need to practise safely and effectively within their scope of practice
- understand the need to maintain high standards of personal conduct
- understand the importance of maintaining their own health
- understand both the need to keep skills and knowledge up to date and the importance of career-long learning.

The Health Professions Council states in its standards of practice for operating depart-ment practitioners:

> An operating department practitioner should understand the principles underpinning the safe and effective utilisation of equipment that is used for diagnostic, monitoring or therapeutic purposes in anaesthesia, surgery, post-anaesthesia care and resuscitation. (3a.1 Standards of proficiency, Health Professions Council 2008)

The Association for Perioperative Practice states: 'Operating department practitioners and registered nurses are required to evidence their continuing professional develop-ment to maintain their professional registration.'

This begs the question, how to do all this? This chapter aims to lay the foundation of understanding on which to build and maintain competence in your role as far as some high-risk equipment safety is concerned. It will do this by describing how diathermy (or electrosurgery) was developed, how it works, some of its dangers and some current/future developments of the technology. In addition, it will seek to do the same for safe management of tourniquets.

As practitioners it is our responsibility to maintain and evidence this basic knowledge and keep abreast of developments. One effective way of doing this is to access the MHRA website education package on diathermy and use the material to assess your knowledge and demonstrate it by completing the online assessment. This can be found at www.mhra.gov.uk. However, this is only a generic based programme and is not com-pany specific. That assessment should be done by the manufacturer of the systems that you use in your own workplace.

Diathermy or Electrosurgery

The diathermy machine is a piece of equipment that is familiar to all who work in an operating theatre, but how many of us know how it actually works, what unintended damage it can do and how as theatre practitioners we can and should avoid the possibility of this happening?

History

In the early eighteenth century, Luigi Galvani discovered that when two different metals came into contact with muscle, the muscle would contract. Allessandro Volta later concluded that electricity could be generated independently of animals and that this property was true of all metals. This form of energy was named 'Galvanic current' in Galvani's honour and it has been suggested is what gave rise to the Frankenstein stories written by Mary Shelley.

As early as 1839, Gustave Crussell began experimenting with electro-cautery following work done by Charles Pravaz which showed how quickly blood could coagulate when electricity was applied to it. Others went on to develop various instruments so that practical applications within surgery could be developed with this discovery, until it was an accepted practice in the removal of skin blemishes such as warts and moles by the 1870s.

However, it was not until George Wyeth developed his endothermic knife that the true value of using this electrosurgical technique instead of the standard scalpel was realised when he demonstrated that he could overcome the problem of cancerous cells spreading during tumour surgery by using it. By 1921, this work had proved so success-ful that Tesla was awarded the Nobel Prize in Medicine for his use of diathermy in the treatment of diseases and tumours.

Diathermy was originally used as a treatment for arthritis, bursitis and other disorders of the tendons and muscles. A short definition of diathermy could be: 'the therapeutic use of heat to body tissues'. Electrodes are used to send an electric current which has the effect of increasing the local blood circulation, therefore accelerating the process of repair to the body. However, because of the high-frequency current used in diathermy, care must be taken to avoid burning the skin.

Understanding diathermy

Several properties of electricity must be understood in order to understand electrosur-gery and this will help the theatre practitioner ensure its safe use on patients.

- Current flow occurs when electrons flow from one atom to an adjacent atom. Voltage is the force that enables the electrons to do this.
- If electrons encounter resistance, heat will be produced and this is known as impedance.
- A complete circuit must be present in order for electrons to flow.
- To complete the circuit the electrons must return to ground. Any grounded object can complete the circuit

In the operating room these properties equate to:

- The electrosurgical generator is the source of the electron flow and voltage.
- The patient's tissue provides the impedance, producing heat as the electrons overcome the impedance.
- The circuit is composed of the generator, active electrode, patient and patient return electrode.
- Pathways to ground are numerous but may include the operating table, stirrups, staff members and equipment.

Electric current and frequency

Standard household electric current alternates at a frequency of 60 cycles per second or Hertz (Hz). Diathermy could function at this frequency, but because the current would

Section 3

be transmitted through body tissue at 60 cycles, excessive neuromuscular stimulation and perhaps electrocution would result. Stimulation of muscles at this frequency is similar to the rate of a heart beating and could therefore potentially cause it to stop.

However this nerve and muscle stimulation ceases at 100 000 cycles/second (100 kHz), and so electrosurgery can be performed safely at frequencies above this. As this is also the frequency at which many radio stations operate, interference can be heard on activating the active electrode while a radio is on in the operating theatre. An electrosurgical generator increases 60 Hz household current to over 200 kHz so enabling electrosurgical energy to pass through the patient with minimal neuromuscular stimulation and no risk of electrocution.

Types of electrosurgery

Bipolar

In bipolar electrosurgery, the functions of both the active electrode and return electrode are performed at the site of surgery. The two tips of the diathermy forceps perform the active and return electrode functions. Only the tissue grasped between them is included in the electrical circuit. Because the return function is performed by one tip of the forceps, no patient return electrode is needed.

Monopolar

There are four components of a monopolar electrosurgical circuit:

- the generator
- the active electrode
- the patient
- the return electrode.

In monopolar electrosurgery, the active electrode (diathermy handpiece) is in the surgical site and the patient return electrode (diathermy plate) is somewhere else on the patient's body. The current passes through the patient as it completes the circuit from the active electrode to the patient return electrode.

Waveforms

Electrosurgical generators are able to produce a variety of electrical waveforms. As these are changed, so the tissue effects change too.

- A constant waveform produces the cut effect in which tissue is vaporised or cut. This waveform produces heat very rapidly.
- An intermittent waveform produces the coagulation effect. Using the coagulation setting causes the generator to modify the waveform so that the duty cycle (on time) is reduced and so produces less heat. Therefore, instead of tissue vaporisation, a coagulum is produced.
- The blend setting is not a mixture of both but rather a modification of the duty cycle. Changing from Blend 1 to Blend 3 on the generator, the duty cycle is progressively reduced thereby producing less heat.
- Blend 1 is able to vaporise tissue with minimal haemostasis.
- Blend 3 is less effective at cutting but has maximum haemostasis.

The only variable that determines whether one waveform vaporises tissue and another produces a coagulum is the rate at which heat is produced.

- High heat causes rapid vaporisation or tissue cutting.
- Low heat creates a coagulum.

Electrosurgical tissue effects

The cut setting divides tissue by focusing intense heat at the surgical site onto a small area. To create this effect the operator should hold the electrode slightly away from the tissue. This produces the greatest amount of heat over the shortest period of time, resulting in vaporisation or cutting of tissue.

The coagulation (or fulguration) setting coagulates and chars the tissue over a wide area and produces less heat. The result is the creation of a coagulum rather than cellular vaporisation. The coagulation waveform uses higher voltage than the cutting setting and as such has implications during laparoscopic surgery.

Alternate site burns

Electrosurgical technology has changed dramatically since its introduction in the 1920s. Originally, generators used grounded (earthed) current from a wall outlet. It was assumed that once the current entered the patient's body it would return to ground through the patient return electrode. But electricity will always seek the path of least resistance so the current will select the most conductive object as the pathway to ground – which may not be the patient return electrode. This may lead to an alternate site burn. Examples could be ECG electrodes or table attachments.

In 1968, the isolated generator was developed to try to minimise the chances of this happening. With these generators, the circuit is completed not by the ground but by the generator. Even though grounded objects remain in the operating room, electrosurgical current will not recognise these objects as pathways to complete the circuit but instead uses the patient return electrode as the preferred pathway back to the generator.

Patient return electrode

The function of the patient return electrode is to remove current from the patient safely. A return electrode burn can occur when the heat produced, over time, is not safely dissipated by its size or conductivity.

To eliminate the risk of current concentration which can lead to a burn, the pad should present a large low-impedance contact area to the patient and placement should be on conductive tissue that is close to the operative site. The only difference between the 'active' electrode and the patient return electrode is their relative size and conductivity.

If the surface area contact between the patient and the return electrode is reduced, or if the impedance of that contact is increased, a dangerous condition can develop. If the contact area of the patient return electrode is reduced, the current flow is concentrated in a smaller area. As this increases, the temperature increases. If the temperature increases enough, a patient burn may result.

Some of the factors that may increase this impedance and so potentially contribute to a patient return electrode burn are:

- excessive hair
- adipose tissue
- bony prominences
- fluid invasion
- adhesive failure
- scar tissue.

Contact quality monitoring was developed to protect patients from burns due to inadequate contact of the return electrode. Generators using this technology actively monitor the amount of impedance at the patient/pad interface and are designed to

Section 3

deactivate the generator before an injury can occur, if it detects a dangerously high level of impedance at the patient/pad interface.

In order to work properly these generators must use a patient return electrode that is compatible and these can be identified by their split appearance and a special plug with a centre pin.

Other Technologies

Radiofrequency ablation

Alternating current through the tissue creates friction on a molecular level. Increased intracellular temperature generates localized interstitial heating. At temperatures above 60°C, cellular proteins rapidly denature and coagulate, resulting in a lesion.

How it works
The system's generator senses tissue impedance and automatically delivers the optimum amount of radiofrequency energy. A unique electrode design prevents charring and allows for maximum current delivery, resulting in a larger ablation zone in less time.

The generator software monitors tissue impedance and adjusts the output accordingly. Pulsed energy delivery allows the target tissue to stabilise, reducing tissue impedance increases. Typical treatments are completed in a 12-minute cycle.

The cooling effect
The electrode's internal circulation of water cools the tissue adjacent to the exposed electrode, maintaining low impedance during the treatment cycle. Low impedance permits maximum energy deposition for a larger ablation volume.

Argon-enhanced electrosurgery

Argon-enhanced electrosurgery has enabled a new element of precision and control in electrosurgical applications. The clinical benefits demonstrated by argon-enhanced coagulation include quick and efficient coagulation, a thinner, more flexible eschar, less charring, less tissue damage and reduced rebleeding.

Argon-enhanced coagulation offers precise energy delivery for efficient, non-contact coagulation over large surface areas. It uses a stream of argon gas to improve the surgical effectiveness of the diathermy current. The properties of argon gas that enable it to do this, are that it:

- is inert
- is non-combustible
- is easily ionised by radiofrequency energy
- creates a bridge between electrode and tissue
- is heavier than air
- displaces nitrogen and oxygen.

Among the advantages of argon-enhanced electrosurgery are:

- decreased smoke, odour
- non-contact in coagulation mode
- decreased blood loss, rebleeding
- decreased tissue damage
- flexible eschar.

Harmonic Scalpel™

The Harmonic Scalpel uses ultrasonic technology that allows both cutting and coagulation at the precise point of impact, resulting in minimal lateral thermal damage. It was introduced commercially in 1993 and is used worldwide for both open and laparoscopic surgery.

As discussed earlier, electrosurgical haemostasis is provided by generation of high temperatures at probe tips, resulting in coagulation necrosis and even charring. Lateral thermal damage and depth of penetration is high in electrocautery. By using an ultrasound wave form instead this is reduced. The Harmonic Scalpel converts electrical energy into ultrasound energy in the hand piece. This ultrasonic wave is transferred to a laparoscopic blade. Cutting speed and coagulation is at the hands of the surgeon and is influenced by varying four factors:

- power
- blade sharpness
- tissue tension
- pressure/grip force.

The Harmonic Scalpel has different power levels. Increasing the power increases the cutting speed and decreases coagulation. In contrast, less power decreases cutting speed and increases coagulation.

How does it work?

Vibrating at 55 500 times per second, the Harmonic blade denatures protein in the tissue to form a sticky coagulum. Pressure exerted on tissue with the blade surface collapses blood vessels and allows the coagulum to form a haemostatic seal. The surgeon controls cutting and coagulation by adjusting the power level, blade edge, tissue tension and blade pressure. By using only mechanical longitudinal vibration at the distal end, no electrical current is passed to or through the patient, and damage to surrounding tissue and nerves is minimised.

Advantages and disadvantages of the Harmonic Scalpel over electrocautery

The advantages of the Harmonic Scalpel are that:

- it has a dual action of coagulation and cutting
- heat generated is low
- there is no lateral tissue damage
- no smoke is produced so visualisation is better
- no current passes through the patient, eliminating the chance of electrical hazard
- there is less tissue damage, so less postoperative pain.

The only disadvantage is the high cost. The high cost of the generator and hand piece and the expense of the disposable probe.

Diathermy in laparoscopic surgery

When electrosurgery is used in minimally invasive surgery, other safety concerns present themselves, including:

- direct coupling
- insulation failure
- capacitive coupling.

Section 3

Direct coupling

This occurs when the user accidentally activates the generator while the active electrode is near another metal instrument, causing it to become energised. This energy will seek a pathway to complete the circuit to the patient return electrode. This can result in significant patient injury.

Do not activate the generator while the active electrode is touching or in close proximity to another metal object.

Insulation failure

Many surgeons routinely use the coagulation setting which has a comparatively high voltage. This voltage can spark through cracked/broken/weak insulation and blow holes in it. Therefore, any breaks in insulation can create an alternate route for the current to flow. If this current is concentrated, it can cause significant injury.

The desired coagulation effect can be achieved without high voltage, simply by using the cut setting while holding the electrode in direct contact with tissue. This technique will reduce the likelihood of insulation failure.

Capacitive coupling

- *Metal cannula system*: A capacitor is created whenever a non-conductor separates two conductors. During minimally invasive surgery procedures, a capacitor may be created inadvertently by the surgical instruments. The conductive active electrode is surrounded by non-conductive insulation. This in turn, is surrounded by a conductive metal cannula. A capacitor creates an electrostatic field between the two conductors and, as a result, a current in one conductor can induce a current in the second conductor. In the case of a minimally invasive surgery procedure, a capacitor may be created by the surgical instruments' composition and placement.
- *Plastic cannula system*: Capacitance cannot be entirely eliminated with an all plastic cannula. The patient's conductive tissue completes the definition of a capacitor. Capacitance is reduced, but is not eliminated.
- *Hybrid cannula system*: The most potentially high-risk situation occurs when a metal cannula is held in place by a plastic anchor (hybrid cannula system). The metal cannula still creates a capacitor with the active electrode. However, the plastic abdominal wall anchor prevents the current from dissipating through the abdominal wall. The current may exit to adjacent tissue on its way to the patient return electrode. This can cause significant injury.

Solutions to avoid complications in minimally invasive surgery

- Inspect insulation carefully.
- Use lowest possible power setting.
- Use the cut setting.
- Use brief intermittent activation vs. prolonged activation.
- Do not activate in open circuit.
- Do not activate in close proximity or direct contact with another instrument.
- Use bipolar electrosurgery when appropriate.
- Select an all-metal cannula system as the safest choice.
- Do not use hybrid cannula systems that mix metal with plastic.

Surgical smoke

This is created when tissue is heated and cellular fluid is vaporised by the thermal action of an energy source – diathermy for example. The Centers for Disease Control in the USA has studied electrosurgical smoke at length. They state:

Research studies have confirmed that this smoke plume can contain toxic gases and vapors such as benzene, hydrogen cyanide, and formaldehyde, bioaerosols, dead and live cellular material (including blood fragments), and viruses.

This would suggest that consideration should be given to a smoke evacuation system when commissioning new generators (Centers for Disease Control 1998).

New products have been introduced to make smoke evacuation easier and more effective. Smoke evacuation devices can now be attached directly to a standard electro-surgical pencil.

Surgical Tourniquets

A tourniquet is a mechanical device that is used during extremity surgery to restrict blood flow, thus creating a 'bloodless' field of vision for the surgeon. All staff involved in the use of tourniquets should understand:

- the anatomy and physiology of the extremity
- the potential dangers to the patient.

These potential dangers include:

- skin damage under a poorly applied cuff
- tissue/nerve damage from overinflation of a cuff
- compromised circulation caused by extended use without releasing the pressure periodically.

The theatre practitioner should be aware of the potential risks when a surgical tourniquet is being used and, as with diathermy and any other medical device, prepare for its use appropriately.

The manufacturer's instructions for use should be followed and prior to surgery this would routinely include ensuring that the cuff is not leaking, connections are not loose, tubing is not worn, the equipment is clean and there is no damage to any of the components.

The widest possible size of cuff should be selected for use as a wider cuff occludes blood flow at a lower pressure (Klenerman 2003) and the cuff should overlap at least 7.5 cm but not more than 15 cm, as too much overlap may cause increased pressure or wrinkling of underlying soft tissue.

The surgical site should be confirmed in accordance with the World Health Organization Safe Surgery Checklist (National Patient Safety Agency 2009).

Types of tourniquet

There are two types of tourniquet in common use in the operating room. These are:

- *leak compensating tourniquets*, which adjust any pressure loss automatically during use and
- *non-leak compensating tourniquets*, which require constant observation and potential adjustment during use. These are now very uncommon.

The recommendations here are based on the use of the leak compensating type.

Application of the tourniquet cuff

Apply under cuff padding to the point of the limb which offers the greatest amount of soft tissue, ensuring that the under cuff padding is the same width as the tourniquet cuff (Meeker and Rothrock 1999).

Section 3

Important points to be aware of when placing the cuff include the following:

- Ensure it is not obscuring the site of surgical incision or placed over a bony prominence.
- On male patients check that genitalia is not caught in the tourniquet cuff when it is placed high on the leg.
- Two qualified practitioners should be available when applying a tourniquet cuff and the under cuff (AfPP 2011).
- The patient's skin should be protected from preparation solutions accumulating under the tourniquet cuff by the application of an occulsion dressing or holding the limb horizontally to the patient's body and alcoholic prep should be avoided where possible due to its inherent risks when pooled.
- When elevating a limb during prepping ensure any excess solution that comes in contact with the tourniquet is dried prior to draping.
- Attach the tubing to the correct pressure regulator on the tourniquet machine (i.e. the left inflation tubing from the left cuff is attached to the left pressure regulator).
- Choice of cuff size should be guided by being approximately half that of the limb diameter and placed over an area of most muscular/fat padding.
- Any prophylactic antibiotics should be given prior to cuff inflation and allow sufficient time to ensure tissue uptake.

Exsanguinate the limb by using one of the following methods:

- a roll cylinder
- limb elevation prior to inflation
- Esmarch bandage as a last resort.

If an Esmarch bandage is to be used it should be applied from the extremity tip towards the tourniquet cuff. The bandage should overlap by 2.5 cm and continuous pressure must be applied during application.

During use

Tourniquet pressure will be selected depending on the patient's systolic blood pressure, patient age and limb size. It is the surgeon's responsibility to approve the tourniquet pressure setting (AfPP 2011). The generally accepted pressures are as follows:

- Upper limb – 50–75 mmHg above systolic blood pressure (AORN 2006) within the range of 250–300 mmHg.
- Lower limb – 100–150 mmHg above systolic blood pressure within the range of 300–500 mmHg. In paediatric patients this would be more in the order of 100 mmHg above systolic blood pressure (Liebermann *et al*. 1997).

The duration of use should be kept to a minimum (Delougrhy and Griffiths 2009) and the maximum time is generally accepted to fall somewhere between 2 and 3 hours (Klenerman 2003, Delougrhy and Griffiths 2009) the tourniquet machine should be visible during the procedure and not occluded by sterile drapes.

Circulating staff should record the time inflation occurred on the theatre count board along with the inflation pressure and the scrub practitioner should inform the surgeon once the tourniquet has been inflated for 1 hour (AORN 2009). This should be repeated every 30 minutes up to the 2 hour point so that the surgeon and anaesthetist can make a clinical decision on the best time to deflate the tourniquet to allow for limb reperfusion for 10–15 minutes prior to proceeding with the surgery.

The ultimate responsibility for the application and release of the tourniquet is that of the operating surgeon. However it is good practice to record the details of the limb, pressure and duration of tourniquet use in the patient's operative notes – medical and nursing (AfPP 2011).

After use

The anaesthetist must be informed prior to the deflation of the tourniquet as the release of toxins on deflation of the cuff may produce a drop in systemic blood pressure.

Once the tourniquet has been deflated the occlusive dressing, cuff and under cuff padding should be removed from the limb because if the cuff remains on the limb venous blood return may be compromised or obstructed.

The following information should be recorded in the patient perioperative care record:

- unit number of the tourniquet machine
- limb – arm/leg
- side – right/left
- pressure
- time of inflation
- time of deflation.

Any damage to the skin underlying the tourniquet cuff must be reported to the surgeon, an incident form completed and a record of the incident placed in the patient's health-care record. An explanation of the incident should be given to the patient (and their family where appropriate) at the earliest opportunity.

Digital tourniquets

The use of digital tourniquets is fraught with dangers, not least of which is the risk of them being left in situ following surgery. De Boer and Houpt (2007) recommend that if they are to be used then they should consist of a brightly coloured disc with a nylon tag attached for easy visualization. Fingers of operating gloves are not recommended due to the risk of being left in place.

If they are to be used then the foregoing principle should, where appropriate, still be adhered to.

Decontamination and maintenance

The cuff, tubing and tourniquet unit should be checked for damage between uses and any soiling cleaned with a neutral hospital detergent diluted into warm tap water. Do not immerse the open end of the tubing in water as this could alter the pressure distribution within the cuff.

All equipment must be dried with a clean disposable cloth following decontamination.

The tourniquet unit must be checked regularly by the biomedical engineering department.

Practice Recommendations

- When purchasing new equipment, try to ensure it is the same unit as is used across the department to prevent potential for accidents by having different makes/models with different user interfaces etc.
- Ensure that a diathermy safety module is included in any new starter's induction package within the medical devices section.
- Ensure that annual or bi-annual updates are part of the clinical mandatory training for theatre staff.

Section 3

- Ensure when buying new equipment that the manufacturer provides good and ongoing post-sales support and training.
- Incorporate the MHRA electrosurgery module within the induction and ongoing updates to training so at least generic knowledge is up to date.

References

AfPP (Association for Perioperative Practice) (2011) *Standards and Recommendations for Safe Perioperative Practice*. Harrogate: AfPP.

AORN (Association of Perioperative Registered Nurses) (2006) Recommended practices for use of the pneumatic tourniquet. In *Standards, Recommended Practices and Guidelines*. Denver: AORN Inc.

AORN (2009) *Recommended Practices For The Use Of The Pneumatic Tourniquet In The Perioperative Practice Setting*. www.tourniquets.org/aorn.php (accessed March 2012).

Centers for Disease Control (1998) *Control of Smoke From Laser/Electric Surgical Procedures*. www.cdc.gov/niosh/hc11.html (accessed March 2012).

De Boer HL and Houpt P (2007) Rubber glove tourniquet; perhaps not so simple or safe? *European Journal of Plastic Surgery* 30: 91–92.

Delougrhy J and Griffiths R (2009) Arterial tourniquets. continuing education in anaesthesia. *Critical Care and Pain* 9(2): 5–9.

Health Professions Council (2008) *Standards of Proficiency: Operating department practitioners*. http://www.hpc-uk.org/assets/documents/10000514Standards_of_Proficiency_ODP.pdf (accessed March 2012).

Klenerman L (2003) *The Tourniquet Manual: Principles and Practice*. London: Springer-Verlag.

Liebermann JR, Staheli LT and Dale MC (1997) Tourniquet pressures on pediatric patients; a clinical study. *Orthopedics* 20(12): 1143–1147.

Meeker M and Rothrock J (1999) *Alexander's Care of the Patient in Surgery*. London: Mosby.

MHRA (Medicines and Healthcare products Regulatory Agency) (2006) *Device Bulletin. Managing Medical Devices. Guidance for healthcare and social services organisations*. DB2006(05). http://www.mhra.gov.uk/home/groups/dts-bs/documents/publication/con2025143.pdf (accessed March 2012).

National Patient Safety Agency (2009) *WHO Surgical Checklist (adapted for England and Wales)*. http://www.nrls.npsa.nhs.uk/resources/?EntryId45=59860 (accessed March 2012).

Nursing and Midwifery Council (2008) *The Code: Standards of conduct, performance and ethics for nurses and midwives*. http://www.nmc-uk.org/Nurses-and-midwives/The-code (accessed March 2012).

CHAPTER 21

Medical Imaging and Radiation

Johnathan Hewis and Sarah Naylor

Chapter Overview

A broad range of different imaging environments or *modalities* are used within a medical imaging department. These include conventional radiography, fluoroscopy, computed tomography (CT), radionuclide imaging (RNI), magnetic resonance imaging (MRI) and ultrasound. Each environment can present potential hazards and challenges for patients and staff.

This chapter will explore basic theory, legislation and practical considerations for the protection of patients and staff when working within medical imaging environments, or when working with patients who are radioactive after medical imaging procedures.

General Principles of Ionising Radiation

The electromagnetic spectrum and radiation

X-Rays exist within an electromagnetic spectrum and share some properties with light; they travel in straight lines and also travel at the same speed (Figure 21.1). Conventional radiography, fluoroscopy and CT all use x-radiation to produce a diagnostic image. RNI uses alpha, beta or gamma radiation to produce an image. X-rays, alpha, beta and gamma radiation all have one thing in common, they all have enough energy to be ionising.

Ionising radiation

Most of the annual ionising radiation dose received by the UK population arises from natural sources of radiation, such as radon gas and cosmic rays. Man-made sources of ionising radiation result from medical exposure and other sources such as radioactive fallout or environmental pollution. Man-made sources account for approximately 15% of the ionising radiation dose received by the UK population each year (Watson *et al.* 2005).

Manual of Perioperative Care: An Essential Guide, First Edition. Edited by Kate Woodhead and Lesley Fudge.
© 2012 John Wiley & Sons, Ltd. Published 2012 by John Wiley & Sons, Ltd.

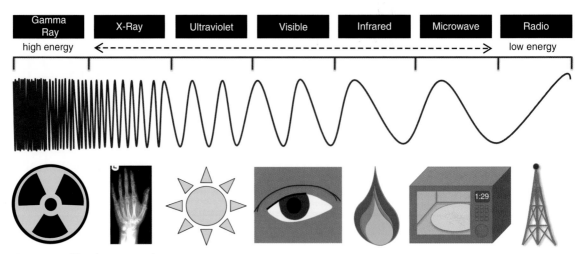

Figure 21.1   The electromagnetic spectrum.

Ionising radiation risks

Ionising radiation can cause biological damage to tissues. Damage is at a cellular level and can be minor and imperceptible, posing no long-term risk. It can also result in more serious biological damage; ionising radiation can trigger abnormal cell growth or differentiation of tissue, leading to cancer. Essential safety measures are required to regulate the medical use of radiation. The Ionising Radiation Regulations 1999 (IRR99) (Health and Safety Executive 1999) and the Ionising Radiation (Medical Exposure) Regulations 2000 (Department of Health 2000) provide clear legal requirements and controls on how ionising radiation is handled and administered in the UK.

Biological damage from ionising radiation can be classified by the potential effect it may have on tissue; the effect can be described using the following terms: somatic and genetic, deterministic and stochastic (ICRP 2007). A *somatic effect* is restricted to the individual who has received the dose of radiation. Cancer and cataracts can be induced by ionising radiation and are examples of a somatic effect. *Genetic effects* are caused by irradiation to the gonads, causing damage to the DNA in the sperm or ovum. Genetic effects do not appear in the person receiving the radiation dose; instead the effects are passed on to their descendants.

The potential for a biological effect is partly dependent upon the amount of the ionising radiation exposure (Figure 21.2). At small levels of exposure, the risk of developing a somatic or genetic effect is tiny, random and unpredictable; this is described as a *stochastic effect*. The probability of a stochastic effect increases with higher radiation doses. Stochastic effects are not immediate; they manifest later and cannot be directly attributed to a specific radiation exposure. When an individual is exposed to very high levels of ionising radiation beyond a known level or threshold, the resultant biological effects can be predicted or determined. These are *deterministic effects* and are normally only associated with therapeutic applications of ionising radiation and not diagnostic procedures. An example of a deterministic effect might be radiation-induced burns or erythema affecting the skin caused by a radiotherapy treatment.

There is a small probability that damage can occur with even the smallest exposure to ionising radiation (e.g. a chest X-ray). There is therefore no such thing as a safe dose of ionising radiation.

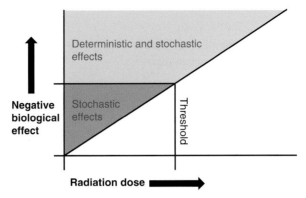

Figure 21.2   Radiation dose versus biological effect (linear model).

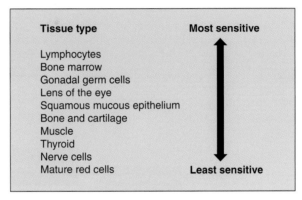

Figure 21.3   Radiosensitivity of tissues. Adapted from Ball *et al.* (2008).

Ionising radiation, tissue sensitivity and pregnancy

Certain tissues are particularly susceptible to biological damage when exposed to ionising radiation and can be described as *radiosensitive*. Generally tissues that have a high rate of cell division or differentiation are the most radiosensitive (Ball *et al.* 2008). Figure 21.3 demonstrates the radiosensitivy of various tissues.

When X-raying a pregnant woman the potential harm to the unborn fetus must be carefully considered and justified using the risk versus benefit principle. The fetus is particularly radiosensitive during the first trimester due to *organogenesis*. Depending upon the examination, the radiographer may need to confirm the pregnancy status of female patients of childbearing age before administering radiation.

Staff working with radiation should also be aware of the risks (Box 21.1).

What is radioactivity?

Radioactivity is a naturally occurring process where a substance composed of unstable atomic nuclei emits ionising radiation as the nuclei decay. As a nucleus decays it can emit three different types of radioactivity: an alpha particle, a beta particle or a gamma ray; all are ionising. Working with a radioactive substance is very different from man-made X-rays. In conventional radiography or CT, X-radiation is only produced when required. However, a radioactive source keeps emitting radiation until all the nuclei have decayed. The time it takes a source to decay is determined by its *half-life*, defined

Section 3

Table 21.1　Examples of radionuclides used in medical imaging.

Radionuclide	Half-life	Clinical uses
Technetium-99 m	6.02 hours	Numerous
Iodine-123	13 hours	Thyroid
Xenon-133	5.27 days	Lung ventilation
Thallium-201	3.1 hours	Heart muscle
Selenium-75	118.5 days	Adrenal glands

From Watson *et al.* (2005).

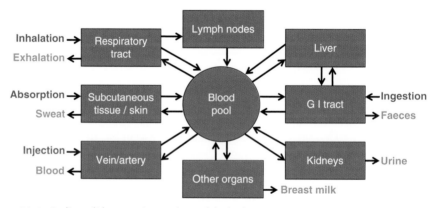

Figure 21.4　Radionuclide routes into and out of the body.

as the time taken to lose half of its radioactivity. The rate of decay cannot be stopped or altered but is determined by the type of radionuclide administered.

Radioactivity and radionuclide imaging

In RNI (or nuclear medicine), radionuclides are manufactured specifically for medical imaging purposes and ideally emit gamma rays that can escape the body rather than alpha or beta particles that cannot. A radionuclide is combined with another pharmaceutical to form a radiopharmaceutical that is administered to the patient, enabling functional imaging of disease. RNI imaging techniques are used to complement the more anatomical diagnostic information gained from other medical imaging modalities such as CT and MRI. Table 21.1 lists some of the commonly used radionuclides in nuclear medicine.

Radiopharmaceuticals can be administered into the body by several delivery methods (Figure 21.4). The patient then becomes an actual source of radioactivity.

> **BOX 21.2**
>
> **How long does a patient stay radioactive after an RNI procedure?**
>
> The amount of time is dependent upon how fast the body removes or excretes the radiopharmaceutical, calculated using a *biological half-life*. Many factors influence the level of radiation emitted by the patient and for how long. The practitioner administering the radiopharmaceutical calculates the time and dose, specific guidance can then be provided for each patient.

Principles of radiation protection

The International Commission on Radiological Protection (ICRP 2007) has identified three basic principles of radiation protection:

- *Justification*: The level of radiation a patient can receive is justified by a *risk versus benefit* principle: the medical benefit should outweigh the radiation risk. There are no medical benefits for staff or public present during a medical exposure.
- *Optimisation*: The dose delivered should be As Low As Reasonably Practicable (the ALARP principle). For a patient receiving a medical exposure, the person administering the radiation will optimise the level of exposure, ideally acquiring the most diagnostic information for the least radiation dose. Staff doses must be reduced to as low as reasonably practicable.
- *Application of radiation dose limits*: There are strict radiation *dose limits* in the UK for people who are exposed to radiation through their work (occupational dose limits) or as members of the general public. Occupational and general public dose limits are imposed by the IRR99 regulations (Health and Safety Executive 1999).

Practical radiation protection

During a medical exposure staff and members of the public are often required to be present. Minimising their radiation dose and keeping within their *annual dose limit* is essential. The radiographer or practitioner administering the radiation dose will optimise and try to reduce unnecessary radiation exposure. They are also responsible for recording and monitoring of radiation doses administered. During an X-ray examination the patient is exposed to a *primary* beam of radiation, however some *photons* of radiation become scattered when the primary beam interacts with the patient to create *secondary* or *scattered* radiation in the surrounding environment (Figure 21.5).

For staff (and the general public) present during a medical exposure there are three methods of practical radiation protection:

- *Time*: The longer you are exposed to radiation the greater your dose and therefore the greater the chance of a negative biological effect. The shorter the duration of your exposure, the better.
- *Distance*: There is an inverse relationship between your proximity to a radiation source and the radiation dose you will receive, a relationship described by the *inverse square law*. Figure 21.6 demonstrates that doubling your distance from a source of radiation reduces your radiation dose by 3/4. The greater your distance from the radiation source, the better.
- *Shielding*: When staff have to be within close proximity to a radiation source (e.g. when fluoroscopic imaging is used during orthopaedic surgery in a theatre environment). Limiting the time of exposure or maintaining a safe distance from the source may not be possible. Various forms of *shielding* can be utilised to absorb or *attenuate* the radiation and act as a physical protective barrier.

Section 3

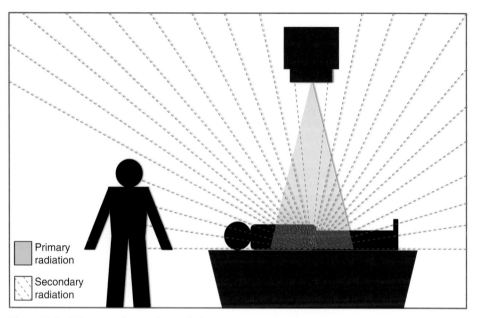

Figure 21.5   Primary and secondary radiation.

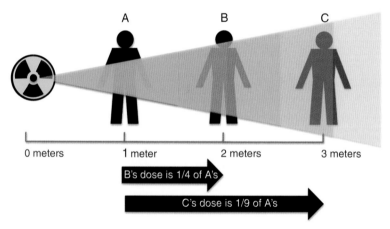

Figure 21.6   Inverse square law and radiation dose.

Radiation shielding and lead

Lead is very effective at absorbing radiation. Lead (or lead equivalent) is used in physical barriers such as lead glass screens and in lead rubber aprons, thyroid protectors, sheets and gloves. It is also used in items like gonad shields, which are used as primary radiation protection for the patient.

It is mandatory that staff always wear the shielding provided and in the correct manner to provide optimum protection to keep radiation exposure within safe limits. Figure 21.7 demonstrates the correct way to wear a lead equivalent apron and thyroid shield. It is important that lead rubber (or lead equivalent material) is stored correctly; if left folded the material can crack, reducing the protective properties.

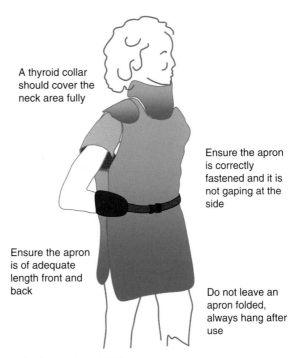

A thyroid collar should cover the neck area fully

Ensure the apron is correctly fastened and it is not gaping at the side

Ensure the apron is of adequate length front and back

Do not leave an apron folded, always hang after use

Figure 21.7   Wearing lead equivalent shielding.

Section 3

Additional radiation protection considerations for radionuclide imaging

The handling, storage and disposal of radioactive substances can potentially be very dangerous. The Administration of Radioactive Substances Advisory Committee provides guidance (ARSAC 2006) and clinicians who justify the radiation doses administered must hold an ARSAC licence.

When dealing with radioactive patients it is important to remember the inverse square law and minimise contact time with a patient. While radioactive, not only the patient but also *all* of their bodily fluids are a source of ionising radiation (see Figure 21.4). It is important to avoid being contaminated by bodily waste, and disposable gloves and aprons should be worn. If your clothing becomes contaminated it should be removed, contaminated skin should be thoroughly washed with water. Depending on the levels of radioactivity, contaminated waste and linen must be stored safely in a sealed contaminated waste bag; this may even be collected for safe storage by the nuclear medicine department.

Specific guidance will be provided by the nuclear medicine department based upon the dose and half-life of the radiopharmaceutical administered. Patients receiving very high doses of radiopharmaceutical for *oblation therapy* are isolated to minimise radiation risk to staff and the general public. Mothers cannot breastfeed for a period of time after receiving radiopharmaceuticals and expressed breast milk during this time must be treated as contaminated waste. Pregnant women and children should not be in contact with radioactive patients.

Local rules

Radiation risk assessments are performed which determine systems of work or local rules for a specific environment that are designed to protect staff and the public from unnecessary radiation exposure. These *must* be adhered to. The radiographer or

> **BOX 21.3**
>
> **I have seen radiographers wearing badges to monitor their radiation dose. Why do I not have a badge and if I don't have one how can you know I am safe?**
>
> Radiation monitoring or *dosimetry* is not a form of radiation protection; it indicates the radiation dose already received by the wearer. Only those individuals who routinely work with radiation or work in high-dose areas require monitoring. Monitored staff rarely reach an accumulative dose that exceeds or approaches their annual dose limit. If you are concerned or would like further advice about personal dosimetry you should speak to your *radiation protection supervisor*.

practitioner administering the radiation exposure has a legal responsibility to enforce these rules. If correctly observed, no member of staff or general public should exceed their annual dose limit.

General Principles of Non-Ionising Radiation

Ultrasound and MRI are two medical imaging modalities that do not use ionising radiation. This makes them ideal imaging options for consideration when radiation exposure is a high concern (e.g. when imaging pregnant patients).

Ultrasound

Ultrasound uses the echoes of inaudible ultrasonic sound waves to create an image. It has been used widely in the management of pregnancy and is also used extensively to image other parts of the body. Ultrasound can cause potential heating of tissue and other negative biological effects but not at the levels used in diagnostic ultrasound if used correctly.

Magnetic resonance imaging

MRI works by placing a patient inside an exceptionally strong magnetic field combined with the use of radiofrequency waves to form medical images from the magnetic relaxation properties of hydrogen protons within tissue. MRI is particularly good at demonstrating soft tissue structures and is used to image the entire body. The magnetic field is typically created using a super-conducting magnet, which is a large electromagnet cooled using helium or nitrogen. Magnetism is measured in the SI units of gauss and tesla; there are 10 000 gauss to 1 tesla.

MRI hazards

MRI creates a unique and highly hazardous environment. Numerous deaths have occurred within this environment.

A super-conducting magnet is ALWAYS turned on; it cannot just be turned off at the end of the day. Therefore, access to the MRI environment has to be strictly controlled at *all* times and *all* staff, patients, visitors and objects entering this environment must first be checked or *screened* by dedicated MRI practitioners.

All substances are affected to some degree when placed inside a powerful magnetic field. Human tissue is only mildly affected (described as *diamagnetic*) and this phenomenon is used beneficially to create MR images. At present there are no large epidemiological studies demonstrating any long-term risk from MRI exposure, but recently some smaller studies have raised concerns so research continues in this area (Shellock 2011).

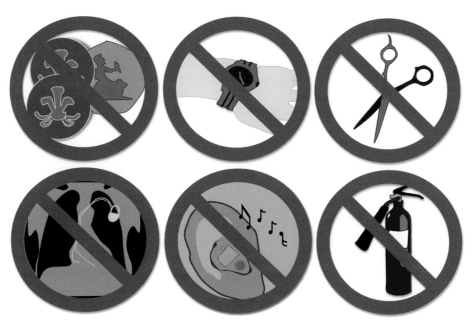

Figure 21.8   Examples of objects that are not safe in MRI.

Certain materials are greatly affected by a magnetic field. If you were to take an iron oxygen cylinder (iron being *ferromagnetic*) into an MRI scan room, strong attractive forces would wrench the cylinder out of your hands and it would fly across the room and eventually stick to the scanner. This *missile* effect poses a significant and common risk. Many everyday objects are not safe to take into the MRI environment and *all* screened individuals entering the scanner room must first remove everyday ferrous objects (Figure 21.8).

Many individuals have implants or medical devices that cannot be removed but may not be MRI safe. Most medical implants, such as orthopaedic implants and vascular stents, are safe. Implants with electrical or magnetic components are typically unsafe. Individuals who have a cardiac pacemaker are NOT safe to enter the MR environment; doing so may result in death. Patients with aneurysm clips also require careful screening. Your MRI department can provide advice and guidance on the safety of a specific medical implant.

MRI uses radiofrequency to transfer energy into the patient to stimulate hydrogen protons to create an image; this energy transfer is called *resonance*. Depositing energy into the patient can increase the patient's core body temperature. This is particularly dangerous in children, the elderly, pregnant women and unconscious or uncommunicative patients. Patients can also develop severe and very deep radiofrequency burns if ferrous objects are left in contact with the skin, such as standard electrocardiogram stickers.

MRI scanning makes a considerable amount of noise, which can exceed 100 decibels, and prolonged exposure to high noise levels can permanently damage hearing (Shellock 2011). All people present in the scan room during this time must wear ear protection.

The aperture of the MRI scanner is fairly restrictive. Larger patients may not physically fit into an MRI scanner, while others can suffer with anxiety or claustrophobia in this enclosed environment.

The MHRA (Medicines and Healthcare products Regulatory Agency) provide safety guidelines for clinical MRI (MHRA 2007).

MRI and pregnancy

Potential heating effects and acoustic noise are both concerns when scanning a pregnant patient, both can be limited to some extent by the MRI radiographer. It is possible to scan pregnant women but elective procedures are normally deferred until after the pregnancy. Scanning is generally avoided in the first trimester due to organogenesis.

References

ARSAC (Administration of Radioactive Substances Advisory Committee) (2006) *Notes for Guidance on the Clinical Administration of Radiopharmaceuticals and Use of Sealed Radioactive Sources.* London: Health Protection Agency.

Ball J, Moore A and Turner S (2008) *Ball and Moore's Essential Physics for Radiographers*, 4th edn. London: Wiley-Blackwell Publishing.

Department of Health (2000) *No. 1059, Ionising Radiation (Medical Exposure) Regulations.* London: Department of Health.

Health and Safety Executive (1999) *No. 3232, Ionising Radiation Regulations.* London: Health and Safety Executive.

ICRP (International Commission on Radiological Protection) (2007) *Radiological Protection in Medicine: ICRP Publication 105.* London: ICRP.

MHRA(Medicines and Healthcare products Regulatory Agency) (2007) *Guidelines for Magnetic Resonance Equipment in Clinical Use.* London: MHRA.

Shellock F (2011) *Reference Manual for Magnetic Resonance Safety, Implants, and Devices: 2011 Edition.* Los Angeles, CA: Biomedical Research Publishing Company.

Watson S, Jones A, Oatway W and Hughes J (2005) *HPA/-RPD-001, Ionising Radiation Exposure of the UK Population: 2005 Review.* Oxford: HPA.

CHAPTER 22

Death in the Perioperative Environment

Kevin Henshaw

Definition of Death

At present in the UK, there is no statutory definition of, death either by natural or unnatural causes.

On the face of it, a definition of death would appear to be quite straightforward. However, with the advancement of medical technologies, the cessation of respiration and of cardiac output now means that death is no longer an inevitable occurrence. The introduction of the stethoscope, for example, enabled physicians to listen more accurately to heart sounds. The introduction of this simple but effective diagnostic tool paved the way for a completely different approach in the treatment of heart disease. The development of the defibrillator meant that even serious cardiac events such as ventricular fibrillation were no longer untreatable. 'Cardiac arrest is no longer accepted as a final diagnosis of death as in some cases resuscitation is successful' (Working Party on behalf of the Health Departments of Great Britain and Northern Ireland 1983).

Developments in mechanical ventilation meant that patients who had previously been incapable of breathing could be kept 'alive'. This advancement in medical technology was another milestone in the blurring of the boundaries between life and death. Youngner *et al.* (1985) described the technique of mechanical ventilation as having the ability to create 'a new class of dead patients'. The need for a more refined definition of 'death' was needed.

In 1976 at the Conference of the Medical Royal Colleges a paper entitled 'Diagnosis of brain death' was presented to delegates. For the first time the term *brainstem death* was introduced into the medical lexicon (Conference of the Medical Royal Colleges 1976). This term referred to an irreversible loss of all use of the brainstem. To all intents and purposes this diagnosis became a working definition of clinical death. It was quickly realised that there was a need for more stringent guidelines to be developed when diagnosing brainstem death. A code of practice entitled 'The removal of cadaveric organs for transplantation' was first distributed to doctors in the UK in January 1983 (Department of Health and Social Security 1979).

The diagnosis of brain death should be made by two medical practitioners who have expertise in this field. One should be the consultant who is in charge of the case and one

Manual of Perioperative Care: An Essential Guide, First Edition. Edited by Kate Woodhead and Lesley Fudge.
© 2012 John Wiley & Sons, Ltd. Published 2012 by John Wiley & Sons, Ltd.

other doctor (or in the absence of the consultant, his deputy who should have been registered for 5 years or more with adequate experience in the care of such cases and one other doctor). The two doctors may carry out their tests separately or together. If the tests confirm brain death they should still be repeated. It is for the doctors to decide how long the interval between the tests should be. It may not be appropriate for the doctors to carry out all the recommended tests. *The criteria are guidelines, not rigid rules.*

The criteria are as follows:

- All brainstem reflexes are absent.
- The pupils are fixed in diameter and do not respond to sharp changes in the intensity of incident light.
- There is no corneal reflex.
- The vestibular-ocular reflexes are absent.
- No motor responses within the cranial nerve distribution can be elicited by adequate stimulation of any somatic area.
- There is no gag reflex or reflex response to bronchial stimulation by a suction catheter passed down the trachea.
- No respiratory movements occur when the patient is disconnected from the mechanical ventilator for long enough to ensure that the arterial carbon dioxide tension rises above the threshold for stimulation of respiration.

Additional recommendations are made as to how some of these tests should be undertaken.

In October 1998 a revised Code of Practice for the diagnosis and confirmation of death was introduced which offered guidance on how best to diagnose and confirm death in patients (Department of Health 1998). This new Code of Practice was designed to reduce the chances of a misdiagnosis and specifically addressed the need to diagnose metabolic, hypothermic and drug-induced comas. The guidelines redefined death as the irreversible loss of the capacity for consciousness, combined with irreversible loss of the capacity to breathe.

The Role of the Coroner

The Coroner is an independent judicial officer who is appointed by local authorities to record and investigate deaths which are unexpected, sudden, violent or unnatural. Coroners are usually qualified as either a doctor or lawyer (or both). Coroners have a statutory duty to establish whether or not the cause of death was due to natural or unnatural causes. In order to arrive at a finding a post mortem may be required. The cause of death and the identity of the body needs to be established before a death certificate can be issued (Urpeth 2010).

All sudden deaths need to be reported to the Coroner. However, the reporting of a death does not automatically mean that a post mortem examination will need to be carried out. Only 22% of all deaths reported to the Coroner result in post mortem examinations and less than 4% require an inquest.

Investigations are dictated by section 8 (1) of the Coroners Act 1988 (Box 22.1).

Organ Donation

Sudden unexpected intraoperative death is, thankfully, a rare event. A sudden unexpected death is one that was *not* anticipated within the preceding 24 hours. Any sudden deaths must be reported to the Coroner as soon as possible. For most perioperative practitioners

> **BOX 22.1**
>
> **Role of the Coroner**
>
> Where a Coroner is informed that a body of a person (the deceased) is lying within his district and there are reasonable grounds to suspect that the deceased:
>
> a) has died a violent or unnatural death
> b) bas died a sudden death of which the cause is unknown
> c) has died in prison or in such a place or in such circumstances as to requite an inquest under any other act
>
> then whether the cause of death arose within his district or not, the Coroner shall as soon as practicable hold an inquest into the death of the deceased either with or without a jury.

contact with dead patients will often take the form of providing perioperative care during organ retrieval. For some practitioners, this can prove to be a challenging and emotive experience (Clay and Crookes 1996).

> Corpses are not warm, they are not pink, they do not move, they are not pregnant – but a person who is brain dead can be all of these things. To all appearances, there is little difference between a person who is brain dead and a person who is asleep. At the same time we ask people if it is OK to remove a beating heart or other living organ from their loved one. (Kellhear 2007)

Taking part in an organ retrieval procedure will involve liaising closely with donor transplant coordinators. Part of the role of the transplant coordinator is to ensure that the best possible management of the donor and their family is provided throughout the donation process. A collaborative approach between the coordinator, critical care staff and perioperative staff is required once the diagnosis of brainstem death has been confirmed. The Coroner is consulted and permission from the Coroner gained before the retrieval process begins.

A crucial point that may sometimes be overlooked by staff new to perioperative practice is that the donor patient will have been diagnosed as brain dead *before* arrival in the perioperative suite. The time of death will have been recorded as whenever the first brainstem diagnosis was carried out.

This may be difficult to come to terms with as often the patients are transferred from critical care units in a 'warm, pink and well perfused state, in sinus rhythm without any visible marks or trauma'. The use of a neuromuscular blocking agent is sometimes used to prevent spinal reflexes from occurring intraoperatively, but their use does not constitute a part of an anaesthetic. To put it bluntly, patients who are brainstem dead do not require an anaesthetic. The role of the perioperative team in this instance then is to help provide support for the organs while maintaining the dignity of the donor.

Restrictions to the organ retrieval may be imposed by the Coroner, such as insisting that a police officer and/or police photographer (taking detailed photos) is present during the organ retrieval.

In all Coroner's cases the lead surgeon should make detailed notes as he or she may be summoned to court at a much later date. Good practice dictates that all perioperative practitioners will also need to be scrupulous with their record-keeping and documentation (Medical Protection Society 2005).

Section 3

Death of a Child

If intraoperative death of a child looks likely to happen, then parents of a Christian faith may ask for an emergency baptism to be carried out while the child is still alive. Ideally this service should be completed by the hospital chaplain. If the child looks likely to die before the attendance of a chaplain then a member of staff (preferably, but not exclusively Christian) can complete an emergency baptism. It is inappropriate to baptise a child after it is dead but baptism during resuscitation can help to provide pastoral support to family members.

If the child dies in the perioperative area then the ward and Coroner need to be informed as soon as possible. The child's body should then be transferred to an appropriate area following discussions with the Coroner. The child's death must be recorded in the appropriate system.

If a newborn baby dies before being registered at birth then both birth and death can be registered at the same time.

Legally, consent is not required for a Coroner to request a post mortem but best practice dictates that family involvement should be encouraged (Goldman 1994).

Patient Care: Last Offices

The practice of Last Offices should be carried out once it has been established that any specific preparations have been addressed. If a post mortem has been requested by the Coroner, then advice from senior staff or the Coroner's office should be sought.

Below are guidelines which may vary, even among members of the same faith. Observation and compliance with local policies and procedures is recommended, together with seeking advice from transplant coordinators, ward staff and family members.

Equipment needed

In general, you will need:

- disposable plastic aprons
- disposable plastic gloves
- bowl of warm water, soap, the deceased's own toiletries and face cloths or disposable washcloths and two towels
- disposable razor or the patient's own electric razor, comb and equipment for nail care
- equipment for mouth care, including equipment for cleaning dentures
- identification labels × 2
- documents required by law and organisation policy (e.g. notification of death cards)
- shroud or patient's personal clothing: nightdress, pyjamas, clothes previously requested by patient, or clothes that comply with family/cultural wishes
- body bag if required (i.e. in event of actual or potential leakage of bodily fluids and/ or infectious disease) and labels for the body defining the nature of the infection/ disease
- gauze, waterproof tape, dressings and bandages if wounds or intravenous/arterial lines and cannulae are present
- disposable or washable receptacle for collecting urine if appropriate
- plastic bags for clinical and household waste
- sharps bin if appropriate
- laundry skip and appropriate bags for soiled linen

- clean bed linen
- record books for property and valuables
- bags for the patient's personal possessions (Dodds 2005).

Religious differences

With all religions, the following points apply:

- All medical devices should be removed unless the patient is to be referred for post mortem, otherwise they should be disconnected, 'capped off' using obturators, and spigotted if appropriate.
- The body should not be left alone and, if possible, a room should be provided to allow watchers to observe a vigil before the burial.

Christian organ donation

Christian doctrine teaches that sacrifice and selfless acts are intrinsically linked to a wider social responsibility. Most Christian denominations will accept Last Offices according to local policy. Items such as rosary beads and religious icons may be asked by family to be placed with the deceased before internment (Howitt 2003a).

Jewish organ donation

If the patient is to be considered for organ donation then no organ can be removed until death has been defined according to Jewish law. Traditionally this can be established by observing the body for approximately 8 minutes and placing a feather onto the nose and lips of the patient to establish apnoea.

The body should be shrouded. Ritual washing and praying will be carried out.

A Rabbi should be contacted by either the family or the hospital chaplain. Practitioners are permitted to touch the body but should handle the patient as little as possible. Gloves should be worn at all times. The body will be washed by the 'Holy Assembly' who will be selected by the family and will ensure a ritual purification *(qahal kadosh)* takes place.

The patient's eyes should be closed and the limbs straightened. The feet should be pointing toward a door.

Bodies should (ideally) be buried within 24 hours (Howitt 2003b).

Islamic organ donation

In 1995 the Muslim Law Council UK issued a *Fatwa* stating that: 'the council supports organ transplantation as a means of alleviating pain or saving life on the basis of the rules of Shariah'.

If possible, the patient should be positioned so that the face points toward Mecca.

The body should be shrouded. Ritual washing and praying will be carried out preferably by another Muslim of the same sex.

Bodies should (ideally) be buried within 24 hours (Open University 2001, Howitt 2003c).

Sikh organ donation

Sikh faith and philosophy encourages acts of sacrifice and emphasises the need to put others needs before your own: 'Where self exists, there is no God. Where God exists, there is no self' (Guru Nanak, Guru Granth Sahib).

Although organ donation is permitted within the Sikh faith, some patients and families may refuse an organ retrieval, as this may be considered as mutilation.

Section 3

The body is washed and dressed by family members (if possible the eldest son will take the lead role in the Last Offices). Sikhs are always cremated (Open University 2001, Howitt 2003d).

Hindu Dharma organ donation

Selfless giving is listed as the 3rd of the 10 virtuous acts (*Niyamas)* in the Hindu scriptures. 'Of all the things that it is possible to donate, to donate your own body is infinitely more worthwhile' (The Manusmruti).

The body is washed and dressed by a family member. The closest family member will circulate the body with burning incense. Hindus are always cremated (Open University 2001, Howitt 2003e).

References

Clay J and Crookes P (1996) Implications of transplantation surgery for theatre nurses: 1. *British Journal of Nursing* 5(7): 400–403.

Conference of the Medical Royal Colleges (1976) Diagnosis of brain death. *British Medical Journal* 1187–1188.

Department of Health (1998) *The Removal of Cadaveric Organs for Transplantation: a Code of Practice.*1998/035. London: HMSO.

Department of Health and Social Security (1979) *The Removal of Cadaveric Organs for Transplantation a Code of Practice.* London: HMSO.

Dodds N (2005) Last Offices. In Dougherty L and Lister S (eds) *The Royal Marsden Hospital Manual of Clinical Nursing Procedures*, 7th edn. Oxford: Wiley Blackwell.

Goldman A (1994) *Care of the Dying Child*. Oxford: Oxford University Press.

Howitt R, Bradford Hospital NHS Trust (2003a) *Christianity and Organ Donation, A guide to organ donation and Christian beliefs*. Bradford: UK Transplant.

Howitt R, Bradford Hospital NHS Trust (2003b) *Judaism and Organ Donation, A guide to organ donation and Jewish beliefs*. Bradford: UK Transplant.

Howitt R, Bradford Hospital NHS Trust (2003c) *Islam and Organ Donation, A guide to organ donation and Muslim beliefs*. Bradford: UK Transplant.

Howitt R, Bradford Hospital NHS Trust (2003d) *Sikhism and Organ Donation, A guide to organ donation and Sikh beliefs*. Bradford: UK Transplant.

Howitt R, Bradford Hospital NHS Trust (2003e) *Hindu Dharma and Organ Donation, A guide to organ donation and Hindu beliefs*. Bradford: UK Transplant.

Kellhear (2007) Call to revamp death definition. BBC News. http://news.bbc.co.uk/1/hi/6987079.stm.

Medical Protection Society (2005) Casebook Vol. 13, no. 4. www.medicalprotection.org.

Urpeth D (2010) Taking and closer look at the role of the coroner. *British Journal of Neuroscience Nursing* 6(7): 131–133.

Youngner SJ, Allen M, Bartlett ET *et al*. (1985) Psychosocial and ethical implications of organ retrieval. *New England Journal of Medicine* 313(5): 321–323.

CHAPTER 23

Postoperative Care

Pat Smedley and Natalie Quine

The Clinical Environment

The Post-Anaesthetic Care Unit (PACU) is an acute specialist clinical environment. Its primary function is to ensure that the patient recovers safely from surgery and anaesthesia. The area should be suitably equipped and appropriately staffed in order to prevent or limit complications that may delay recovery. PACU staff must be knowledgeable and skilled with a patient-centred focus to the care they deliver. It is essential that the PACU, together with its staff, are available on a 24-hour basis to ensure cover for the emergency theatre workload.

There are very clear guidelines pertaining to the layout and space necessary to recover patients in the NHS Estates Guidance Health Building Note 26 (NHS Estates 2004). This is influenced by infection control, patient safety and the space needed to manage an emergency situation. It is essential that there is easy access to assistance in the event of an emergency. There must be 360-degree access around the bed. There should be an agreed method for summoning necessary help through a call system. There should also be a telephone available for summoning help via the cardiac arrest paging system. It is essential that the environment is well lit to allow PACU staff to observe subtle changes in the patient condition (i.e. pallor). Because of the use of anaesthetic gases and the need to care for staff health there should be a regularly tested scavenging system to remove expired anaesthetic gases from the environment. Each bay will need ceiling-mounted curtains; in an ideal world this would be suitable for X-ray protection curtains, but should as a minimum maintain patient privacy and dignity. These must not reduce overall general visibility in recovery and should be used as needed rather than continuously.

Each PACU will require a 'dirty utility' or sluice for the disposal of linen, clinical waste and other used items. Sharps disposal units are needed either at the bedside or as a mobile box for bedside sharps disposal. A sharps bin will also be needed in the medication preparation area. A larger bin will be needed within the environment for the disposal of used giving sets and fluid bags.

Manual of Perioperative Care: An Essential Guide, First Edition. Edited by Kate Woodhead and Lesley Fudge.
© 2012 John Wiley & Sons, Ltd. Published 2012 by John Wiley & Sons, Ltd.

The PACU should be easily accessible from all theatres. The area should be self-contained within the theatre complex. Patients should not pass through the PACU to access theatre routinely. There should be a defined flow through PACU, patients entering through one door and exiting through another, to ensure there is no conflict between patients leaving and coming into the PACU.

The NHS Estates Guidance HBN 26 (NHS Estates 2004) states there should be a minimum of two recovery bays per theatre. The number of beds per theatre will be influenced by the length of surgery and the anticipated length of stay for each patient in recovery.

Equipment at the Bedside

Each PACU bed should be equipped separately for air, oxygen and suction through a pipeline supply. In addition, the following equipment should be available:

- A double oxygen flow meter, one port is used directly for the patient oxygen administration and the second is available for use in an emergency. This emergency port can be used for oxygen delivery via a hand ventilation circuit.
- Wall-mounted variable pressure suction equipment is essential, with a large-bore suction catheter attached. The choice of suction catheter will be dependent on the situation. A variety of long suction catheters, suitable for use via tracheal tubes, should also be available.
- If the PACU recovers paediatric patients there must be a variety of suitable paediatric equipment available for the purposes of suction, emergency hand ventilation and general oxygen administration postoperatively (NHS Estates 2004).

Each recovery bay should have:

- monitoring equipment that as a minimum records, blood pressure, pulse, ECG, oxygen saturation and temperature on a continuous basis
- capnography and invasive monitoring equipment readily available so that staff can set it up, use it and interpret the observations (BARNA 2005, ASPAN 2010a, Royal College of Anaesthetists 2010)
- a variety of oral pharyngeal airways
- nasopharyngeal airways
- vomit bowls
- incontinence pads
- a syringe for deflating cuffs on endotracheal tubes and laryngeal mask airways if necessary.

Within the department there should be:

- a selection of analgesics for a variety of routes
- a variety of antiemetics
- emergency re-intubation medications
- reversal agents for muscle relaxants
- latex-free anaphylaxis medication box
- wide variety of intravenous fluids in a variety of volumes.

Within the theatre complex there will be a latex-free cardiac arrest trolley equipped with a defibrillator that is compliant with hospital policy and is checked on a regular basis to ensure that the equipment is in date. With regular checking the staff will become familiar with the contents. Equipment should be available for managing a difficult intubation, including a variety of laryngoscope blades and tracheostomy equipment.

Staff Training and Competence

Staff working in the PACU should be appropriately trained and competent. They are very often working outside the direct supervision of an anaesthetist and as such should be competent to manage an emergency until medical help arrives. The recovery practitioner will constantly assess the patient's condition and respond to any changes in an appropriate manner, ensuring that help and advice is sought from the anaesthetist as it is needed.

In the event of an emergency the recovery practitioner is expected to respond and manage the situation while summoning immediate help. The recovery practitioner is an individual who remains calm and focused on the patient and their safety at all times. PACU staff should have attended a recognised recovery course; this course will ideally cover all aspects of recovery including:

- applied anatomy and physiology of all body systems
- principles of airway/respiratory management
- principles of haemodynamic management including fluid management
- thermoregulatory management
- pain management
- management of postoperative nausea and vomiting
- management of emergencies (anaphylaxis, malignant hyperpyrexia, respiratory and cardiac arrest, suxamethonium apnoea and laryngeal spasm)

Staff new to the unit should be fully orientated and competence assessed through locally and nationally established competency packages. Assessments should be undertaken by a competent member of staff who holds the appropriate teaching and assessing qualification and has been regularly updated. Students working in the clinical area should be supervised on a one to one basis for all clinical practice.

Staff should attend courses on:

- basic life support
- immediate life support
- manual handling
- locally nominated mandatory training.

If the environment caters for paediatrics then the appropriate paediatric resuscitation courses should be completed. Consideration should be given on an individual basis to the need for staff to complete advanced life support training, particularly those who undertake on calls and out of hours working where the number of staff available diminishes. For areas managing children, the paediatric equivalent should be undertaken (BARNA 2005, Royal College of Anaesthetists 2009, ASPAN 2010a).

Staffing and Skill Mix

Recovery staffing is a complex issue, depending on skill mix, patient acuity and patient numbers. Whenever there is a patient in recovery there should be a minimum of two registered practitioners who are trained in recovery present (Royal College of Anaesthetists 2009). When a patient is unconscious there must be one nurse to one patient until the patient has regained their protective reflexes and are able to maintain their own airway (Royal College of Anaesthetists 2009). There can be one nurse to two patients who are stable and maintaining their own airway and one nurse to three patients who are recovered sufficiently to return to the ward for the continuation of their longer term postoperative care. A patient who is unstable, under 8 or requiring

Table 23.1   Minimum staffing summary.

Patient condition/special considerations	Number of registered recovery practitioners per patient
Unconscious	1 nurse to one patient
Alert/orientated/stable	1 nurse for two patients
Unstable/under 8 or requiring ITU/HDU level care	2 nurses to one patient

Note: When there is a patient in PACU there must be two recovery practitioners present.
From Royal College of Anaesthetists (2009), British Anaesthetic and Recovery Nursing Association (2005) and ASPAN (2010a).

intensive care/high dependency care will require two staff to one patient ratio (BARNA 2005, Royal College of Anaesthetists 2009, ASPAN 2010a). Minimum staffing levels are summarised in Table 23.1.

The evidence supporting PACU staffing numbers is limited and in the majority of incidences, relates to 'expert opinion' and 'best guess' scenarios. The PACU is an unpredictable environment that is further complicated with the delays in discharging patients back to the ward or critical care facility. These delays can impact on the ability of the department to admit new patients, causing a bottleneck and slowing the patient pathway through theatre (Smedley 2010). It is essential to keep the patient pathway through theatre, recovery and return to the ward as smooth as possible to avoid bottlenecks and delays. The key to this smooth running is communication between areas and an understanding of each others' needs and issues and ensuring that the patient's safety is the fundamental issue.

Daily Equipment Checking

All bedside equipment should be checked prior to the patient's arrival in recovery. Checks should include the following:

- Oxygen flow should be checked by switching the oxygen on and ensuring there is uninterrupted flow.
- Suction should be checked to ensure that it maintains and increases pressure when the tubing is kinked or suctioning fluids.
- Bedside emergency ventilation equipment should be tested to ensure that there are no leaks in the bag or obstructions in the oxygen flow.
- Equipment should be changed as each patient is discharged, and the area and non-disposable equipment wiped down as per hospital infection prevention and control policies.

All emergency equipment should be checked on a daily basis or as per the department schedule to ensure that it is in full working order. When the equipment is used, it must be replaced as soon as possible so that it is ready for next use.

Patient Transfer from Theatre to PACU/Handover of Patient

The patient will be accompanied to the PACU by the anaesthetist and an operating room practitioner. Oxygen is delivered en route and must be attached to wall delivery on arrival in PACU. The patient should be received by two PACU practitioners to ensure safe transfer of care, management of monitoring systems, intravenous infusions, drains and urine bags (BARNA 2005). Handover will include patient name, relevant medical history, anaesthetic technique and drugs, intraoperative complications and operative detail including sutures, dressing and drains. Instructions for postoperative care from both surgeon and anaesthetist are detailed at this time. At this point the PACU practitioner will rapidly assess the patient in order of clinical priority of airway, breathing and circulation. The anaesthetist should remain to assess that the patient is breathing spontaneously and the PACU practitioner is ready to take over care (AAGBI 2002). Clinical guidelines may be given based on patient's baseline observations, anaesthetic and surgical history. Documentation is completed as soon as the patient is stable.

Risk Assessment of Patient in Planning Care

The patient undergoes dynamic physiological changes in this initial postoperative period due to the profound impact of anaesthesia and surgery on normal body function as illustrated in Table 23.2. Planning patient care follows risk assessment in order to evaluate potential complications associated with the patient's medical history, surgical and anaesthetic process. The PACU practitioner will gather information both from anaesthetic/ theatre handover, together with use of the anaesthetic record and surgeon's notes.

While risk assessment alerts the practitioner to potential complications, it is by rigorous continual physical assessment of all body systems followed by rapid intervention and reassessment that safe patient outcomes are achieved. Baseline recordings of airway

Table 23.2 Anaesthetic and surgical risk factors.

Anaesthetic/surgical process	Risk of complications in PACU
Induction agents	
Induce unconscious state	Propofol may leave mild hypotension
Airway maintenance: laryngeal mask airway, endotracheal intubation	Intubation potentiates risk of laryngospasm
Maintenance agents	
Maintain unconscious state	Opioids, failure to wake, respiratory depression, airway obstruction Volatile anaesthetic agents, failure to wake, respiratory depression, vasodilation and hypotension, airway obstruction Muscle relaxants, residual respiratory muscle weakness, residual paralysis if not reversed, airway obstruction
Reversal agents	
Reverse muscle relaxant (neostigmine)	Inadequate dose of neostigmine results in residual paralysis
Hypothermia	Mild to profound hypothermia delays recovery
Fluid loss	Clear fluid/blood loss – will result in circulatory disturbance
Pain	Pain causes distress and stimulation of sympathetic nervous system – tachycardia and potential cardiac stress

Section 3

patency, respirations, blood pressure, level of consciousness, core temperature, sedation/pain and nausea scoring are noted. Monitoring of pulse oximetry, electrocardiogram and the use of non-invasive blood pressure are now routine (AAGBI 2007). Central venous pressure, arterial blood gas results may be used dependent on the complexity of the procedure and patient medical history. Capnography is recommended by the AAGBI (2009) for all intubated patients and those whose airway is maintained by supraglottic or other similar airway devices.

Intraoperative fluid balance is noted, taking into consideration actual drainage into urinary catheter bags and drains. Observations are routinely noted every 10 minutes while the patient is in the PACU. The early stages of patient recovery are when the patient is most vulnerable to sudden clinical changes. While progression towards full recovery and homeostasis is the norm, at any stage the patient's condition may deteriorate and complications set in.

Airway: the First Priority

Multiple anaesthetic agents as shown in Table 23.2 can lead to delayed return to consciousness with loss of normal airway protective mechanisms (swallow, cough and gag reflexes) combined with upper airway muscle weakness. The delicate structures of the upper airway function normally to allow the free passage of air to and from the lungs.

Upper airway structures

The tongue is a large muscular organ which helps in the mastication of food before swallowing. The adult pharynx is a 13-cm-long muscular channel comprising the nasopharynx, oropharynx (throat) and hypopharynx, communicating with the oesophagus and larynx (Figure 23.1). Food and water pass via the oropharynx and, on swallowing, are diverted to the oesophagus, which lies posterior to the trachea en route to the stomach. The epiglottis (a leaf-like cartilage) folds over the vocal cords on swallowing to ensure that food does not pass into the trachea. The vocal cords are narrow ligaments contained in the larynx which allow speech and the free flow of air to the lungs.

From the induction of anaesthesia until the patient is awake (with the return of muscle tone and vital reflexes) these structures are at risk of malfunction, leading quickly to airway obstruction (Table 23.3).

Airway assessment

Airway obstruction in the immediate post-anaesthetic phase is a common and potentially dangerous complication in the semi- or unconscious patient whose protective reflexes have not returned. Risk factors for obstruction should be assessed in planning care. Use of narcotics, muscle relaxants, surgical procedures and obesity may all cause obstruction. Complications are avoided by rigorous continuous physical assessment, recognition of early derangement from the norm and rapid appropriate intervention. The PACU practitioner uses the 'look, listen, feel' method to comprehensively assess the airway as in Table 23.4.

Airway management

Airway management may be considered in three stages commencing with the use of routine manoeuvres to prevent or relieve obstruction.

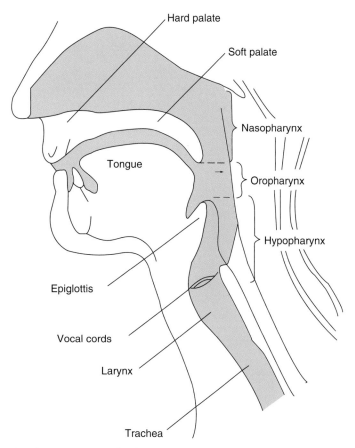

Figure 23.1 The pharynx is a muscular channel comprising the nasopharynx, oropharynx and hypopharynx.

Table 23.3 Effect of general anaesthesia on normal airway function.

Anatomical point	Surgery/anaesthetic risk	Potential for airway obstruction
Nasopharynx: nostrils	Ear, nose and throat (ENT) surgery: nasal intubation	Highly vascular area – bleeding may obstruct airway
Oropharynx: tongue/oral cavity	Anaesthetic agents: muscle weakness ENT/dental surgery	Tongue floppy – falls to back of oropharynx Foreign body (throat/dental pack) blocks airway Bleeding from oral cavity/saliva
Laryngeal structures Epiglottis Vocal cords (glottis)	Anaesthetic agents relax the larynx leaving the airway unprotected Clumsy intubation causes risk of laryngospasm	Loss of epiglottal function: aspiration of food/fluid into trachea Partial or total obstruction caused by irritation to vocal cords

Table 23.4   Airway assessment.

	Indicators for obstruction	Normal airway	Obstructive signs
Look	Patient colour	Pink	Pallor leading to cyanosis a sign of hypoxia
	Saturation of oxygen	SaO$_2$ 96–100%	Falling saturation of oxygen
	Level of consciousness	Conscious and alert	Unconscious/semi-conscious state
	Mask misting	Mask misting	Limited misting on mask
	Breathing pattern	Regular breathing pattern	Irregular breathing pattern indicates obstruction
	CVS – tachycardia may be a sign of hypoxia	CVS within normal parameters (unless primary CVS disorder)	Use of accessory muscles
Listen	Sound of breathing Noisy breathing indicates partial obstruction	Quiet breathing NB: absolute silence may denote total obstruction as no air flows through airway	Snoring indicates tongue obstructing airway Gurgling: obstruction by fluid in oral cavity Crowing – laryngospasm Wheezing – constricted lower airways
Feel	Feel of expired air at nose and mouth	Breath felt from nose/mouth	Limited feel of breath from nose/mouth

Stage 1: Routine airway manoeuvres

A variety of techniques are used to ensure the airway remains clear. While unconscious, the tongue constitutes a major risk of obstruction. The laryngeal mask airway (LMA) left in situ is a valuable airway adjunct which prevents the tongue from occluding the oropharynx and should not be removed until the patient is waking and no longer able to tolerate it. The LMA may be withdrawn along with secretions if the cuff is left inflated where possible. If the LMA is not in situ and partial obstruction by the tongue is indicated by snoring, the use of the head tilt and chin lift may ease the obstruction. If this fails, jaw thrust manoeuvre is indicated (Figure 23.2). It may be necessary to insert a Guedel airway and if this fails to relieve obstruction the next step would often be reinsertion of LMA. Careful suctioning or placing the patient in recovery position, head down, can relieve obstruction by fluids in the oral cavity. Examination of the oropharynx will reveal obstruction by foreign body (tooth, dental pack). Oxygen is turned up to full flow if there is any sign of obstruction. Ongoing physical assessment confirms whether any of the above manoeuvres has successfully cured the obstruction. If clinical deterioration is seen, anaesthetic help must be sought immediately and an attempt to force oxygen into the airway by positive pressure bagging should be performed. If airway obstruction is sustained for many minutes brain death may follow.

Stage 2: Bagging patient using bag–valve–mask

It may require two practitioners to use the bag–valve–mask – one to hold the mask, the other to perform bagging while waiting for the anaesthetic team to take over management of this critical situation (Figure 23.3). With an oxygen reservoir bagging may open up the airway and deliver 96% O$_2$. PACU staff must have the emergency

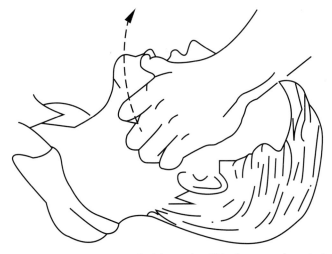

Figure 23.2   Jaw thrust. The mandible is pushed forward and lifts the tongue from the back of the oropharynx.

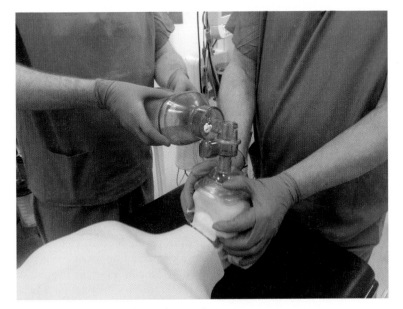

Figure 23.3   Bagging patient using bag–valve–mask.

intubation trolley ready with equipment and drugs that may be needed by the anaesthetist.

Stage 3: Patient intubation

If the above manoeuvres fail to remove the obstruction then endotracheal intubation will be necessary. It is often difficult in emergency situations to identify the prime cause of obstruction. Prior to intubating the patient the anaesthetist may try to alleviate the condition by administration of reversal drugs (neostigmine/naloxone/doxapram) (see Table 23.6). If the patient fails to respond then the role of the PACU team is to assist the anaesthetist in patient intubation.

Laryngospasm

Laryngospasm is the partial or complete spasm of laryngeal muscles preventing the free flow of air to and from the lungs. Clumsy intubation, secretions (blood/saliva) are common causes of spasm. A crowing noise is the classic sign of stridor, together with agitation, decreased oxygen saturation, use of accessory muscles and irregular breathing pattern if spasm severe. Laryngospasm must always be treated as a clinical emergency and anaesthetic help must be sought immediately. Spasm may worsen, leading to complete closure of the glottis and onset of severe hypoxia. Positive pressure ventilation with 100% oxygen should open up the cords and careful suction may relieve spasm caused by blood or secretions. Steroids, lignocaine or epinephrine may be used to decrease airway irritation. Failure to relieve spasm may require administration of muscle relaxants and re-intubation.

Aspiration

Aspiration of foreign body, blood or gastric contents into the lungs in the unprotected airway may occur while the patient is returning to full consciousness. Those at high risk include patients who are obese, pregnant or suffering from hiatus hernia. Coughing, bronchospasm, airway obstruction with resulting hypoxia may indicate aspiration. Any sign of aspirate dribbling from the mouth should be taken seriously and anaesthetic help summoned. The patient should be laid in the recovery position, head down to drain secretions, and suction applied. Airway maintenance and prevention of hypoxia are key management objectives. Potential damage to the lungs from food particles and acid secretions depends on the size and nature of aspirate. Further management includes a chest X-ray, possible use of antibiotics and/or steroids and the patient should be followed up in the high dependency area.

Breathing: the Second Priority

External respiration is the act of inhaling air into the lungs on inspiration and exhaling carbon dioxide on expiration via an unobstructed airway.

All body cells require a constant supply of oxygen to maintain normal cell function. Oxygen is consumed by the tissues in the process of internal respiration. Failure to deliver oxygen to the cells results in hypoxia and acidosis caused by anaerobic metabolism, both causing cell death. Carbon dioxide (CO_2) must also be eliminated constantly. A build-up of CO_2 in the blood causes acidosis. Normal acid level (pH) for cell function is 7.35–7.42. This narrow margin must be maintained for normal cell function. Patients routinely receive oxygen while in the PACU via a Hudson mask at 40% to ensure optimal oxygen levels in the blood. If the patient has lung disease a Venturi system is used which delivers a constant fixed percentage of oxygen appropriate for the patient's condition.

Control of breathing

The respiratory centre in the medulla of the brain is the control centre for breathing and stimulates inspiration (Figure 23.4). Peripheral chemoreceptors in the arteries sense rising levels of CO_2 in the blood while central chemoreceptors monitor increased acidity

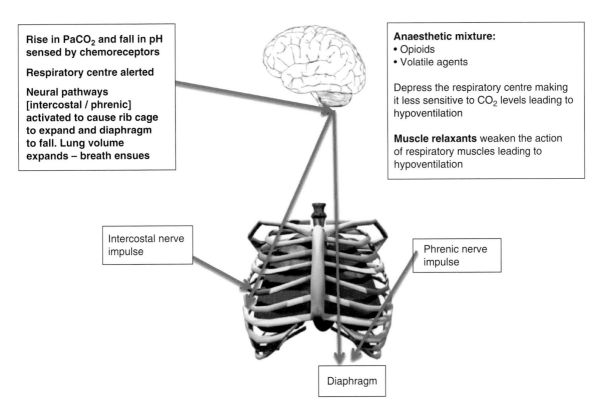

Rise in PaCO₂ and fall in pH sensed by chemoreceptors

Respiratory centre alerted

Neural pathways [intercostal / phrenic] activated to cause rib cage to expand and diaphragm to fall. Lung volume expands – breath ensues

Anaesthetic mixture:
• Opioids
• Volatile agents

Depress the respiratory centre making it less sensitive to CO₂ levels leading to hypoventilation

Muscle relaxants weaken the action of respiratory muscles leading to hypoventilation

Intercostal nerve impulse

Phrenic nerve impulse

Diaphragm

Figure 23.4   Action of the respiratory centre.

Section 3

of cerebral spinal fluid. The primary stimulus to breathe is to exhale carbon dioxide and maintain the pH level within its narrow margins. Oxygen lack, detected via the chemoreceptors, is a secondary stimulus to breathe.

Mechanics of breathing

With rising CO_2 levels the respiratory centre stimulates the intercostal nerves to contract, lifting the ribcage wall upwards and outwards. Simultaneously the diaphragm contracts downwards, both these effects expanding the lung volume. At this point the pressure in the lung is lower than atmospheric pressure. Gases always travel from an area of higher to lower pressure. Air containing oxygen is sucked into the lungs until the pressures are equal. On expiration the ribcage wall collapses down and the diaphragm pushes upwards, contracting the lung volume. Lung pressure is higher than atmospheric and CO_2 is exhaled to the atmosphere. In post-anaesthetic care the use of muscle relaxants together with opioids and volatile agents leads to residual weakness of respiratory muscles, making a degree of hypoventilation a risk factor.

Effect of general anaesthesia on normal respiratory function

As seen in Table 23.5 the agents used in general anaesthesia affect breathing to a greater or lesser degree. The primary danger to the patient in the post-anaesthetic phase is hypoventilation, when the exchange of gases in the lungs is insufficient to provide sufficient oxygen to be transported to the cells, and to allow adequate elimination of carbon dioxide. The combination of induction and maintenance agents may prove to be a lethal mixture, especially to the elderly patient who has limited respiratory reserve, or

Table 23.5   Effect of anaesthetic drugs/surgery on breathing.

Drug group/surgical effect	Residual effect on breathing in PACU
Induction agent	Combines with maintenance agents to reduce respiratory drive and bring about delayed return of consciousness
Maintenance agents:	
Opioids Volatile agents	Opioids/volatile agents: render respiratory centre less sensitive to CO_2 levels, resulting in hypoventilation and delayed return of consciousness
Muscle relaxants	Muscle relaxants: weaken intercostal muscles affecting respiratory excursion. If not reversed profoundly affect muscle function
Surgical effect	Pain may discourage deep breathing (in thoracic/abdominal surgery)

those with coexistent lung disease. These agents impact on normal respiratory function and by prolonging the unconscious state they increase the risk of airway obstruction.

Consideration of the risk factors shown in Table 23.5 will alert the PACU practitioner to the importance of taking preventative action to avoid hypoventilation. Multiple risk factors increase the risk of hypoventilation. For example the elderly, obese patient, with possible coexistent lung disease, undergoing a prolonged abdominal or thoracic procedure represents a high risk for hypoventilation and should be very carefully assessed and managed.

Assessment of breathing

'Look, listen, feel' technique is employed for full respiratory assessment which includes airway indicators as in Table 23.4. The rate, depth and pattern of breathing, SaO_2 and level of consciousness are examined. The normal adult respiratory rate at rest is around 12–15 breaths per minute (bpm) with a volume per breath of 500 mL of air, although due to dead space only 350 mL is used in gas exchange. The volume of air exchanged over 1 minute is around 5 litres and this is known as minute volume.

Central respiratory depression

Falling respiratory rate and/or shallow breathing indicates primary failure of the depressed respiratory centre to sustain a minute volume sufficient to deliver oxygen to the tissues and eliminate CO_2. Note that a respiratory rate of 8 bpm may not be serious if the tidal volume is adequate. Pulse oximetry is an essential monitoring tool, oxygen saturation falling below 95% as a general rule must be queried. Placing the hand over the abdomen is useful to check respiratory movement, together with signs of the face-mask misting. The unconscious patient is also at risk of obstruction so primary airway management is essential.

Management of central respiratory depression

Clearing the airway must be the first priority, while at the same time using a stir-up regime, stimulating the patient to wake up by calling his or her name while all the time assessing conscious level and breathing rate and pattern. If the patient is unresponsive and displays signs of deterioration, positive pressure bagging and call for help is essential. The emergency intubation trolley, equipment and drugs should be prepared for possible intubation.

Table 23.6   Action of reversal drugs.

Drug	Action	Effect
Neostigmine/ glycopyrrolate	Reverses long-acting muscle relaxants	Patient recovers muscle strength
Narcan (naloxone)	Opioid antagonist	Opioids reversed; patient awake; respirations restored however patient may be in considerable pain
Dopram (doxapram)	Stimulates respiratory centre	Patient wakes, and breathing rate and depth increased

The anaesthetist may administer naloxone or doxapram to reverse the effect of the drugs that have caused delayed return of consciousness and respiratory depression as seen in Table 23.5. The response to naloxone/doxapram is often immediate; the patient wakes up, takes deeper breaths to restore his or her minute volume. Naloxone, an opioid anatagonist, may cause the return of pain, and other non-opioid analgesia should then be introduced (Table 23.6).

Residual paralysis

Hypoventilation may also be caused or exacerbated by the use of muscle relaxants intraoperatively. These agents paralyse all the muscles, including the respiratory muscles normally essential to ensure strong respiratory excursion. If neostigmine/glycopyrrolate has not been effective, the patient may be left with residual paralysis which may be mild to severe. Acute anxiety follows in the awake patient who feels he or she has no control over breathing. Residual paralysis may be recognised by twitchy muscles, discoordination of muscle function, irregular breathing and signs of hypoxia if severe. Failure of the patient to stick out their tongue, raise their head from the pillow and squeeze with their hand confirms this diagnosis. Residual paralysis must be reported to the anaesthetist urgently and neostigmine/glycopyrrolate administered. Careful nursing is required to ease patient anxiety and teach the patient how to coordinate breaths.

Circulation: the Third Priority

Assessment and management of circulation is the third essential priority. The heart and circulatory system deliver oxygen-rich blood to the tissues, and transport carbon dioxide to the lungs for exhalation. If airway and breathing are not functioning, there is little point in trying to establish circulation.

Blood pressure is the result of the relationship between the volume of blood in the circulation (cardiac output) pushing against a degree of resistance in the arteriole system (systemic vascular resistance).

$$\text{Blood pressure (BP)} = \text{Cardiac output (CO)} \times \text{Systemic vascular resistance (SVR)}$$

The normal adult blood or circulatory volume is 5 litres. The resistance in the arteriole system is controlled by the sympathetic nervous system. Cardiac output depends on the relationship between stroke volume (blood ejected on one contraction) multiplied by heart rate over 1 minute. Stroke volume is around 70 mL and heart rate around 70 bpm, making a total of 4900 mL. Stroke volume is greatly affected by preload or the volume

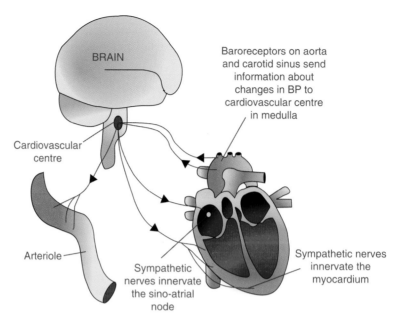

Figure 23.5   Control of blood pressure.

of blood returned to the right heart and measured by central venous pressure. With healthy heart muscle, as a rule the greater the preload, the greater the myocardial stretch and the more blood pumped out in cardiac output. In perioperative practice loss of circulating fluid (i.e. in haemorrhage) can rapidly diminish preload, myocardial stretch, cardiac output and ultimately blood pressure.

Heart rate/rhythm is another key determinant of cardiac output. Sinus rhythm of around 70 bpm is the normal heart rate, which allows time for the ventricles to fill in diastole to sustain a healthy stroke volume and ultimately blood pressure. Bradycardia (slow heart rate) and tachycardia (fast heart rate) should be treated in the PACU if compromising blood pressure. Bradycardia may be caused by the administration of neostigmine alone, again by hypothermia and hypoxaemia. The cause of the problem should addressed, and atropine given where indicated. Tachycardia may be due to pain, anxiety, hypoxaemia or raised temperature, hypovolaemia and also hyperthyroid state. The cause should be treated.

Systemic vascular resistance

Blood pressure is controlled by the cardiovascular centre in the medulla oblongata (Figure 23.5). Specialised cells called baroreceptors situated in the arteries detect hypo/hypertensive states, relaying this message to the cardiovascular centre. If blood pressure is low the cardiac (sympathetic) nerves stimulate the heart to contract faster and harder to boost cardiac output. Simultaneously the sympathetic nerves vasoconstrict the arteriole bed, raising the systemic vascular resistance. Blood pressure goes up. If blood pressure is high this sympathetic stimulus will tail off. The heart rate falls, beats less forcibly and arterioles dilate. Blood pressure falls. The use of epidural or spinal anaesthesia causes vasodilation and loss of systemic vascular resistance. The patient should have intravenous fluids *in situ* to fill the dilated vessels and ephedrine may be given to vasoconstrict and conserve the blood pressure. The effects of surgery and general anaesthesia on blood pressure are summarised in Table 23.7.

Table 23.7 Effect of surgery and general anaesthesia on blood pressure.

Anaesthetic/surgical effect	Residual effect on blood pressure in PACU
Maintenance:	
Opioids	Depress myocardium; diminish cardiac output; hypotension
Volatile agents	Depress myocardium; diminish cardiac output; hypotension
Reversal agent: neostigmine (although this is usually combined with glycopyrrolate)	Vasodilate; diminish vascular resistance; hypotension Causes bradycardia; diminishes cardiac output; hypotension
Regional anaesthesia: epidural/spinal	Vasodilate; diminish systemic vascular resistance; hypotension
Fluid loss (blood or clear fluids)	Diminishes preload; loss of cardiac output; hypotension
Pain	Increases sympathetic nervous activity; speeds up heart rate and contraction; hypertension

Table 23.8 Assessment of circulation.

Organ	Signs of hypoperfusion	Measureable circulatory parameters
Brain (cerebral hypoxia)	Agitation, confusion leading to drowsiness, semi to unconscious state	Patient observation
Heart (ischaemia)	Angina, ECG changes, pallor, diaphoresis	12-lead ECG, blood for cardiac enzymes
Kidney	Urine output less than 0.5 mL/kg/h – leading to oliguria	Hourly calculation of urine output
Peripheral vascular circulation	Cool peripheries, pallor, diaphoresis, faint thready pulses, increased capillary refill time	Physical examination

Section 3

Risk analysis of the above variables

As with airway and breathing, the PACU practitioner must risk assess the patient to avoid circulatory complications. Again, multiple risk factors increase the danger to the patient. For example, transurethral resection of prostate (TURP) represents a high risk of bleeding (with loss of cardiac output). This procedure is usually performed under spinal anaesthesia with associated vasodilation and loss of systemic vascular resistance. These two risks may cause the patient profound hypotension with insufficient blood volume to fill the dilated arteriole bed. For these patients intravenous therapy is essential. Again, if the patient has a cardiac history (ischaemic heart disease) the danger of stressing the heart by overloading the patient with fluid is clear.

Assessment of the circulation

Rigorous assessment using physical examination and monitoring equipment is essential to detect early small changes in cardiovascular performance and correct them before they become a significant complication. Treatment should follow analysis of trends, not single readings of blood pressure, pulse. Clear signs of hypoperfusion to the major organs and tissues can be seen in Table 23.8.

Table 23.9   Reasons for hypotension in the PACU.

Physiological rationale	Anaesthetic/surgical cause	Management
Loss of preload	Haemorrhage/loss of clear fluid	Fluid replacement as appropriate-: crystalloids/colloids (including blood products) using in line fluid warming Careful inspection of wound/drains: communicate with surgical team. Possible return to theatre
	Massive haemorrhage	Fluid replacement/coordinate resuscitation efforts with laboratory for blood replacement/platelets/FFP. Repeat bloods Hb, FBC, coagulation through resuscitation
Loss of systemic vascular resistance	Use of volatile agents which cause vasodilation Use of epidural/spinal: vasodilation	Fluids via intravenous route to fill up dilated arteriole bed Use of ephedrine IV to vasoconstrict arterioles
Heart rate: arrhythmias		ECG monitoring – antiarrhythmic drugs if indicated
Bradycardia	Neostigmine	Glycopyrrolate/atropine speeds up heart
Myocardial damage/loss of contractility	Myocardium overstretched (stress/fluids?)	12-lead ECG: bloods, nitrates, opioids Transfer to ICU or CCU

Hypotension is a common post-anaesthetic complication and may vary on a continuum from mild (as a result of mix of anaesthetic agents) to severe (haemorrhage) leading to shock. For all degrees of hypotension the patient requires high flow oxygen as the heart is failing to deliver enough blood containing oxygen to the tissues. The patient needs to be kept warm, and placed supine and flat with legs elevated if necessary to improve preload. Monitoring of physical signs, blood pressure, SaO$_2$, ECG and central venous pressure are all indicated. Beyond these measures the management should be directed at the cause, which may be simple (bradycardia) or complex (fluid loss combined with the vasodilating effect of regional anaesthesia). Table 23.9 gives some management guidelines.

Fluid balance

Estimating fluid balance accurately is an essential component of cardiovascular management. The most common cause of hypotension is fluid deficit. While haemorrhage and resulting loss in circulatory volume is an obvious cause of hypotension, clear fluid depletion may be contributory or the main cause of this. Normal fluid input and output over 24 hours is around 2500 mL. It is important to remember that the surgical patient will not be ingesting water, but will still be losing fluid in expired air, through the skin and in the urine. Some surgical procedures cause massive loss of clear fluid such as major abdominal surgery where fluid is lost to the atmosphere from the open gut. Effective anaesthetic management will allow for fluid deficit and the role of the PACU practitioner is to administer IV fluids, measure and document fluid balance and observe for signs of hypovolaemia. Hypervolaemia may be a complication. Circulatory overload may lead to breathlessness, pulmonary oedema and tachycardia, all serious signs which require urgent anaesthetic management.

Hypertension, indicated by a blood pressure 20–30% above baseline, is another common complication in the PACU. Risk factors include pain, anxiety, hypoxaemia, hypercarbia, hypothermia, bladder distension, fluid overload or existing history of hypertension. Patients with cardiac history are particularly at risk of myocardial damage if the pressure is not controlled.

Management of hypertension

A sustained systolic pressure above 180 mmHg or diastolic over 105 mmHg or any ventricular premature beats or ischaemic changes on ECG should indicate active management under anaesthetic instructions. Respiratory causes of hypertension must be prioritised and managed. The patient is best treated sitting up, ECG monitoring attached to look for signs of ischaemia. Pain must be treated as a priority and the patient reassured if anxious. Antihypertensive therapy such as a vasodilator (nitroglycerin, hydralazine) or beta-blocker (labetolol) or calcium channel blocker (nifedipine) may be administered to treat the hypertension. Overtransfusion should be treated urgently with diuretics.

Delayed Emergence

Delayed emergence is commonly caused by prolonged drug effects as the combination of drugs used in general anaesthesia are eliminated from the body. Metabolic problems such as hypo/hyperglycaemia, hypothyroidism and hypovolaemia may exacerbate this condition. Risk factors also include hypothermia and liver or renal disease, all of which delay metabolism and excretion of drugs. Management includes rigorous assessment (pupil reaction is a good indicator of returning conscious level) and management of the cause and contributory factors. If opioids are the cause of delayed emergence, and if respiratory depression is also present, the patient's airway must be supported and ventilation maintained while naloxone may be administered. Hypothermia and metabolic disturbances must be corrected.

Neurologic injury is a serious but rare cause of delayed emergence. Brain damage may be sustained following a stroke, cerebral hypoxia or emboli. If the patient does not move one side, or has a dilated or non-reacting pupil on one side or change in rate and pattern of breathing, then brain damage must be suspected. The patient should be very carefully monitored using the Glasgow Coma Scale and immediate surgical and anaesthetic help solicited.

Postoperative Nausea and Vomiting

Postoperative nausea and vomiting (PONV) is a very common postoperative complication and, along with pain, is highly unpleasant for the patient. PONV can range from feeling nauseated to active vomiting, and if the vomiting is prolonged can lead to severe dehydration and delay recovery time. Regurgitation in the semi/unconscious patient may lead to aspiration of vomitus into the lung and cause aspiration pneumonitis. PONV is also associated with hypotension, bradycardia and may damage the operative site.

Risk assessment in PONV is now an important recognised guideline to management and is recommended by the American Society of Peri-Anesthesia Nurses (ASPAN 2006). Certain types of procedures, for example gynaecological laparoscopic surgery, ENT and ophthalmic surgery are high risk. Children are more at risk for PONV. Drugs used in anaesthesia may add to risk, many induction and inhalation agents cause PONV together with opioids. In the PACU severe pain, hypotension, hypoxia and hypovolaemia are all known factors associated with PONV. Motion, for instance when the trolley is moved, may also bring on an attack.

Table 23.10   Antiemetic therapy.

Group	Drug	Best for
Phenothiazines	Promethazine, prochlorperazine	Opioid-induced PONV
Antihistamine	Cyclizine	All PONV
5-HT3 antagonist	Ondanestron, granisteron	Gut and gynaecological surgery Major tissue damage
Steroids	Dexamethosone	All PONV
Benzamide	Metoclopramide	Gut and gynaecological surgery
Butyrophenones	Droperidol	All PONV
Anticholinergic	L-Hyposcine (scopolamine)	Opioid-induced PONV

From Hatfield and Tronson (2009).

The key to good management is risk assessment and risk scores are being used more frequently. By identifying those most at risk, antiemetics may be given prophylactically. Maintenance of fluid therapy by intravenous route is another important factor in eliminating PONV. Antiemetic drugs are divided into different classes of drug and may relieve the symptoms. Multi-modal antiemetic therapy is the treatment of choice since different classes of drug act on the complex mesh of centres in the brainstem responsible for PONV. Table 23.10 lists the main elements of antiemetic drug therapy. If drugs do not work, additional fluids may relieve the distressing condition. Empathetic nursing care, mouthwashes and cool compresses will enhance patient comfort.

However, despite careful management, PONV is difficult to eradicate altogether in the high-risk patient and the incidence of PONV remains high.

Discharge Criteria

Patients should be discharged when they meet the local discharge criteria. The Association of Anaesthetists of Great Britain and Ireland (AAGBI 2002) recommend that agreed criteria for discharge should be in place. A summary of these criteria include:

- fully conscious state without excessive stimulation
- airway patent with protective reflexes
- respiration and oxygenation satisfactory
- stable cardiovascular status
- pain and emesis controlled
- temperature within acceptable limits.

Transferring patients to the ward is the responsibility of a registered practitioner. If transferring the patient back to a ward using a lift, portable oxygen and suction should be available in case of an emergency arising in the lift. There should be at least one registered practitioner who is appropriately trained to manage an emergency (BARNA 2005, Royal College of Anaesthetists 2010) Moving patients around in beds or on trolleys always requires two staff. In an ideal world, to reduce risk to staff a motorised bed/trolley device would be available for the purposes of moving patients to and from their wards.

Transfer to an Acute Setting

When transferring patients to the intensive care unit (ICU), they should always be accompanied by an anaesthetist (Royal College of Anaesthetists 2010). For the purposes of the transfer all the necessary equipment and medications needed for a re-intubation or medical emergency should be readily available. Portable oxygen and suction will be required and the patient should be continuously monitored using invasive and non-invasive monitoring techniques for the duration of the transfer. A registered practitioner will participate in the transfer and will be available to assist in any emergency. In addition, an extra person should participate to assist with moving the bed and patient with the anaesthetist at the head of the bed to ventilate the patient throughout the transfer (Royal College of Anaesthetists 2010).

For transfers to the high dependency unit (HDU) there will be a minimum of two staff, one of whom must be a registered practitioner who can deal with an emergency if needed. Oxygen and suction should be available for the transfer and depending on the patient's condition, it may be appropriate to transfer them while they are being monitored.

For all transfers from recovery a full handover of care is essential, particularly in relation to surgical procedure, medications administered, fluid balance and any issues experienced or noted during the recovery phase of care. All documentation should be completed and transferred with the patient. Patients should not routinely leave recovery without:

- a surgical record of procedure and surgical instructions
- a completed anaesthetic record
- a prescription chart with the appropriate analgesia, antiemetics and fluids prescribed as needed
- all documentation in relation to patient care in recovery and the record of observations and fluid chart as appropriate.

Any patient requiring transfer out of recovery and to another hospital by ambulance will have different needs depending on the reason for transfer and general preoperative health. If the patient is intubated, they will require an anaesthetist to accompany them as per an ITU transfer.

This chapter has given a brief overview of the main guidelines to managing the patient in the PACU. It is a challenging area where the patient's clinical status changes rapidly. Planning care based on consideration of known risk factors together with ongoing physical assessment ensure that complications do not routinely occur. The PACU practitioner performs a semi-autonomous role working alongside the surgical and anaesthetic teams. An excellent knowledge of applied anatomy and physiology, understanding of the intraoperative experience including surgical procedures, anaesthetic drugs and techniques is essential in order to ensure the safe recovery of all patients in this dynamic area.

References

AAGBI (Association of Anaesthetists of Great Britain and Ireland) (2002) *Immediate Postanaesthetic Recovery*. http://www.aagbi.org/sites/default/files/postanaes02.pdf (accessed 17 April 2012).

AAGBI (2007) *Recommendations for Standards of Monitoring during Anaesthesia and Recovery*, 4th edn. http://www.aagbi.org/sites/default/files/standardsofmonitoring07.pdf (accessed 17 April 2012).

AAGBI (2009) *AAGBi Safety Statement: Capnography Outside the Operating Theatre*. http://www.aagbi.org/sites/default/files/AAGBI%20SAFETY%20STATEMENT_0.pdf (accessed 17 April 2012).

Section 3

ASPAN (American Society of Peri-Anesthesia Nurses) (2006) *ASPAN's Evidence-Based Clinical Practrice Guideline for the Prevention and/or Management of PONV/PDNV*. http://www.aagbi.org/sites/default/files/AAGBI%20SAFETY%20 STATEMENT_0.pdf (accessed 17 April 2012).

ASPAN (2010a) *Position Statement on Minimum Staffing*. Cherry Hill, NJ: American Society of Peri-Anesthesia Nurses. www.aspan.org

ASPAN (2010b) *Standards of Practice*. Cherry Hill, NJ: American Society of Peri-Anesthesia Nurses. www.aspan.org

ASPAN (2010c) *Evidence-based Clinical Practice Guideline for the Prevention and/or Treatment of Postoperative Nausea and Vomiting and Post Discharge Nausea and Vomiting in Adult Patients*. Cherry Hill, NJ: American Society of Peri-Anesthesia Nurses. www.aspan.org

BARNA (British Anaesthetic and Recovery Nursing Association) (2005) *Standards of Clinical Practice*. London: BARNA. www.barna.co.uk

Hatfield A and Tronson M (2009) *The Complete Recovery Book*, 4th edn. Oxford: Oxford University Press.

Litwack K (1999) *Core Curriculum for Perianesthesia Nursing Practice*, 4th edn. Philadelphia, PA: WB Saunders.

NHS Estates (2004) *HBN 26: Facilities for Surgical Procedures*, Volume 1. Health Building Notes, Health Technical Memoranda and Model Engineering Specifications. London: Department of Health, HMSO.

Royal College of Anaesthetists (2010) *Guidance on the Provision of Anaesthesia Services for Post-Operative Care*. http://www.rcoa.ac.uk/docs/GPAS-Postop.pdf (accessed 17 April 2012).

Smedley P (2010) Safe staffing in the post anaesthetic care unit: no magic formula. *British Journal of Anaesthetic and Recovery Nursing* 11(1): 3–8.

Tortora GJ and Grabowski SR (2003) *Principles of Anatomy and Physiology*, 10th edn. Hoboken NJ: John Wiley and Sons.

Woodhead K and Wicker P (2005) *A Textbook of Perioperative Care*. Edinburgh: Elsevier Churchill Livingstone.

CHAPTER 24

Pain Management

Felicia Cox

Introduction

Pain is a subjective experience that cannot be objectively measured using a bedside test. Pain is defined by the International Association for the Study of Pain (IASP) as an 'unpleasant sensory and emotional experience associated with actual or potential tissue damage' (Merskey and Bogduk 1994, p. 209). What someone experiences and expresses as pain is a result of their previous history, genetics, gender and a plethora of other variables, including culture and the context of that pain. Pain may be acute or chronic, with the only difference being the duration. Acute pain is usually defined as lasting for less than three months and usually results from an injury or surgery.

Persistent Post-Surgical Pain

A proportion of patients may experience pain that persists after surgery even after wound healing has occurred. The incidence of persistent post-surgical pain is difficult to measure as there is no consensus on what to report and when (Cox 2011). Estimates of prevalence suggest that 2–3% of patients experience this type of pain and it is mostly underrecognised. Certain surgical incisions and types of surgery are known to be associated with persistent pain and these include amputation, thoracotomy, inguinal hernia repair and breast surgery.

Persistent post-surgical pain results from either ongoing inflammation or more frequently from damage to the nerves supplying the area of the incision. Pain which arises from nerve damage is known as neuropathic pain. Neuropathic pain can be the result of physiological (e.g. or nerve compression from sutures) and pathological (e.g. nerve division/destruction during surgery) processes.

Barriers to effective acute pain management

Acute pain arises from recently damaged tissues but there are many barriers to effectively managing acute pain. Carr (2009) reports that patients often have a poor understanding regarding their pain management, thus low expectations of relief from pain, while healthcare professionals have inadequate undergraduate education about pain which

Manual of Perioperative Care: An Essential Guide, First Edition. Edited by Kate Woodhead and Lesley Fudge.
© 2012 John Wiley & Sons, Ltd. Published 2012 by John Wiley & Sons, Ltd.

results in inappropriate knowledge, attitude and skills. Barriers can also result from failing to use a structured approach to pain assessment and not recognising that procedures can result in unrelieved pain, especially post-procedure (e.g. drain removal and tracheal suctioning). Local policy on analgesia storage or the failure of the prescriber to prescribe pro re nata (prn) medicines can hinder efforts to provide the patient with effective and timely interventions.

How one asks a patient about their pain has a direct impact. Asking an open question such as 'Tell me about your pain' will provide more useful information than asking 'Do you have pain?' which is likely to result in an either yes or no answer. Pain assessment needs be structured so that it is known where the pain is, what it is like, how strong is it, what makes it worse and what makes it better. Pain in the recovery room and on the ward should be seen as the fifth vital sign and should be assessed and treated alongside observations of blood pressure, pulse, respiratory rate and temperature. As the patient's advocate you need to ensure that appropriate medicines (including an appropriate dose and frequency) are prescribed for regular and prn use and that they are administered.

Acute pain arises from recently damaged tissues and we tend to think that acute pain results predominantly from surgery. Failure to identify other commonly occurring acute pain, such as that arising from tissue biopsies and leg ulcer dressings, leads to undertreatment and may have adverse effects on the person experiencing it.

Acute pain is a warning sign and left untreated it can delay wound healing, increase the risk of venous thromboembolism (VTE), affect sleep, induce fear and increase anxiety, thus delaying the patient's recovery. A patient unable to cough efficiently is at risk of pneumonia, while a patient unable to mobilise early is at greater risk of VTE. Both may result in an increased length of hospital stay. It has been suggested that undertreated pain implies poor quality of care, and thus could be construed as a form of torture.

A structured approach to pain management

In 1986 the World Health Organization (WHO) introduced the 'Analgesic Ladder' (Figure 24.1) to improve cancer pain management in the developing world. This ladder has been adapted for use in acute pain and provides a clear structure for prescribing and relies upon regular assessment of pain and reviewing the impact of interventions. The basic principle is that if pain persists or increases, the practitioner needs to move up the

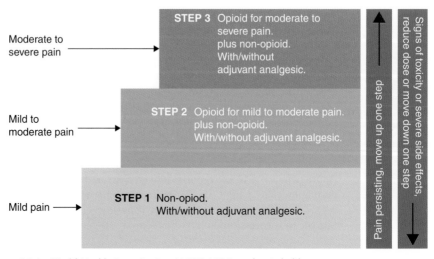

Figure 24.1   World Health Organization (WHO 1986) analgesia ladder.

ladder. This ladder, however, makes no mention of non-pharmacological techniques such as distraction, massage, the application of heat or cold or the use of transcutaneous electrical nerve stimulation (TENS) to relieve pain.

Extensive work has also been undertaken by the Oxford Pain Research Group (www.medicine.ox.ac.uk/bandolier/painres/PRintro.html) and the Australian and New Zealand College of Anaesthetists and Faculty of Pain Medicine (ANZCA 2010) who regularly publish guidance on the evidence for acute pain management.

Physiology of Acute Pain

Pain may be considered as either nociceptive or neuropathic. Nociceptive is a term that describes the normal physiological processes relating to tissue damage, while neuropathic relates to pain caused by damage to or dysfunction of the nervous system (Briggs 2010). What a patient perceives as pain is a complex mix of physiology, previous experiences, culture and emotion.

Nociceptive pain

This type of pain has a protective function and alerts the person experiencing it to potential damage. It provides a reminder to postoperative patients to limit their movements and actions while their wound is healing. A painful stimulus (the surgical incision) is converted to an electrical signal in the nerve cells, which is known as transduction. Damaged cells release a number of chemical neurotransmitters including prostaglandins, serotonin and histamine, which sensitise these nerve endings. The electrical signal is then relayed to the dorsal horn in the spinal cord by two types of peripheral nerves (A-delta and C fibres). A-delta fibres are myelinated and quickly carry sharp, stabbing pain signals. Dull and throbbing pain is carried by the slower unmyelinated C fibres. This process is known as transmission.

These electrical signals are assisted by neurotransmitters so that the signal passes up the spinothalmic and spinoreticular tracts (ascending pathways) in the spinal cord to the brainstem and the thalamus in the brain (Briggs 2010). The information is then processed and relayed to other brain regions. The brainstem produces an autonomic response which can be seen in the patient and is illustrated in Table 24.1.

Repeated exposure to noxious stimuli such as cannulation can sensitise patients to further painful interventions. The body is able to modulate the pain experience by

Table 24.1   Multi-dimensional effects of acute pain.

Physiological effects	Cognitive and emotional responses
• Increased heart rate but decreased myocardial blood flow • Increased blood pressure • Increased respiration rate but decreased depth of inspiration • Elevated blood sugar levels • Decreased gut motility • Nausea and vomiting • Increased sodium and water retention • Muscle spasms and 'splinting' of wound	• Urge to obtain pain relief • Reduced cognitive function • Anxiety • Fear • Irritability and/or aggression • Reduced appetite • Reduced mobility

Adapted with permission of RCN Publishing from Briggs (2010).

producing naturally occurring substances that can inhibit pain. These endogenous opioids include endorphins, enkephalins and dynorphins (Bromley 2005).

The descending pathways from the brain into the dorsal horn of the spinal cord can act as a gate (Melzack and Wall 2008). Opening the gate amplifies the pain signal while closing the gate can reduce the pain signal. Modulation of pain is not just reliant upon electrical signals and the action of analgesics as sensory input (e.g. distraction or relaxation) can reduce the intensity of the pain experience.

Neuropathic pain

This pain is often described by patients as burning, stinging, pricking, tingling or numbness. Neuropathic pain arises from dysfunction of the nerves. Patients may also report paroxysmal pain that may be shooting, stabbing or jabbing in nature. Neuropathic post-surgical pain may also be associated with allodynia (pain evoked by a normally non-painful stimulus such as clothing lightly touching the skin), hyperalgesia (an exaggerated pain response) and autonomic dysfunction (e.g. changes in skin temperature, blood flow and sweating). There are a number of validated tools to screen and diagnose neuropathic pain (Bouhassira and Attal 2011).

Pain Assessment

Hagger-Holt (2009) reminds us that pain is a subjective experience and is influenced by psychosocial factors and a patient's previous experience of pain. Quantifying pain, using a unidimensional tool which looks at only one aspect of the patient's pain experience, that is pain intensity using a numerical rating scale (where 0 = no pain, 10 = worst pain imaginable) is useful but alone does not provide sufficient information to determine the nature and properties of the pain nor its impact upon activities.

Pain after surgery at rest is usually moderate (i.e. 3–4 out of 10) for the initial two to three days, even when parenteral analgesia has been given. Pain at rest tends to resolve in the seven days after surgery, but pain on movement can be moderate or severe and persist for many weeks after surgery (Brennan 2011).

A multi-dimensional tool should be used at each patient assessment. A multidimensional tool is likely to assess the following factors:

- pain intensity (how strong is the pain?)
- location (where is the pain?)
- radiation
- triggers (what makes it worse?)
- alleviators (what makes it better?)
- pattern (brief, intermittent, constant)
- nature (e.g. dull, aching, sharp, stabbing).

An example of a multi-dimensional pain assessment tool is shown in Figure 24.2. Using the same tool at each assessment will determine whether the patient has experienced any improvement in their pain and functional ability. An ideal tool should has the following properties (Brown 2009). It should:

- be understood by patient and staff
- be quick to apply
- be consistently applied and evaluated with patient input
- give consideration to context and behavioural signs
- offer sensible, reliable and valid measures.

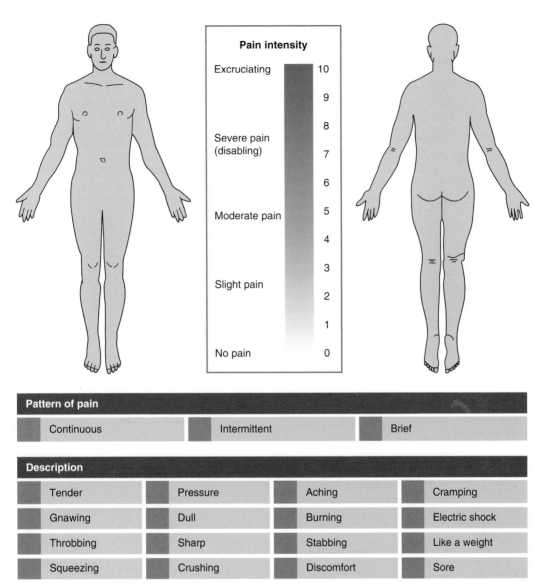

Figure 24.2 An example of a multi-dimensional pain assessment tool. Top part adapted from Melzack R (1975) The McGill Pain Questionnaire: major properties and scoring methods. *Pain* 1: 277–299. Lower part adapted from Bourbonnais F (1981) Pain assessment: development of a tool for the nurse and the patient. *Journal of Advanced Nursing* 6(4): 277–282.

Pain assessment ideally should involve the patient but this can be challenging in non-verbal patients. Assessing pain in neonates requires the use of an observational tool that categorises behaviour (crying, grimacing) and physiology (heart rate, blood pressure). Chapters 25 and 26 describe the specific care of neonates and paediatrics.

Brown (2009) states that assessing pain in patients with moderate to severe cognitive impairment such as an older person with dementia necessitates observation of:

- physiological changes (vital signs, colour, sleep pattern, guarding, loss of appetite)
- body language changes (agitation, aggression, increased or decreased movement) and
- behavioural changes (facial expression, assuming the fetal position).

Patients may be unable to adequately express their pain verbally so the practitioner should observe behaviours to gain an understanding of the patient's pain. The perioperative care of older people is described in Chapter 28.

The Biopsychosocial Model of Pain

Cognitive behaviour therapy (CBT) remains the most important contemporary psychological treatment for pain and is a class of treatments because it includes psychological and sociological aspects of the pain experience. It explores the meaning, behaviours and distress associated with pain by individual patients. Preoperative preparation and information giving can impact positively upon the patient's experience and outcome. Preoperative preparation can consist of information about sensations (what can be expected, the nature and duration of pain), what behaviours will promote recovery (early mobilisation) and cognitive coping training (thoughts and worries a patient has and ways to manage them) (Hagger-Holt 2009).

Pharmacology

Analgesia can be defined as relief from pain, thus analgesics are medicines that relieve pain. How much relief an analgesic provides results from the cause and nature of the pain, a patient's previous pain history, gender and ethnicity (Cox 2010a).

Pharmacology describes the analgesic's action and its interaction with the patient. It has four main divisions:

- pharmacodynamics – what the analgesic does to the body (e.g. reduces inflammation by inhibiting enzyme production)
- pharmacokinetics – what the body does to the analgesic (how the medicine is absorbed, distributed, metabolised and excreted)
- pharmacoeconomics – the cost and benefit ratio compared to other analgesics
- pharmacovigilance – how safe is the analgesic?

Perioperative Analgesic Medicines

Information on all licensed medicines can be found in a document called the Summary of Product Characteristics (SPC). The most up-to-date SPC can be found in the electronic Medicines Compendium (eMC) and downloaded at www.medicines.org.uk. All licence and dose information that follows has been provided from this source unless otherwise indicated.

Paracetamol

Paracetamol is one of the world's most commonly used analgesics. It is understood that this centrally acting analgesic interacts with the cyclo-oxygenase (COX) system, endogenous opioids and serotonergic inhibitory pathways (Mattia and Coluzzi 2009). The oral formulation is well tolerated and very cheap. One gram of paracetamol in combination with codeine 60 mg produces greater analgesia than paracetamol alone. The intravenous formulation is now widely used during and after surgery (ANZCA 2010). A lower dose than the recommended 4 g daily maximum should be used in patients who have renal impairment.

Table 24.2   Non-steroidal anti-inflammatory drugs (NSAIDs) and cyclo-oxygenase inhibitors (COX-2) properties for acute pain.

	Type	Presentations	Cautions
Diclofenac	NSAID	Injection (IV or deep IM) Tablets (IR or PR) Dispersible tablets (IR) Suppositories	Pregnancy Breastfeeding Hypersensitivity to aspirin or other NSAIDs
Keterolac	NSAID	Injection (IV or IM)	Severe heart failure
Flurbiprofen	NSAID	Capsules (PR) Tablets	Older people Bleeding
Ketoprofen	NSAID	Capsules Forte tablets Suppositories Injection (gluteal only)	Renal or hepatic impairment Previous or active peptic ulceration
Ibuprofen	NSAID	Tablets Syrup	
Parecoxib	COX-2 inhibitor	Injection (IV or deep IM)	Contraindicated in patients with ischaemic heart disease, cerebrovascular disease, peripheral arterial disease, moderate to severe heart failure

IV, intravenous; IM, intramuscular; IR, immediate release; PR, prolonged release.

Non-steroidal anti-inflammatory drugs (NSAIDs) and cyclo-oxygenase-2 inhibitors (COX-2)

NSAIDs reduce pain and inflammation in response to injury and inhibit the formation of both COX-1 (protective) and COX-2 (inducible) enzymes (McGavock 2005). COX-1 has many functions and protects the gastric mucosal lining, maintains renal sodium and water balance and platelet aggregation (clumping) (Macintyre and Schug 2007). Examples of non-selective NSAIDs include diclofenac, keterolac and ibuprofen. Using NSAIDs can producing an opioid-sparing effect.

Table 24.2 illustrates the properties of NSAIDs and COX-2 medicines. Caution must be used perioperatively when administering NSAIDs, as contraindications include active peptic ulceration and impaired renal function. A dehydrated or hypovolaemic patient may have renal function dependent upon prostaglandins. Serum urea and creatinine should be checked and the patient's urine output must be in excess of the recommended 0.5 mg/kg per hour so for a patient weighing 70 kg their hourly urine output should exceed 35 mL/h.

Diclofenac 100 mg produces more pain relief than a 50 mg dose for acute pain (Bandolier 2007). Ketorolac is an injectable NSAID that is only licensed for acute post-operative pain. It has a long time to peak effect, between 1 and 2 hours after administration (Smith *et al.* 2000). The maximum daily dose for an adult is 90 mg over 24 hours but this should be reduced for older people to 60 mg over 24 hours.

There has been a debate about the safety of COX-2 inhibitors because of an increased incidence of thromboembolic events in long-term users. Parecoxib is an injectable COX-2 inhibitor licensed for acute pain that can be used intra-operatively as it does not impair platelet aggregation, in contrast to diclofenac and keterolac.

Section 3

Table 24.3 Opioids; receptors and their effects.

Property	Mu (μ) MOP1	Kappa (κ) KOP1	Delta (δ) DOP1
Analgesia	✓	✓	✓
Respiratory depression	✓	✓	✓
Euphoria	✓	✗	✗
Dependence	✓	✗	✓
Gut motility	✓	✗	✗
Sedation	✗	✓	✗
Dysphoria	✗	✗	✗
Hallucinations	✗	✗	✗
Delusions	✗	✗	✗

Opioids

Opioids are a group of medicines that includes opiates derived from the opium poppy (codeine and morphine) and synthetic and semi-synthetic medicines (e.g. oxycodone, fentanyl, remifentanil and tramadol) which are derived from other sources. Opioids exhibit much variation in their properties, potency and unwanted effects (Bromley 2005).

In addition to prostaglandins, the body produces endogenous endorphins that bind with opioid receptors (thereby acting as an agonist) to produce analgesia by inhibiting substance P's transmission of pain signals. Substance P is a neurotransmitter produced by the body in response to a painful stimulus like surgery and it assists the transmission of the pain signal. Opioid agonists such as morphine mimic the effect of the naturally occurring endorphins (Cox 2010b).

Different opioids produce different effects for the different receptors (Table 24.3). The affinity that an opioid has for a certain receptor determines its analgesic effect alongside its onset and duration of action.

Diamorphine is synthetically produced and is the pro-drug of morphine and is converted by tissue esterases to become pharmacologically identical to morphine (Bromley 2005). Codeine is metabolised to morphine by a process known as demethylation (enzyme pathway CYP2D6), but there is a genetic variability in the process as up to 10% of the Caucasian population may have a polymorphism that results in them lacking the ability to convert codeine to morphine thus not gaining any analgesia from codeine. These patients are known as codeine non-responders.

Morphine is the most widely available opioid. It is an effective analgesic in most perioperative patient populations and is very cost effective. In common with other opioids, morphine can cause sedation and respiratory depression but these adverse effects can be reversed using incremental doses of the opioid antagonist naloxone. Morphine can also activate the chemoreceptor trigger zone and cause nausea and vomiting. It is commonly used for patient-controlled analgesia (PCA) (described below). Preservative-free morphine can be administered into the subarachoid (spinal/intrathecal) space to provide analgesia.

Fentanyl has a rapid onset of action (Chumbley and Mountford 2010) and can be useful in patients with renal impairment because, unlike morphine, it does not have any active metabolites than accumulate and cause toxicity (Macintyre and Schug 2007). It is used at induction, may be used in PCA systems and is commonly used in combination with a local anaesthetic for epidural use.

Table 24.4 Local anaesthetics summary for infiltration (field blocks).

	Concentration (mg/mL)	Dose plain (mL)	Dose plain (mg)
Lidocaine	10	0.5–30	5–300
Ropivacaine	7.5	1–30	7.5–225
Bupivacaine	2.5	<60	<150
Levobupivacaine	2.5	1–60	2.5–150

All data obtained from Summary of Product Characteristics from eMC at www.medicines.org.uk.

Oxycodone may also be used intraoperatively as it has a longer duration of action than fentanyl and, like fentanyl, lacks any active metabolites.

Alfentanil is an analogue of fentanyl which has short duration of action. It is usually administered by a continuous infusion and has a lower incidence of respiratory depression compared with morphine (Wicker and Bocos 2010).

Remifentanil is an ultra short-acting opioid often used for total intravenous anaesthesia (TIVA) and also in combination with propofol in the recovery room and intensive care unit. Patients need to have a loading dose of a longer acting opioid (e.g. morphine) approximately 30 minutes before reducing the remifentanil infusion rate in a step-wise fashion. A loading dose is given to avoid pain because the context-sensitive half-life of remifentanil is less than 2.5 minutes.

Tramadol is a weak opioid agonist but it also provides analgesia by inhibiting the reuptake of serotonin and norepinephrine. Its metabolism also relies upon the CYP2D6 enzyme and it has an active metabolite which has stronger receptor affinity than the 'parent' molecule (tramadol).

Local anaesthetics

Peripheral and central blockade using local anaesthetic medicines is described in Chapter 9. Local anaesthetic medicines can be used for field/nerve blocks, as infiltration, as continuous infusions or applied topically to surgical wounds before closure. Both motor and sensory nerves may be blocked, depending on the agent used and where the agent is applied. Local anaesthetic medicines have differing potency, toxicity and duration of action. A comparison of doses for local anaesthetics for infiltration or field block are shown in Table 24.4.

Intermediate duration (lidocaine, prilocaine)

Of the amide group of local anaesthetics, lidocaine is the most widely used as it has a short onset of action and good tissue penetration (Viscomi 2004) and is used as a dental anaesthetic and for procedural pain. Lidocaine acts locally and causes stabilisation of the membrane of the neurone by inhibiting the movement of Na^+ ions that are necessary to initiate and conduct the impulse (Scott 2009). It is metabolised by the liver and excreted by the kidneys. It should be used with caution in patients with liver dysfunction as the half-life may be prolonged. It can be infiltrated before cannulation and in minor surgery to provide a field block. As it can be effectively absorbed from mucous membranes it is used as a surface anaesthetic. EMLA® cream consists of a mix of lidocaine and prilocaine. Lidocaine is sometimes combined with epinephrine (adrenaline) to reduce bleeding. Plain lidocaine is available in a wide variety of presentations including sprays, gels and a topical liquid.

Long duration (bupivacaine, levobupivacaine and ropivacaine)

These three medicines are available in ampoules for infiltration and block use and infusion bags for continuous infusion for peripheral and central blocks. Recent guidance outlines the care of patients receiving epidural analgesia in the hospital setting (Faculty of Pain Medicine 2010).

Bupivacaine hydrochloride is an amide local anaesthetic principally used for spinal or epidural analgesia. It is a racemic mixture which has the potential for cardiotoxicity thus is not used for intravenous analgesia. Bupivacaine is metabolised by the liver, therefore patients with severe liver disease are at risk of toxicity. It has a longer onset of action compared to lidocaine taking up to 30 minutes for full effect. It is often used in epidural analgesia for acute pain and labour. Bupivacaine may be combined with epinephrine (adrenaline) as epinephrine causes local vasoconstriction, thus reducing the rate of absorption and increasing the duration of action of nerve blocks (e.g. intercostal nerve blocks). Combinations of local anaesthetics and epinephrine should never be used for digit (finger or toe) blocks as vasoconstriction is likely to impair the blood supply to the digit.

Levobupivacaine is a chiral mixture and has anaesthetic and analgesic properties similar to bupivacaine but with fewer adverse effects. Levobupivacaine is used for pain management as a continuous or patient-controlled epidural infusion, for the management of postoperative pain and labour analgesia.

Ropivacaine is indicated for surgical anaesthesia including epidural blocks for surgery including Caesarean section. It is also used for major nerve field blocks and in continuous and intermittent epidural infusions. In common with other amide local anaesthetic medicines, ropivacaine is metabolised by the liver and must be used with caution in patients with hepatic disease.

Methods of Analgesia Delivery

Intramuscular injections of opioids were the mainstay of postoperative analgesia until the widespread adoption of patient-controlled analgesia in the late 1980s. Injections can be painful and result in poor-quality analgesia as they are intermittent and may result in peaks and troughs as illustrated in Figure 24.3. The initiation and administration of continuous central (spinal/epidural) and peripheral blocks are described in Chapter 9.

Patient-Controlled Analgesia

Patient-controlled analgesia (PCA) is often associated with intravenous opioids but it does refer more widely to patient initiated dosing of medicines. This includes peripheral local anaesthetic blocks, epidural analgesia or subcutaneous opioids. This section describes solely intravenous opioid PCA for moderate to severe postoperative pain as this is the most common technique, although the principles are transferable.

PCA requires a functional cannula, an infusion device (pump), a giving set with a one-way valve, a reservoir of opioid, and a patient demand button. Patients must be educated about PCA, agree to use this analgesia system and be capable of pressing the button prior to commencement (Chumbley and Mountford 2010). Chumbley *et al.* (2002) identified from focus groups that patients were concerned about the dangers and side-effects of morphine, support from staff, what the system looked like and suggestions for how to use to use PCA. Information showing images of the system and suggestions for use together with details of the medicine and potential side-effects should be provided to the patient preoperatively. Practitioner-administered analgesia may be more suitable for patients who have a cognitive impairment or where there are communication difficulties.

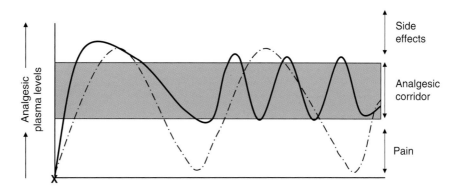

Figure 24.3   Analgesia associated with intramuscular (IM) injections and intravenous patient-controlled analgesia (PCA). The dashed line illustrates the peaks and troughs of analgesia associated with IM injections with a significant proportion of time spent below the analgesic corridor which indicates pain. The unbroken line demonstrates that once the PCA loading dose administered by the recovery staff has worn off then patients become aware of pain. Patients may tend to only press the bolus button when they become aware of pain in the future as they are not instructed about PCA prior to surgery. The cross (×) indicates the administration of the PCA loading dose and the initial IM injection.

In theory, PCA provides immediate access to analgesia and allows the patient to titrate analgesia against side-effects, but the patient must be awake and alert to use this system. It has been suggested that staff are less likely to question patients about their pain as immediate access implies adequate analgesia.

Prescriptions for PCA must state the medicine concentration, loading dose, bolus dose, lockout period and 4-hourly limit. The loading dose (in milligrams or micrograms) is the initial dose usually administered in recovery which 'loads' the patient with the medicine prior to the patient assuming control of the system. This loading dose ensures the patient has effective analgesia before discharge from recovery. The bolus dose is the pre-programmed dose defined within the prescription that a patient self-administers when they make a demand for analgesia by pressing the button. This dose may vary because of age, weight, previous opioid exposure and other individual factors. The lockout period is a pre-set time (in minutes) also defined within the prescription that a patient must wait after administering a dose before the device will deliver a subsequent dose. Most devices have the ability to determine the maximum amount of medicine that a patient may receive in any 4-hour period but there is no evidence to support the use of this limit (ANZCA 2010).

Pain in Special Circumstances

The care of patients across the age spectrum (from neonates to the older person) is described in Chapters 25–28. Acute postoperative pain can be challenging to manage in patients with chronic pain, in known or suspected substance misusers and in patients who are opioid dependent such as patients with cancer pain. Further reading on the patient groups is listed below.

Summary

Pain is a complex and individualised phenomenon. Previous experiences will influence the patient's perception and expression of pain. Using a structured approach to pain

Section 3

assessment coupled with an understanding of the most appropriate pharmacological and non-pharmacological techniques to manage acute pain will improve the patient experience of this multidimensional phenomenon.

References

ANZCA (Australian and New Zealand College of Anaesthetists) (2010) *Acute Pain Management: Scientific Evidence*, 3rd edn. Canberra: Australian and New Zealand College of Anaesthetists and Faculty of Pain Medicine. http://www.anzca.edu.au/resources/books-and-publications/Acute%20pain%20management%20-%20scientific%20evidence%20-%20third%20edition.pdf

Bandolier (2007) *Oxford League Table of Analgesics in Acute Pain.* http://www.medicine.ox.ac.uk/bandolier/booth/painpag/Acutrev/Analgesics/Leagtab.html (accessed 29 March 2011).

Bouhassira D and Attal N (2011) Diagnosis and assessment of neuropathic pain: The saga of clinical tools. *Pain* 152(3S): S74–83.

Brennan T (2011) Pathophysiology of postoperative pain. *Pain* 152(3S): S33–40.

Briggs E (2010) Understanding the experience and physiology of pain. *Nursing Standard* 25(3): 35–39.

Bromley L (2005) Opioids and codeine. In Jagger S and Holdcroft A (eds) *Core Topics in Pain.* Cambridge: Cambridge University Press, pp. 269–276.

Brown D (2009) Principles of acute pain assessment. In Cox F (ed.) *Perioperative Pain Management.* Oxford: Wiley Blackwell, pp. 17–44.

Carr E (2009) Barriers to effective pain management. In Cox F (ed.) *Perioperative Pain Management.* Oxford: Wiley Blackwell, pp. 45–63.

Chumbley G and Mountford L (2010) Patient-controlled analgesia infusion pumps for adults. *Nursing Standard* 25(8): 35–40.

Chumbley G, Hall GM and Salmon P (2002) Patient-controlled analgesia; what information does the patient want. *Journal of Advanced Nursing* 39(5): 459–471.

Cox F (2010a) An overview of pharmacology and acute pain: part one. *Nursing Standard* 25(4): 35–38.

Cox F (2010b) An overview of pharmacology and acute pain: part two. *Nursing Standard* 25(5): 35–39.

Cox F (2011) Persistent post-surgical pain. *Independent Nurse* 2 May, 34–35.

Faculty of Pain Medicine, Royal College of Anaesthetists, Royal College of Nursing *et al.* (2010) *Best Practice in the Management of Epidural Analgesia in the Hospital Setting.* London: FPM. http://www.britishpainsociety.org/pub_prof_EpiduralAnalgesia2010.pdf (accessed 29 March 2011).

Hagger-Holt R (2009) Psychosocial perspectives of acute pain. In Cox F (ed.) *Perioperative Pain Management.* Oxford: Wiley Blackwell, pp. 64–80.

Macintyre PE and Schug SA (2007) *Acute Pain Management: A Practical Guide*, 3rd edn. Edinburgh: Saunders Elsevier.

Mattia C and Coluzzi F (2009) What anesthesiologists should know about paracetamol (acetaminophen). *Minerva Anestesiologica* 75(11): 744–653.

McGavock H (2005) *How Drugs Work: Basic Pharmacology for Healthcare Professionals*, 2nd edn. Oxford: Radcliffe Press.

Melzack H and Wall PD (2008) *The Challenge of Pain*, 2nd edn. London: Penguin Books.

Merskey H and Bogduk M (eds) (1994) *Classification of Chronic Pain*, 2nd edn. Seattle WA: International Association for the Study of Pain Taskforce on Taxonomy. IASP Press. http://www.iasp-pain.org/AM/Template.cfm?Section=Pain_Definitions&Template=/CM/HTMLDisplay.cfm&ContentID=1728 (accessed 29 March 2011).

Scott K (2009) How analgesics work. In Cox F (ed.) *Perioperative Pain Management.* Oxford: Wiley Blackwell, pp. 95–107.

Smith LA, Carroll D, Edwards JE, Moore RA and McQuay HJ (2000) Single dose ketorolac and pethidine in acute post-operative pain: systematic review with meta-analysis. *British Journal of Anaesthesia* 84(1): 48–58.

Viscomi CM (2004) Pharmacology of local anaesthetics. In Rathmell JP, Neal JM and Visconi CM (eds) *Regional Anesthesia. The Requisites in Anesthesiology.* Philadelphia, PA: Elsevier Mosby.

Wicker P and Bocos A (2010) Perioperative pharmacology. In Wicker P and O'Neill J (eds) *Caring for the Perioperative Patient.* Oxford: Wiley Blackwell, pp. 101–133.

World Health Organization (1986) *Analgesic Ladder.* http://www.who.int/cancer/palliative/painladder/en/ (accessed 29 March 2011).

Further Readings

British Pain Society (2007) *Pain and Substance Misuse: Improving the patient experience.* London: British Pain Society. http://www.britishpainsociety.org/book_misuse_patients.pdf

Section 3

British Pain Society (2010) Management of acute pain in cancer patients. In *Cancer Pain Management*. London: British Pain Society. http://www.britishpainsociety.org/book_cancer_pain_v5_ch12.pdf

Kumar A and Allcock N (2008) *Pain in the Older Person*. London: Help the Aged. http://www.britishpainsociety.org/book_pain_in_older_age_ID7826.pdf

Royal College of Nursing (2009) *The recognition and Assessment of Acute Pain in Children*. London: RCN Publishing. http://www.rcn.org.uk/__data/assets/pdf_file/0004/269185/003542.pdf

Section 4

Different Patient Care Groups

CHAPTER 25

Neonatal Surgery

Helen Carter

Neonatal surgery covers the preterm infant to the first month of post normal gestational life. In practice this means from 24 weeks gestation to 44 weeks gestation and beyond. The extreme preterm infant requiring surgery may weigh between 500 g and 1 kg, less than a bag of sugar. Many neonates who have not been home post birth will remain on the neonatal surgical unit until they gain enough weight, generally reaching 3–3.5 kg depending on local protocols/guidelines, before being cared for on the conventional paediatric ward. Neonatal surgery is conducted in supraregional centres by experienced paediatric surgeons with specially trained, highly skilled staff with excellent support from other services, such as knowledgeable nurses, paediatric theatre practitioners, neonatologists, paediatric radiologists, physiotherapists, microbiologists, occupational therapists, pharmacists and dieticians, to name but a few.

Most centres use a retrieval service to safely transport neonates requiring surgery from hospitals which do not have these services. As many neonates require surgery within the first few days of birth, the mother may not be in the same hospital. This raises issues about consent for surgery, which sometimes this has to be done over the phone. This is not ideal. Many congenital deformities can be identified during pregnancy. In this case the parents will have had counselling from their obstetrician and a paediatric surgeon so they have some idea of what to expect. It is a stressful and emotional time for the family when a baby is born, but when they have surgery to cope with as well it becomes even more difficult. This is all happening when a mother should be bonding with her baby, but we may be starving the infant for surgery, and parents often worry about touching their newborn child following surgery in case they hurt them. It is a time where the parents need a lot of support and understanding.

To many theatre practitioners, involvement in neonatal surgery is a daunting prospect. The difference from adult practice is vast, from the obvious contrast in size to the wide variety of surgical procedures the practitioner needs to become familiar with. The bulk of work in the adult field involves surgery to repair the body from the effects of disease or trauma, whereas in the neonate most surgery is carried out to repair congenital deformities due to interruption of normal embryological development or to correct the complications due to prematurity. Table 25.1 shows the incidence of a number of congenital abnormalities. The neonate may go on to need further surgery into

Table 25.1   Incidence of congenital abnormalities per live births (approx).

Congenital heart defect	1:125
Hypospadias	1:300
Talipes	1:1000
Congenital diaphragmatic hernia	1:2500
Gastroschisis	1:2000
Tracheoesophageal fistula/oesophageal atresia	1:3500
Anorectal malformations	1:5000
Duodenal atresia	1:7500
Biliary atresia	1:15 000

childhood and on into adulthood. A good knowledge of normal anatomy is required in order to be able to understand the altered anatomy caused by congenital abnormalities.

Because of the size of these patients the environment and equipment in the operating room needs careful consideration. Neonates do not have the same physiological ability to regulate their temperature as the adult or older child. Fluid maintenance during surgery differs, as does method of administration. Haemoglobin in the neonate changes from fetal to adult. Medication requirements differ because of the immature hepatic enzyme system and reduced renal function following birth, which can drastically increase the half-life of some medications. Appropriate instrumentation should be selected due to the nature of the tissues and the scale of the operative site. Magnification in the form of surgical 'loupes' or microscopes may be necessary. Consideration is needed of the draping materials because of their weight, method of keeping in place and material (i.e. disposable versus reusable). Disposable drapes are generally lighter but usually have an adhesive edge to adhere the drape to the patient, which may remove the delicate skin of the newborn patient.

Neonatal surgery is complicated not just because of the wide range of abnormalities but also the need for prudent planning for each individual patient from transfer from the ward, through induction of anaesthesia, operation and how the neonate is transferred back to the ward and which ward area is appropriate. Decisions as to whether they require neonatal intensive care or the surgical neonatal ward post surgery will need to be taken. Communication between the theatre practitioners, the ward nurses and neonatologists, the anaesthetist and the operating surgeon are key to ensuring a safe, effective procedure with no delays to the surgery, which may affect the overall outcome for the patient.

Blood loss/Haemostasis and Fluid Requirements

A newborn baby's body comprises 75% water at term (Bhatia 2006), more if preterm, and reduces to 60% by adulthood. In the neonate most of this water is extracellular fluid (ECF), so they do not cope well with fluid loss. In the premature neonate the ratio of ECF to intracellular fluid (ICF) is even higher. In the adult patient ICF is higher than ECF. Electrolyte imbalance during the neonatal period can be a significant problem and should be monitored perioperatively by use of blood gases. This helps the anaesthetist to calculate intravenous (IV) fluid amount and type required.

Neonatal blood volume is around 80 mL/kg so a term baby weighing 3 kg will only have a circulating volume of 240 mL. Prior to surgery, vitamin K should be given.

Vitamin K is necessary for the production of prothrombin, a crucial part of the normal clotting cascade. Preoperative bloods should be taken for full blood count, urea and electrolytes. The infant requires a maternal cross-matched blood sample up to the age of four months (there are exceptions to this, e.g. unusual maternal antibodies). This is because the neonate's haemoglobin is composed of fetal haemoglobin, which has a different oxygen-holding capacity, and there is a gradual change to adult haemoglobin over the first four months of life. General principles for the requirement for transfusion are the same as for adults (i.e. ≥15% of blood volume lost). Therefore a term neonate weighing 3 kg may require transfusion following a loss of only 36 mL during surgery. When dealing with such small volumes it becomes imperative to keep a note of blood loss on swabs through weighing (blood has a similar specific gravity to water, therefore 1 g = 1 mL) and through suctioning, recorded and communicated to the anaesthetist. Syringe drivers can be used for blood transfusion in neonates as long as a 170–200 µm filter is incorporated into the infusion (McClelland 2007). Small Paedipaks containing 40 mL can be obtained.

The need for careful haemostasis is paramount when operating on the neonate. This means gentle tissue handling, acting quickly to stop bleeding and the use of precise diathermy to coagulate even minimal bleeding points. Bipolar diathermy is widely used in neonatal surgery due to the accurate nature of the application and lack of thermal spread found with monopolar diathermy. When dealing with such small, closely located structures this prevents unwanted tissue damage.

Airway Management

Neonates breathe mainly through the nose. This should be remembered when positioning a mask and care should be taken not to apply too much pressure which can obstruct the nasal passages. The larynx is higher and more anterior in the neonate than in the older child and adult. The epiglottis is more floppy and elongated. These differences can make the neonate more difficult to intubate. The narrowest part of the upper airway is at the cricoid ring compared to the larynx in the post-pubertal child and adult. The cricoid ring forms a natural cuff, and for this reason uncuffed endotracheal (ET) tubes are used. These allow an air leak that prevents mucosal oedema which could block a small airway. In the neonate requiring prolonged ventilation, this could lead to subglottic stenosis.

Use of the correct size of ET tube is essential to prevent damage. The ET tube size formula (age in years/4 + 4) does not work for the infant under 1 year. As a guide, for the neonate use the following internal diameter (ID) tubes:

- < 1000 g: 2.5 mm ID
- 1000–2000 g: 3.0 mm ID
- 2000–3000 g: 3.5 mm ID
- > 3000 g: 3.5–4.0 mm ID.

A tube size down and up from the one anticipated should be prepared. Neonatal laryngoscopes have a straight blade but not all anaesthetists like this pattern. For oral intubation some anaesthetists prefer the tube to have a stilette inserted. If required it should be ensured the stilette is 1 cm inside the distal end of the ET tube to prevent damage on insertion.

Prior to intubation and postoperatively, to keep the airway open the neonate's head should be placed in a neutral position, preventing their relatively large head flexing on their comparatively short neck and avoiding blockage of the airway. If the tongue is occluding the airway a chin lift may also be necessary. Newborn babies will be observed

Section 4

overnight following surgery up to 52 weeks gestational age, or 60 weeks for premature babies, because they are prone to apnoea post anaesthetic due to immature respiratory control.

Temperature Regulation

Neonatal and premature infants have a large surface area to body mass ratio compared to adults. This means that they are more inclined to lose heat by evaporation, convection, radiation and conduction than older children or adults. Healthy term neonates maintain their temperature by peripheral vasoconstriction in response to their surroundings, but in premature babies this response is poorly developed. Anaesthesia also dulls this response. Neonates are unable to shiver, a mechanism used by older children and adults to trap air beneath body hair to retain a warm air layer next to the skin. They also have very thin skin and little insulating fat. During induction of anaesthesia the neonate is often exposed for intubation, IV access and pain-controlling blocks. In order to minimise heat loss during this time the use of an overhead heater, heated mattresses, warm ambient room temperature and increased humidity can help.

During surgery it is not usually possible for the surgeon to operate under an overhead heater, therefore other heating adjuncts should be used such as Bair Huggers™, heated mattresses, plastic sheeting covering the non-operative site, baby bonnet, warmed prepping and washing solutions and a warm ambient theatre temperature. Care should be taken not to leave the baby exposed for too long during prepping the operative site and draping. Using modern water-repellent material drapes and disposable waterproof drapes reduces the chance of losing heat with wet drapes being in contact with the baby's skin for long periods.

Instrumentation

Theatre practitioners will find that the instrumentation used for neonatal surgery looks very similar to that used for adults but the tips of instruments are finer to cope with the small delicate structures. The small size sutures used necessitate delicate needleholders designed to hold and not damage size 5/0, 6/0 and smaller sutures, and the instruments are shorter because in general in neonatal surgery the surgeon is not 'a long way down a deep gaping hole'. That is not to say that there are not times when longer instruments are required but these tend to have a slimmer body to manage the access through small incisions (e.g. if a long artery forceps is required then a Kilner or Kelly forceps which is less bulky and finer pointed rather than a Spencer Wells would be appropriate). Malleable copper retractors are widely used to provide good visualisation of the operative field and when deeper retractors than cats' paws are needed, Ragnell's or small Langenbeck's are used.

Neonatal Emergencies

Gastroschisis

Gastroschisis is a herniation of the abdominal contents through a full thickness defect in the baby's abdominal wall, in the region of the umbilicus, usually to the right (see Figure 25.1). It is generally recognised during pregnancy and the mother delivered in a centre with facilities for neonatal surgery, to prevent the bowel being exposed for a

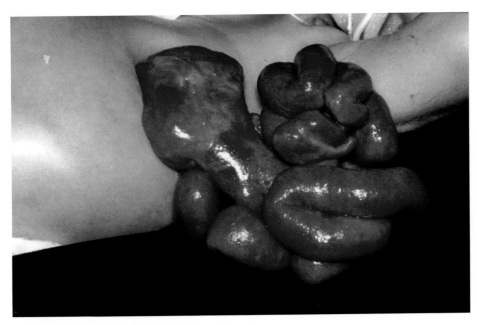

Figure 25.1 Baby born with gastroschisis.

prolonged period post delivery. Immediately after delivery, the baby's abdomen including the exteriorised contents are wrapped in a plastic protective wrap to prevent heat and fluid loss from the exposed bowels. There was a time when all neonates with gastroschisis were operated on within a few hours of birth to reduce the bowel back into the abdomen or to place the bowel into a handfashioned silo to allow the protected contents to be reduced over the next few days. The neonate would then return to the operating theatre to formally close the abdomen. Current practice in many centres is to apply a preformed silastic silo on the neonatal unit without the use of general anaesthetic, as described by Owen *et al.* (2006). The bowel is slowly reduced and the abdomen closed without the need for suturing. This is not possible for all babies with gastroschisis and the theatre practitioner working in neonatal surgery will continue to see these neonates coming through the operating theatre.

Oesophageal Atresia

The most common configuration of this condition is oesophageal atresia with distal tracheoesophageal fistula (85%) as shown in Figure 25.2. If not identified on ultrasound examinations during pregnancy the baby presents with excessive salivation, choking, coughing and respiratory distress or problems if passing of a nasogastric tube is attempted. Many of these neonates will also have other associated congenital abnormalities. This congenital condition requires surgery to close the fistula, thus preventing over gastric dilatation as the baby breathes, which can lead to gastric perforation, and anastomosis of the two ends of the oesophagus to effect continuity to allow oral feeding and prevent aspiration. After birth a Replogle tube is inserted into the upper pouch of the oesophagus via the nasal route. This tube has two lumens, one inside the other, to allow small quantities of saline to be inserted via the outer tube to soften salivary secretions and suction to be applied to the shorter inner tube to prevent overflow of secretions into the lungs without getting blocked by sucking against the mucosa of the upper pouch. If the neonate requires artificial ventilation this

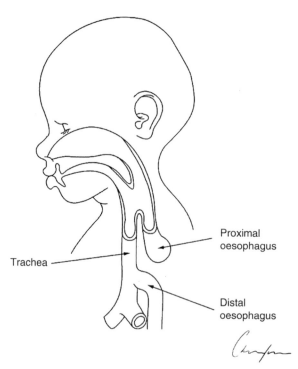

Figure 25.2 Baby born with oesophageal atresia and distal tracheoesophageal fistula. Image courtesy of David Crabbe, Consultant Paediatric Surgeon.

should be performed with low pressures to lower the risk of gastric perforation and surgery becomes more urgent.

The procedure is usually carried out through a right thoracotomy unless the neonate has an abnormally positioned aortic arch. It is possible to block the fistula using a small Fogarty embolectomy catheter inserted through the fistula with use of a rigid broncho-scope. This is of temporary benefit while performing the thoracotomy. In the very unstable neonate it may be necessary to perform a crash thoracotomy and just ligate the fistula, bringing the baby back to theatre a few days later to formally close the fistula and anastomose the oesophagus.

Some neonates with this congenital deformity will require multiple trips back to theatre to deal with further complications, such as the gap between the two ends of the oesophagus being too far apart to anastomose, requiring either gastric transposition or interposition of colon or small bowel to the gap. They can go on to develop tracheo-malacia, oesophageal strictures at the anastomosis site, food blockages in the oesopha-gus and gastro-oesophageal reflux requiring surgery.

Malrotation with volvulus

Malrotation of the gut is a congenital deformity where the distance between the duo-denojejunal flexure (DJ flexure) and the caecum is small, leaving the mid-gut mesentery on a narrow pedicle. The DJ flexure should sit to the left of the spine in line with the pylorus of the stomach and the caecum should sit down in the right ileac fossa. In this normal configuration the mid-gut mesenteric base is wide and extremely unlikely to twist. If the caecum is high and the DJ flexure to the right of the spine the mid-gut can twist, termed a volvulus (Figure 25.3), which cuts off the blood supply to much of the

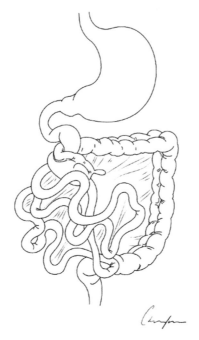

Figure 25.3 Malrotation with volvulus.

small bowel. This is a real surgical emergency and, if not treated expeditiously, can lead to much of the bowel needing to be removed and a life of living with short bowel syndrome for the baby with complications of parenteral nutrition, malabsorption issues, bowel lengthening procedures and liver and small bowel transplant prospects for the future if the baby survives the initial period.

Surgery involves a laparotomy, untwisting the gut, straightening and bringing forward the duodenum, division of Ladd's bands, widening the mesenteric base and inversion appendicectomy. The appendix is removed because at the end of the procedure the caecum is positioned on the left of the abdomen and if in later life the child has appendicitis it could go unrecognised due to the non-anatomical position. This is called a Ladd's procedure. If any of the bowel is ischaemic and does not show signs of improvement following untwisting, excision of the dead segment is required.

Conclusion

Survival rates for neonates with congenital deformities are increasing due to improving neonatal services and advances in anaesthetic and surgical techniques. Babies born with oesophageal atresia in the 1960s had a survival rate of 60–70% whereas in the twenty-first century a survival rate of 90–100% is the norm (Johnson 2005). Duro *et al.* (2008) report a survival rate for short bowel syndrome of 73–89%. Improvements in introducing enteral feeding and caring for these patients using a multi-disciplinary approach have enhanced outcomes. Progress in paediatric liver and bowel transplantation gives hope for better results in the future.

The theatre practitioner will find neonatal surgery to be constantly challenging as new treatments and our ability to perform new techniques, such as thorascopic surgery, on small premature babies evolves.

Section 4

References

Bhatia J (2006) Fluid and electrolyte management in the very low birth weight neonate. *Journal of Perinatology* 26: S19–S21.

Duro D, Kamin D and Duggan C (2008) Overview of pediatric short bowel syndrome. *Journal of Pediatric Gastroenterology and Nutrition* 47: S33–S36.

Johnson PRV (2005) Oesophageal atresia. *Infant* 1(5): 163–167.

McClelland DBL (ed.) (2007) *Handbook of Transfusion Medicine*. London: The Stationery Office.

Owen A, Marven S, Jackson L *et al.* (2006) Experience of bedside preformed silo staged reduction and closure for gastroschisis. *Journal of Pediatric Surgery* 41(11): 1830–1835.

CHAPTER 26

Paediatric Surgery

Helen Carter

Children are not small adults. This certainly adds to the interest of this speciality. A laparotomy performed for bowel obstruction on a six-month-old infant is very different to the same procedure on a 13-year-old child, requiring a different approach to the child from anaesthetic room, through the operating theatre and on to care in the recovery room. Different instrumentation is required for what is essentially a similar operative procedure. Differential diagnosis for bowel obstruction would also vary depending on age and previous medical history. High on the list for a six month old would be intussusception, whereas this would be very unlikely in the 13 year old.

Ideally, children should be cared for in child-only areas that meet the needs of children, parents and families by suitably trained staff who are able to maintain their skills (Department of Health 2004). In practice this means children's theatres should be isolated from adults; however this is not always possible in many Trusts. There are measures that can be taken to ensure the environment is appropriately managed, such as having child-only theatre lists or putting children first on the list, making the anaesthetic room child friendly, decorated with pictures, having toys and suitably age-related books available, screening off an area in the recovery room to keep children separate to adult patients and ensuring that theatre and recovery staff have regular exposure to caring for children. Theatre complexes performing paediatric surgery should employ child branch nurses, and operating department practitioners (ODPs) should possess child-specific skills to deal with this diverse group of patients. Training for these theatre personnel needs to include paediatric life support, safeguarding children and communication skills.

Consent

The parents usually give consent for surgery performed on children under the age of 16 years unless the parents do not have parental responsibility for the child, in which case the legal guardians consent is sought. Children should be involved in the consent process along with someone with parental responsibility (General Medical Council 2008). For children born after 1 December 2003 in England and Wales (Northern

Manual of Perioperative Care: An Essential Guide, First Edition. Edited by Kate Woodhead and Lesley Fudge.
© 2012 John Wiley & Sons, Ltd. Published 2012 by John Wiley & Sons, Ltd.

Ireland 15 April 2002, Scotland 04 May 2006), where both parents are cited on the child's birth certificate, they can both legally give consent for surgery. For children born before this date, if the parents are not married, only the mother has parental responsibility and therefore the right to give consent for the child. If a child under 16 years is deemed competent to make this decision they can provide their own consent. In order to be deemed competent they should be able to show they have the maturity and understanding needed to be able to make an informed decision regarding the treatment required. However if a patient under 18 years, although deemed competent, refuses treatment and that refusal puts their health in danger, they are not legally allowed to reject treatment (General Medical Council 2007).

For the theatre practitioner to ensure the correct procedure is to be performed on the right child they should follow the WHO Surgical Safety Checklist (World Health Organization 2008), endorsed by the National Patient Safety Agency in 2009, before the theatre session begins and then subsequently for each patient listed. The identity of the child should be checked by their name bands and by communicating with the adult with parental responsibility that accompanies the child to theatre. Good practice dictates that the practitioner in the anaesthetic room asks the accompanying adult, and the child if appropriate, if they understand the procedure the child is to undergo.

Children with Chronic Conditions

Children with chronic conditions such as cerebral palsy, inflammatory bowel disease, cystic fibrosis and cancer may well require many periods of hospitalisation, including several trips to theatre during their childhood. If not managed well, their theatre visits can become extremely traumatic for them and their family. Careful planning is essential to make the episodes as easy to cope with as possible. Many procedures these children go through are unpleasant, but with good communication they can understand what is going to happen and how they are likely to feel. Anticipated stress is easier to cope with than the unknown.

Familiar environments and friendly, honest staff can be beneficial as they can build up a rapport and trust with them. Allowing children to wear their own clothes to theatre can reduce anxiety. If this is sanctioned, the parents should be informed beforehand that the clothes should be clean, to avoid infection issues, and they should be loose fitting and easy to remove when the child is asleep. Tops with a front or back opening are easier to remove than those that need to be taken off over the child's head, not an uncomplicated manoeuvre when the child is intubated! This is not always appropriate, for example, the larger child or teenager requiring major surgery or screening colonoscopy where a hospital gown may be more suitable due to the likelihood of the clothes becoming soiled.

If the child does not require premedication to reduce worry and concern, they should be able to walk to theatre, brought in a pushchair or wheelchair or be carried in their parent's arms instead of being transported by hospital trolley. Some centres provide motorised toy vehicles for children to drive themselves to theatre. Asking the child how they wish to go to theatre can give them a sense of inclusion, independence and control just by giving them a decision they can make themselves. If not contraindicated, the anaesthetist will often allow the child to decide on method of induction of anaesthesia (i.e. gas or intravenous). All children having general anaesthesia will have a cannula inserted but this can be performed following gas induction if preferred. Parents accompanying their child in the anaesthetic room need to be aware of their role. They are there to support their child and can be extremely helpful in utilising distraction techniques during cannulation if well informed in advance.

All the points in this section also apply to all children coming to theatre, in order to make the experience as least disturbing as possible. A visit to hospital for surgery can be a satisfactory experience if handled well.

Gastrointestinal Endoscopy in the Paediatric Patient

In contrast to the adult patient, most centres perform gastrointestinal (GI) endoscopy in children under general anaesthetic. Much adult GI endoscopy is looking for cancers, whereas in children most is performed to diagnose conditions such as gastro-oesophageal reflux, *Helicobacter pylori*, chronic conditions such as Crohn's disease or ulcerative colitis, and screening programmes for premalignant conditions such as familial adenomatous polyposis (FAP).

As adults are awake it is possible to encourage them to move when their position needs changing. In the anaesthetised child care should be taken to support joints on changes required to position and pressure points should be protected throughout the procedure. Moving and handling skills are required to ensure safe positioning of the child and also to protect the theatre practitioner. Upper GI endoscopy in an anaesthetised patient puts the position of the endotracheal tube (ET tube) at risk of becoming dislodged with movement of the scope. The practitioner should be aware of this possibility, and ensure the ET tube remains in the correct position. The ET tube needs to be secured to the side of the mouth to enable the endoscope to be easily inserted. The child's lips should be protected to make sure they do not get dragged across the teeth if a mouthguard is not used.

As with all surgery, the theatre practitioner should make certain the child's privacy and dignity is protected at all times, by only exposing the child when required and by making sure the child is clean and comfortable at the end of the procedure.

Paediatric Emergencies

Intussusception

Intussusception is a potentially life-threatening condition most commonly affecting infants aged three months to one year of age. Eighty per cent of cases are seen in children less than two years old. The distal small bowel telescopes into the colon (Figure 26.1). Most intussusceptions occur for unknown reasons, however following a viral illness the lymphoid tissue (Peyer's patches) in the distal ileum become more prolific, which is thought to contribute to the reason this occurs. Some intussusceptions do have what is known as a 'lead point' such as a polyp or Meckel's diverticulum.

These infants present with abdominal colicky pain, worsening over time. They may experience abdominal distension and vomiting. As the process worsens they might pass 'redcurrant jelly' stool, but this is a late sign of intussusception. Initial treatment involves fluid resuscitation followed by attempted air enema reduction under radiological control. This is successful in about 84% of cases (Lui *et al.* 2001). For those patients who fail air enema reduction, laparotomy is the only course of action.

Laparotomy is performed through a right transverse incision above the level of the umbilicus. The affected part of the bowel is delivered and the bowel gently squeezed to push out the intussuscepted portion. If it is not possible to reduce the intussusception completely or if the bowel is necrotic then a resection of the affected portion is necessary. Paediatric bowel is anastomosed with interrupted sutures to allow growth of the anastomosis site, therefore preventing stenosis as the child grows.

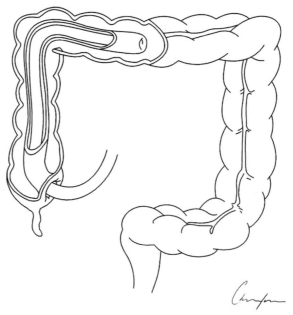

Figure 26.1   Intussusception.

These patients require close monitoring in the post-anaesthetic care unit (PACU) as they can collapse due to reperfusion injury following reduction of the intussusception.

Foreign body in the airway

Small children are prone to put things in their mouth and sometimes they either swallow them or occasionally inhale them. Toys have warning messages on them to inform parents and carers of the appropriate age the toy is intended for, and those toys with small removable parts are recommended for children over three years of age. Food does not generally carry the same warning messages and infants can choke on small hard items such as pieces of carrot or nuts. Peanuts are particularly irritant if lodged in the airway and should not be left long even if the child appears to not be distressed. The anatomy of the airway is such that the right main bronchus is slightly larger and at less of an angle to the trachea than the left, therefore a peanut would be most likely to pass through the trachea and become lodged in the right main bronchus as shown in Figure 26.2.

Removal of the peanut involves the infant undergoing an emergency bronchoscopy under general anaesthetic. Some surgeons will initially insert a flexible bronchoscope either through an ET tube or through a laryngeal mask to ascertain the presence of a foreign body. In order to remove the peanut a rigid bronchoscope and optical forceps are required. The rigid bronchoscope is inserted into the airway with the aid of a laryngoscope following the spraying of local anaesthetic to the vocal chords. The quality of vision through a rigid bronchoscope far exceeds that of the flexible bronchoscope, making visualisation much better. The child can be ventilated through the bronchoscope once the side-vents on the scope have passed through the chords and cricoid cartilage. The optical forceps are then passed down the bronchoscope and the peanut grasped, removing the whole scope, optical forceps and the peanut from the child in one movement. Airway control is then passed back to the anaesthetist. The bronchoscope is then reinserted to ensure no fragments remain. Due to the vocal chord's being sprayed with local anaesthetic the child cannot eat or drink until the effect has worn off, usually a couple of hours.

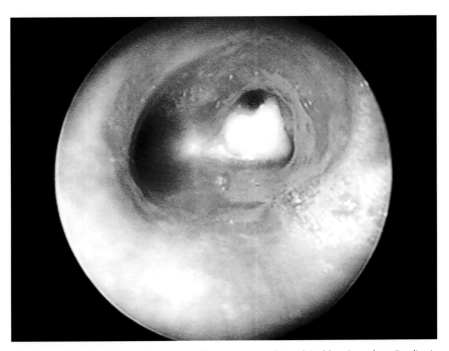

Figure 26.2 Peanut in right main bronchus. Photo courtesy of David Crabbe, Consultant Paediatric Surgeon.

Advances in Paediatric Surgery

Surgery has advanced over the years and paediatric surgery is no exception. Breakthroughs in technology and scientific research have changed the way we manage surgical procedures. For example, for pyloric stenosis, a condition where the pyloric sphincter, the outlet of the stomach, is hypertrophied (Figure 26.3), the surgical approach has changed dramatically. Surgery involves splitting the pyloric sphincter muscle from the stomach to the duodenum, leaving the mucosa intact. Pyloric stenosis has a strong familial pattern of inheritance and as such different generations of the same family may have undergone essentially the same procedure, but through a different approach. In the past, most babies with pyloric stenosis underwent a Ramstedt's pyloromyotomy through a right upper transverse incision (see incision A Figure 26.4) but more recently surgeons perform the pyloromyotomy through a cosmetically appealing supra-umbilical incision (see incision B Figure 26.4). Many centres are now adopting a laparoscopic approach to this surgery, using delicate 3 mm laparoscopic instrumentation. With the laparoscopic approach the incisions (see incisions C Figure 26.4) are so small that in a year's time it is difficult to even see the scars.

With increased use of laparoscopic surgery in paediatrics, reducing the need for large disfiguring incisions, many procedures are now carried out with much improved cosmetic results. For many years there has been evidence that laparoscopic surgery can decrease the likelihood of adhesion formation as shown by Lundorf *et al.* (1991). Advances in technology have aided the development of robotic laparoscopic surgery, commenced in adult surgery and found to be enormously useful for prostatectomy among other procedures. In recent years, as robotic equipment (ports and instrumentation) has become smaller this surgery has been introduced into paediatric practice and

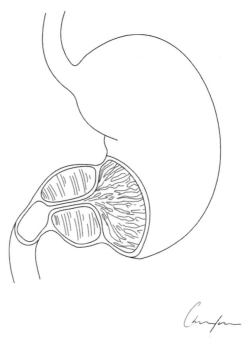

Figure 26.3 Pyloric stenosis.

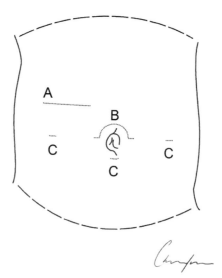

Figure 26.4 Pyloromyotomy incisions.

is suitable for many varied procedures (Najmaldin and Antao 2007). It has the benefits of increased magnification, three-dimensional vision and greater, more precise movement of the instrumentation than conventional laparoscopic surgery. It is particularly useful for those laparoscopic procedures where a large amount of suturing is required (e.g. pyeloplasty). Laparoscopic suturing is extremely time-consuming and the use of the robot can make this much quicker. A robotic surgical procedure on a child is shown underway in Figure 26.5.

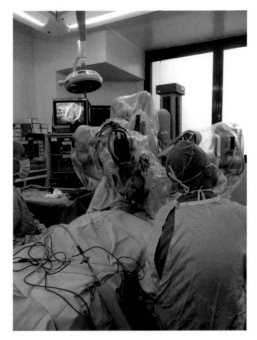

Figure 26.5   Robotic surgery.

Conclusion

Many theatre practitioners will work with children even if most of their patient group are adults. In district general hospitals children will undergo minor surgical procedures such as insertion of grommets, tonsillectomy and emergency surgery, for example appendicectomy or manipulation under anaesthetic of fractures. Most complicated surgery is performed in large teaching hospitals with paediatric surgery departments. ODPs may need to accompany anaesthetists to the accident and emergency department to assist with airway maintenance of children; therefore it is important that the practitioners have the appropriate skills.

Paediatric surgery is an interesting and diverse area, demanding outstanding knowledge and skills. Unlike adult specialities where surgery tends to be confined to one part of the body or body system, the practitioner may be involved in surgery to any part of the body; for example, a general paediatric surgeon may in one day perform a thoracotomy, an inguinal hernia repair, a wedge excision of great toenail, a gastrostomy and a release of tongue tie, thus operating 'top to toe'. For this reason the theatre practitioner needs to be able to plan and adapt to different situations. For those practitioners working mainly with adults, they must not overlook the differences required when they are faced with a child on their theatre list.

References

Department of Health (2004) *National Service Framework for Children Young People and Maternity Services*. London: Department of Health.
General Medical Council (2007) *0–18 years: Guidance for all doctors*. London: GMC.
General Medical Council (2008) *Consent: patients and doctors making decisions together*. London: GMC.

Section 4

Lui K, Wong H, Cheung Y, *et al.* (2001) Air enema for diagnosis and reduction of intussusception in children: Clinical experience and fluoroscopy time correlation. *Journal of Pediatric Surgery* 36(3):479–481.

Lundorf P, Hablin M, Kallfelt B, Thorburn J and Lindblom B (1991) Adhesion formation after laparoscopic surgery in tubal pregnancy: a randomised trial versus laparotomy. *Fertility and Sterility* 55(5): 911–915.

Najmaldin A and Antao B (2007) Early experience of tele-robotic surgery in children. *International Journal of Medical Robotics and Computer Assisted Surgery* 3(3): 199–202.

World Health Organization (2008) *Second Global Patient Safety Challenge: Safe surgery saves lives.* Geneva: WHO.

CHAPTER 27

Care of the Adolescent in Surgery

Liz McArthur

Early work by pioneers such as Robertson (1953a) and Bowlby (1973) highlighted the needs of the child in hospital and the anxiety that extended far beyond their hospital stay. 'Have we moved forward as a country?' Kennedy (2010) cited a 2007 UNICEF report in which the UK ranked bottom of 25 industrialised countries for the wellbeing enjoyed by children. What has changed? There appears to be clear and measurable effort by the government that the views of the users – children, young people and their families – in the delivery of their healthcare must be sought and taken into account. Kennedy (2010) made 39 recommendations to take forward the agenda 'getting it right for children and young people' and overcoming cultural barriers in the NHS so as to meet their needs.

Two areas outlined the involvement of the stakeholders: no. 9 stated that 'the Local Partnership must create structures whereby the views of children and young people can be sought and taken into account of in the planning and delivery of health and healthcare services' and no. 33 'NHS services for children and young people should be designed, organised and delivered from the perspective of the child, young person and parent or carer.' These recommendations were echoed in *Equity and Excellence* (Department of Health 2010), which outlined the importance of seeking and involving children and young people in decision-making: 'no decision about me without me'. When reviewing the literature and guidance both at a local and at a national level, what remains unchanged is the hostile and unknown environment of both hospitals and theatres in the eyes of this group.

The Royal College of Nursing standard (RCN 2011) states that there needs to be a separate area in the operating department reception and recovery areas and the opportunity for parents/carers to accompany the adolescent to theatre.

The World Health Organization 'Safe Surgery' initiative was undertaken to introduce a systematic way of organising theatres to address the issues around anaesthetic practices, surgical infection and poor communication (WHO 2008). This work is being adopted in many settings and provides a framework that many are familiar with. Communication is seen as one of the vital areas. This should extend not only to the theatre environment itself but also to the perioperative care of the patient.

Manual of Perioperative Care: An Essential Guide, First Edition. Edited by Kate Woodhead and Lesley Fudge.
© 2012 John Wiley & Sons, Ltd. Published 2012 by John Wiley & Sons, Ltd.

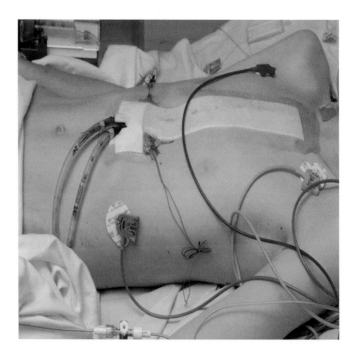

Figure 27.1   An adolescent patient.

Communication with Young People

Adolescence defined by the WHO acknowledged the transitional nature of this life stage and the inherent variation between biological and emotional maturity and socio-cultural contexts (RCN 2008).

A hospital-wide consultation carried out in 2002 in a paediatric teaching hospital (Alder Hey 2002) involving 219 young people over the age of 12 years identified a number of areas that are pertinent to the preoperative adolescent patient:

- a dedicated area for adolescents
- pain relief when they needed it
- knowing what is said and written about them
- knowing the rules of the institution
- privacy and dignity to be maintained.

Christie and Viner (2005) discussed the specialised communication skills that are required when communicating with young people to ensure that the outcomes were agreeable to both parties, and outlined the following practical points for communicating and working with adolescents.

- See young people by themselves as well as with their parents. Do not exclude parents completely, but make it clear that the adolescent is the centre of the consultation. Do this routinely as a way of respecting their healthcare rights.
- Be empathic, respectful and non-judgemental, particularly when discussing behaviours such as substance misuse that may result in harm to the adolescent. Assure confidentiality in all clinical settings.

HAVE YOU ASKED THE QUESTIONS BELOW ? IF NOT PLEASE DO NOW!

Name
DOB
Hospital No:
Procedure

CLINICAL – MEDICAL/ SOCIAL

Information to be obtained preoperatively

- Parental input (degree of input to be negotiated)
- Privacy and dignity to be observed at all times especially when sensitive information or examination is being undertaken
- Personal information (areas that might be pertinent preoperatively – require discretion – sexual activity, medication i.e. pill.
- Medical history including allergies
- Mental health history
- Anaesthetic history
- Pain history
- Medication
- Maintenance of glycaemic control
- Antibiotic prophylaxis required
- Site of surgery to be discussed
- Baseline set of observations
- Relevant bloods, investigations inc radiological) to be ordered
- Age and ability appropriate explanations to be provided re all the necessary invasive procedures
- Would they like a pre-operative visit to the area they are being admitted to?

COMMUNICATION/ CONSENT

- Clear guidelines on where and at what time the appointment will be
- Staff who will be present – to identify who they are and what their role is
- Developmental level of understanding
- Disabilities/hearing/ sight/complex needs
- Wheel chair use
- Reading ability
- Language
- Mental health status
- Behavioural issues – ADHD, ASD
- Asylum seekers and refugee +/- history
- Young offender status
- Sexual orientation
- Language being used
- Consent discussed, obtained and documented.

PRE OP INFORMATION
How would you like to be contacted? E mail, letter, text.

- Where to go
- What do they need to bring in – i.e. medication/clothes/toiletries?
- Pre existing medical condition – i.e. colostomy do they need supplies?
- What do they have to wear to theatre?
- What about earrings/tattoos/nail varnish?
- How long do they have to fast for?
- What equipment is going to be used?
- Who is allowed to accompany them?
- Rules and regulations of area
- Do they need money?

DISCHARGE INFORMATION

- How do they get home?
- What do they need at home regarding medication – antibiotics, analgesics
- Who might visit them to check on wound etc?
- When can they go out/go to school?
- When is the next appointment?
- Who can they contact and how if there are problems?
- What to expect when they get home?

COORDINATION

PREOPERATIVE PREPARATION

- Level of understanding/ disabilities
- Mental health status / does the young person require to be restrained/ psychologist?
- What medication are they on – can it be omitted?
- Where is the surgery taking place?
- What time is the surgery?
- When were they fasted from?
- Who is carrying out the surgery?
- Who is the anaesthetist?
- Is there a named nurse?
- Has the site been marked (WHO checklist)?
- Who is accompanying them to theatre?
- How long will the operation take?
- Is a pre med required, has it been prescribed?
- Is local anaesthetic cream to be applied?
- Has venous thrombo-embolism (VTE) prophylaxis been undertaken?

POSTOPERATIVE

- Are recovery staff aware of any issues around communication, mental health, fear/anxiety

Section 4

Figure 27.2A Perioperative adolescent checklist – 3 Cs. Adapted and modified from the World Health Organization.

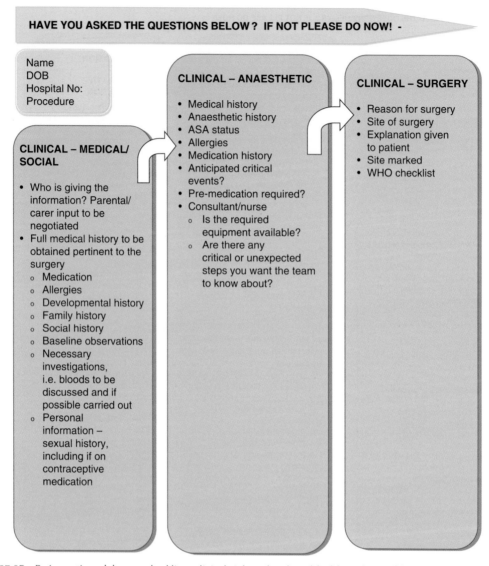

HAVE YOU ASKED THE QUESTIONS BELOW ? IF NOT PLEASE DO NOW! -

Name
DOB
Hospital No:
Procedure

**CLINICAL – MEDICAL/
SOCIAL**

- Who is giving the information? Parental/carer input to be negotiated
- Full medical history to be obtained pertinent to the surgery
  - Medication
  - Allergies
  - Developmental history
  - Family history
  - Social history
  - Baseline observations
  - Necessary investigations, i.e. bloods to be discussed and if possible carried out
  - Personal information – sexual history, including if on contraceptive medication

CLINICAL – ANAESTHETIC

- Medical history
- Anaesthetic history
- ASA status
- Allergies
- Medication history
- Anticipated critical events?
- Pre-medication required?
- Consultant/nurse
  - Is the required equipment available?
  - Are there any critical or unexpected steps you want the team to know about?

CLINICAL – SURGERY

- Reason for surgery
- Site of surgery
- Explanation given to patient
- Site marked
- WHO checklist

Figure 27.2B   Perioperative adolescent checklist – clinical. Adapted and modified from the World Health Organization.

- Be yourself. Don't try to be cool or hip – young people want a healthcare professional, not a friend.
- Try to communicate and explain concepts in a manner appropriate to their development. For young adolescents, use only 'here and now' concrete examples and avoid abstract concepts ('if ... then') discussions.

While these are general guidelines, modification will ensure that the concepts can be utilised in the theatre setting.

Communication and environment are two areas identified by a Department of Health document, *You're Welcome*, published in 2011, which acknowledged the growing requirement that to meet the needs of young people services had to both communicate

HAVE YOU ASKED THE QUESTIONS BELOW? IF NOT PLEASE DO NOW! –

Name
DOB
Hospital No:

**COMMUNICATION/CONSENT –
PREOPERATIVE**

Sign in (entering room)

- Have all team members introduced themselves by name and role?
- Has the patient confirmed his / her identify, site, procedure and consent (if patient is unable to confirm an identified advocate must be present i.e. parent / carer)
- Is the checklist complete?
- Does the patient have a known allergy?
- Have the risk factors for bleeding been checked?
- Has the patient confirmed transport home?
- Is the monitoring equipment and medications check complete?
- WHO checklist?
- Are there any drains, catheters to be in place following surgery?

**COMMUNICATION/CONSENT –
OPERATION**

Time out (on the table)

- All team members verbally confirm:
- What procedure site and position are planned?
- Has the site been marked?

**COMMUNICATION/
CONSENT –
POSTOPERATIVE**

- Has the patient's medication/supplies been organised if appropriate?
- Is information regarding the procedure available?
- Has a follow-up appointment been made?
- Has transport been discussed?
- Has a contact number been given if problem or questions arise?
- Has the community nursing team been informed and a contact number available?
- Are there any drains, catheters to be in place following surgery?
- Are they going home with any of these interventions?
- Are dressings required?

Section 4

Figure 27.3 Perioperative adolescent checklist – communication/consent. Adapted and modified from the World Health Organization.

with them on what they required and also to act on the outcomes. 'Doctors see the illness before they realise that I am actually a young person' (WHO 2009).

The WHO 'Safe Surgery' initiative was undertaken to introduce a systematic way of organising theatres to address the issues around anaesthetic practices, surgical infection and poor communication (WHO 2008). This work is being adopted in many settings

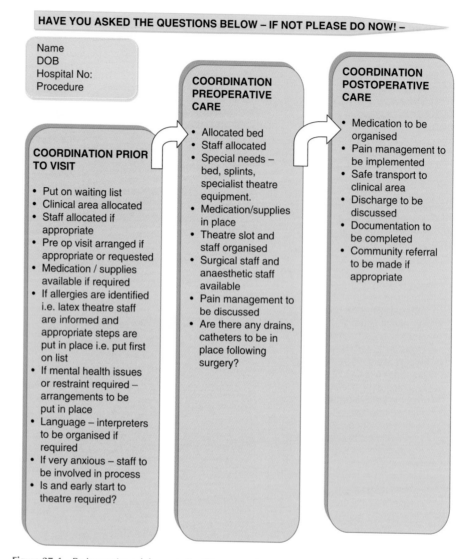

HAVE YOU ASKED THE QUESTIONS BELOW – IF NOT PLEASE DO NOW! –

Name
DOB
Hospital No:
Procedure

COORDINATION PRIOR TO VISIT

- Put on waiting list
- Clinical area allocated
- Staff allocated if appropriate
- Pre op visit arranged if appropriate or requested
- Medication / supplies available if required
- If allergies are identified i.e. latex theatre staff are informed and appropriate steps are put in place i.e. put first on list
- If mental health issues or restraint required – arrangements to be put in place
- Language – interpreters to be organised if required
- If very anxious – staff to be involved in process
- Is and early start to theatre required?

COORDINATION PREOPERATIVE CARE

- Allocated bed
- Staff allocated
- Special needs – bed, splints, specialist theatre equipment.
- Medication/supplies in place
- Theatre slot and staff organised
- Surgical staff and anaesthetic staff available
- Pain management to be discussed
- Are there any drains, catheters to be in place following surgery?

COORDINATION POSTOPERATIVE CARE

- Medication to be organised
- Pain management to be implemented
- Safe transport to clinical area
- Discharge to be discussed
- Documentation to be completed
- Community referral to be made if appropriate

Figure 27.4   Perioperative adolescent checklist – coordination. Adapted and modified from the World Health Organization.

and is providing a framework that many are familiar with. Communication is seen as one of the vital areas. This should extend not only to the theatre environment itself but also to the perioperative care of the patient.

Five flowcharts that echo the layout of the WHO checklist format but are specific for adolescents are shown in Figures 27.2–27.5.

YOUR INFORMATION CHECKLIST

Name: WHAT DO YOU LIKE TO BE CALLED?
How old are you?

CLINICAL – MEDICAL/SOCIAL

- Do you feel confident that the conversation and examination is private?
- Have the doctor/nurse introduced themselves?
- Do you need to note things down or tape things for future reference?
- Do you understand what is being discussed?
- What observations are they going to carry out?
- What is a medical history - what information do they want?
- Do you want access to what is written down?
- Are you allergic to anything?
- What medicines are you on?
- What investigations do they need before your operation?
- Do you need to visit the area before your operation?

COMMUNICATION/CONSENT

- What do you like to be called?
- Do you have any problems with communication for instance hearing or sight issues?
- Do you know what consent is?
- Are you worried or anxious about what is about to happen?

COORDINATION

Pre-op visit
- Where are you going?
- What time is your appointment?
- Who are you going to see?
- What are you going for?
- What is fasting?
- What time do you need to take your last drink and something to eat?

Visit for surgery
- Who do you want to come with you?
- What do you need to bring in – clothes, toiletries, and medicines?
- What equipment is being used?

Going home – when you leave?
- What medicine are you on?
- Do you need to bring them in with you?
- Do you need any supplies such as bandages?
- Do you need any dressings for a wound?
- Who is going to see you from the community nursing team?
- Do you have a contact number for help or advice?

Section 4

Figure 27.5 Perioperative adolescent checklist – information for the patient. Adapted and modified from the World Health Organization.

References

Alder Hey (2002) *Listening to Children and Young People.* The Alder Hey Consultation.
Bowlby J (1973) *Attachment and Loss*, Vol. 2: *Separation.* New York: Basic Books.
Christie D and Viner R (2005) Adolescent development, *British Medical Journal* 330(7486).
Department of Health (2010) *Achieving Equity and Excellence for Children.* London: Department of Health.

Department of Health (2011) *You're Welcome: Quality criteria for young people friendly health Services*. London: Department of Health.

Kennedy Sir Ian (2010) *Getting it Right for Children and Young People – Overcoming cultural barriers in the NHS so as to meet with needs*, a review by Professor Sir Ian Kennedy. September 2010.

RCN (Royal College of Nursing) (2003, 2008, 2010) *Restraining, Holding Still and Containing Children and Young People – Guidance for nursing staff*. London: RCN.

RCN (2008) *Adolescents: Boundaries and Connections – An RCN guide for working with young people*. London: RCN.

RCN (2011) *Health Care Service Standards in Caring for Neonates, Children and Young People*. London: RCN.

Robertson J (1953a) *A Two Year Old Goes to Hospital*. London: Tavistock Child Development Research Unit.

WHO (World Health Organization) (2008) *Implementation Manual Surgical Safety Checklist*, 1st edn. Geneva: WHO.

WHO (2009) *The Respect of Childrens' Rights in Hospital: An Initiative of the International Network of Health Promoting Hospitals and Health Service*. Geneva: WHO Collaborating Centre.

Further Readings

Janke E, Chalk V and Kinley, H (2002) Pre operative assessment – setting a standard through learning. University of Southampton.

Shields L (2010) *Perioperative Care of the Child – a nursing manual*. Oxford: Wiley Blackwell.

Watson D (2011) *Perioperative Safety*. Edinburgh: Mosby Elsevier.

Wicker P and O'Neill P (2010) *Caring for the Perioperative Patient*, 2nd edn. Oxford: Wiley Blackwell.

Woodhead K and Wicker P (2005) *A Textbook of Perioperative Care*. Edinburgh: Elsevier, Churchill Livingstone.

CHAPTER 28

Care of the Elderly Patient

Rita Hehir

The elderly patient coming to the operating theatre has very specific clinical needs and the perioperative practitioner needs to be cognisant of this fact and have the clinical knowledge permitting them to implement a plan of care that meets the elderly patient's needs. Many factors need to be taken into consideration (Box 28.1).

The numbers of people living into old age is constantly increasing due to improved social conditions and advances in medicine (Office for National Statistics 2011). Despite this overall enhancement in the health status of the elderly, there remains a substantial proportion of the elderly population who experience deterioration of their health solely as a consequence of life-long poverty or poverty experienced in their old age. A geographical divide still exists within the UK, with recent research showing that life expectancy is much shorter in the north of England than in more affluent parts of the south of England (Age UK 2012).

The recent publication of four separate reports which highlight the lack of respect, care and right to basic human dignity accorded to elderly patients in hospital serves to point out how vulnerable this patient group are and how effortlessly a culture of neglect can develop. Once this culture becomes a reality and is embedded, it negates the rights of the elderly to even a fundamental standard of care. Both the Nursing and Midwifery Council and the Health Professions Council (2008) instruct that every patient must be treated with respect and dignity regardless of ethnicity, sexual orientation, health status, disability or age. The ill-treatment of the elderly also breaks the law of the land, being illegal under the terms of the Equality Act 2010 (www.direct.gov.uk 2011).

Old age may appear to be an easy thing to define. Chronological age is used as a measure, individuals who are in receipt of the state pension, or those with any degree of disability tend to be labelled as old. As Victor (2006) points out, this is a subjective and limited definition of old age and one that does not allow for the range of individual characteristics which make older people a far from homogeneous group. In a time when people are living longer and healthier lives, the improving health status of older people is influenced not just by chronological age but by education, life chances and type of employment, socio-economic status and living conditions (Joseph Rowntree Foundation 2011).

Manual of Perioperative Care: An Essential Guide, First Edition. Edited by Kate Woodhead and Lesley Fudge.
© 2012 John Wiley & Sons, Ltd. Published 2012 by John Wiley & Sons, Ltd.

> **BOX 28.1**
>
> **How we treat the elderly**
>
> - Demographic trends
> - Socio-economic influences on health
> - Preoperative assessment
> - Pre-existing morbidities
> - Potential complications for the elderly in perioperative care.

The Francis Report (Francis 2010) detailed the indignity suffered by elderly patients in the Mid-Staffordshire Hospital, where they were denied the basic courtesy of being addressed by their given name, allowed to lie in their own excrement, and left to become dehydrated and malnourished. For these patients hospital care became synonymous with declining health not healing. Evidence of the standard of elderly care as chronicled in this report has more resonance with accounts of nineteenth-century workhouses than healthcare delivery in the fifth richest country in the world, in the twenty-first century.

Similar dreadful and unacceptable events were recounted in the Health Ombudsman's Report *Care and Compassion?* (Abraham 2011). This Report records the ill-treatment, neglect and abuse of ten elderly patients over the previous year who had the misfortune to require primary or acute care interventions from the NHS. Their maltreatment ranged from a failure to diagnose a condition through to failure to note that an elderly man was minutes away in the waiting room while his wife died alone, failure to respond to requests for medical consultations, and weighting the anticipated prognosis for an elderly patient against the cost of surgical intervention and choosing to deny active treatment. These all suggest that the media headlines pronouncing the elderly as a 'burden' are accepted as a societal truth. The report makes for sobering and distressing reading.

The findings of the Care Quality Commission (2011) following unannounced visits to a number of NHS hospitals investigating the standard of care and nutrition for the elderly found additional evidence to illustrate the level of indifference, neglect and denial of dignified care to elderly patients. The Report highlights a situation in one hospital in which doctors resorted to prescribing water for elderly patients in an effort to get staff to give patients a drink of water and prevent dehydration.

In all the cases cited in these three reports there exist two common denominators:

- the patients afflicted by the callous lack of care and repeated indignities were the elderly and
- being elderly, these patients became invisible to healthcare practitioners.

The report by the King's Fund (Foot 2011) clearly highlights the disparity in outcomes for the elderly who required surgical intervention for cancer in the UK versus a similar demographic in Scandinavia, Canada, Australia and some countries within mainland Europe. Indications are that the elderly in the UK fare less well (Foot 2011).

The National Confidential Enquiry in Patient Outcomes and Death (NCEPOD 2010b) reveals a lack of appropriate management of the elderly in hospitals. NCEPOD reports failures in having clinical assessments carried out by experienced doctors from a range of clinical specialities, in particular doctors trained in the care of elderly patients. Errors in the management of hydration and nutrition leading to delays in surgery which in turn led to placing the patient in more danger and the failure to provide suitable pain relief were found to be the greatest deficits in care of the elderly.

While recognising both the vulnerability of the elderly and the fact that the number of over 80-year-old patients coming to theatre is set to increase, the Association of

> **BOX 28.2**
>
> **American Society of Anestheologists Grading (Robinson and Hall 2007)**
>
> - ASA 1 A healthy patient with no illness
> - ASA 2 A patient with a mild systemic illness
> - ASA 3 A patient with a server, incapacitating illness
> - ASA 4 Illness which is a constant threat to life
> - ASA 5 A seriously ill patient who will not survive without surgical intervention.

Anaesthetists of Great Britain and Ireland (AAGBI) stipulate that with an experienced, well-trained perioperative team, age in itself does not constitute a reason to avoid surgical intervention (AAGBI 2001).

A vital prerequisite to elective surgical intervention is a thorough and comprehensive preoperative assessment of the patient. This should include an extensive search of the patient's medical history, blood chemistry profile, physical examination for scars for evidence of previous surgery and accurate recording of the patient's medication history (Hehir 2005).

The physiology of ageing dictates that the efficiency of the body systems deteriorates. The majority of elderly patients will be graded as ASA 2 under the American Society of Anesthesiologists grading system shown in Box 28.2.

Preoperative Assessment

Prior to surgery a detailed medical history is essential, which necessitates having access to the patient's medical notes. These will provide the anaesthetist with reliable and up-to-date information on the patient's health status, knowledge of concurrent conditions and intelligence on the current management of any existing conditions, including any drug regime the patient may require (Hudsmith *et al.* 2004). Access to contemporary medical notes will negate the possibility of the patient omitting details of current conditions and treatment but also forgetting to mention episodes of illness or surgical intervention which may have occurred in excess of 60 or 70 years previously.

A difference can be found to exist in how individuals react to any drug. These idiosyncratic responses are likely based on 'ethnicity, existing co-morbidity and drug interactions'. The elderly more commonly have a propensity to be adversely affected by drugs due to changes in how the body handles pharmaceutical materials. Polypharmacy is characterised as a patient being prescribed multiple drugs for a variety of pathologies, and may also include the use of over-the-counter drugs, which in turn increases the risk of adverse drug interactions (Tabernacle *et al.* 2009). According to Dodds *et al.* (2007), 'Organ function declines at an average rate of 1% a year from the age of 40'.

The Cardiovascular System

As many as 50–65% of elderly patients have a cardiovascular deficit. The probability of any patient having coronary artery disease is elevated in the case of elderly patients. Disorders such as hardening of the arteries, reduced cardiac output and atrial fibrillation is frequently present. It is quite urgent to consider fluid management due to the change in the capacity for venous return, which can lead to bigger changes in ventricular preload and cardiac output (Hardle 2006).

The Respiratory System

The lungs are hard-working organs proficient in functioning over the human lifespan but can be damaged by factors such as environment and lifestyle, in particular tobacco smoking. When subjected to adverse conditions the lungs diminish in their capacity to function normally. Age-related changes in the elasticity of lung tissue, lack of movement of the chest wall and a loss of force in the muscles of the respiratory muscles all contribute to less than optimal functioning (Dodds *et al.* 2007).

In the elderly patient it is not uncommon to find existing problems of breathlessness that may be attributed to lifestyle. Bronchial cancer, especially in an older patient who has smoked all their adult life, may be a primary presenting symptom or may be diagnosed following admission to hospital. The presence of chronic obstructive pulmonary disease (CODP) can further complicate the anaesthetic management of the patient.

Adults under 70 years of age normally have oxygen saturation between 96% and 98% at rest, whereas the patient over 70 years old is more likely to be closer to 94% when awake.

A further issue to be aware of is the administration of oxygen. In the case of the patient with 'chronic carbon dioxide retention, oxygen administration may cause further increases in carbon dioxide and respiratory acidosis' (British Thoracic Society 2011).

Endocrine System

The most significant disorder of the endocrine system is diabetes. Statistics suggest that an estimated 2.8 million people in the UK were diagnosed as having diabetes in 2010. A more bewildering statistic states that over 1 million people risk damaging their health in order to keep their diabetes a secret, because of anxiety about being discriminated against or in certain circumstances being considered abnormal (Diabetes UK 2011a).

The elderly patient with diabetes presents specific concerns to the perioperative team, with increased risk of renal insufficiency, cardiovascular disease, hypertension and neuropathy. Other complications of diabetes include gastroenteritis, a condition which causes delayed emptying of the stomach. Since gastroparesis makes stomach emptying unpredictable, a person's blood glucose levels can be erratic and difficult to control (Diabetes UK 2011b). The perioperative mortality rate may be 50% higher in diabetic than in non-diabetic patients. To lessen the risk of complications, fasting time can be reduced by placing diabetic patients first on the operating list. The perioperative team having a good knowledge of diabetes is crucial to the keep the patient with diabetes safe and avoid mistakes and omissions that frequently give rise to longer stays in hospital, increased infection rates and death.

Inadvertent Hypothermia

Inadvertent hypothermia is defined as a core body temperature below 36 °C. It is a preventable condition and should not be part of any complications incurred during surgery (NICE 2008). Ward staff, porters, reception staff and all perioperative practitioners can play a vital, minimal cost role in ensuring the elderly patient does not become cold. This can be simply done by covering the patient with an additional blanket during the transfer from ward to theatre. Applying a warm blanket during a waiting period or in the anaesthetic room can prevent a loss of body temperature.

A common feature of the deteriorating physiological function in the elderly is the inability to thermoregulate. Other factors are temperature reduction due to dehydration, vasodilatation resultant from the administration of regional or local anaesthetic agents and other environmental factors. This situation can be remedied by the use of forced air warming devices. The use of warm fluid from a cabinet controlled at 38–40 °C for irrigation of an open cavity as well as blood and fluid warmers are required.

A psychological consequence is an increased sense of vulnerability due to being cold. Complications include delayed pain relief due to poor circulation, an increased risk of infection due to lack of oxygenated blood to the wound site and the danger of elderly patients developing cardiac arrhythmias brought about by the response of the muscles to shivering (NICE 2008).

Skeletal Considerations

Arthritis and osteoarthritis of the skeletal system is commonly diagnosed in the elderly. Both are painful conditions, which is very relevant to the care given by the perioperative practitioner. A simple procedure such as extending the hand to facilitate peripheral venous access at the dorsal flexure can cause what may appear to be a disproportionate amount of pain to the patient. Moving and handling of patients with arthritic conditions needs to be carefully conducted using best practice protocols. The practitioner needs to be mindful of the implications of cervical spine degeneration which may limit neck movement, thereby making intubation difficult. Arthritic hips or patients having had hip replacement surgery may make it difficult to position the patient in lithotomy stirrups; requiring manual support of the legs for urology or gynaecological procedures.

Elderly patients with arthritis will most likely be prescribed a mixture of drugs possibly including preparations that contain steroid substances.

Delivering the Appropriate Standard of Care for the Elderly in the Operating Theatre

The elderly patient does not require a complete change in the management of postoperative pain treatment but rather an adaptation of the usual practice to meet the specific requirements in this population (Dodds *et al.* 2007).

Patients are the reason for the existence of a healthcare team. They look to the perioperative team to fulfil the diverse needs during the preoperative, intraoperative and postoperative phases of care. The patient is always the centre of attention – not just when under the operating room spotlight (Phillips 2007).

Achieving delivery of appropriate care to the elderly is very simple and does not require millions of pounds of investment. The Health Ombudsman's Report (Abraham 2011) and the Francis Report (2010) clearly illustrate what was lacking in the care of the elderly were the basics of human decency and professional responsibility:

- kindness
- respect
- dignity
- empathy
- compassion.

What your elderly patients require from you is that you adhere to your professional Code of Conduct, Performance and Ethics. Treat them with respect, it is to their vision and valour we owe the existence of the NHS. Provide dignity by allowing them access to their dentures, hearing aid and spectacles for as long as it is safe to do so.

Section 4

Most discrimination has its origins in the belief that some element within a given society are unworthy of equity due to their inferior status, especially those who lack economic power. Be mindful that all care in the NHS is free at the point of delivery and the elderly have paid in more than their fair share over a lifetime even if they end up as social welfare recipients.

References

AAGBI (Association of Anaesthesia Great Britain and Ireland) (2001) *Anaesthesia and Peri-Operative Care of the Elderly.* http://www.aagbi.org/sites/default/files/careelderly01.pdf (accessed 25 May 2011).

Abraham A (2011) *Care and compassion? Report of the Health Service Ombudsman on ten investigations into NHS care of older people.* London: HMSO.

Age UK (2012) Agenda for Later Life 2012. Policy priorities for active ageing. Chapter 6, Health and care. www.ageuk.org.uk/documents/en-gb/for-professionals/policy/chapter%207%20dignity%20in%20care%20and%20support.pdf?dtrk=true (accessed June 2012).

British Thoracic Society (2011) *What's In The New COPD Guidelines.* www.brit.thoracic.org.uk (accessed 2 July 2011).

Care Quality Commission (2011) *Dignity and Nutrition for older people.* London: Care Quality Commission.

Diabetes UK (2011a) One million risk health. Media release. www.diabetes.org.uk/About_us/Media-centre/One-million-risk-health-by-keeping-diabetes-a-secret/.

Diabetes UK (2011b) Gastroparesis. What happens if I've got gastroparesis? www.diabetes.org.uk/Guide-to-diabetes/Complications/Nerves_Neuropathy/Gastroparesis/What-happens-if-Ive-got-gastroparesis/.

Dodds C, Kumar C and Servin F (2007) *Anaesthetics for the Elderly Patient.* Cambridge: Cambridge University Press.

Foot C (2011) *Cancer Performance in England behind Other Countries Confirms New Review.* www.kingsfund.org.uk/press/press_releases/cancer_performance.html (accessed 24 July 2011).

Francis R (2010) *Report into Mid-Staffordshire NHS Foundation Trust Inquiry.* http://www.dh.gov.uk/en/Publicationsandstatistics/Publications/PublicationsPolicyAndGuidance/DH_113 (accessed 5 May 2011).

Hardle C (2006) The patient with cardiac disease undergoing non-cardiac surgery. In McConachie I (ed.) *Anaesthesia for the High-Risk Patient.* Cambridge: Cambridge University Press, pp. 299–331.

Health Professions Council (2008) *Standards of Conduct, Performance and Ethics.* http://www.hpc-uk.org/assets/documents/10002367FINALcopyofSCPEJuly2008.pdf (accessed 15 June 2011).

Hehir R (2005) Care of the elderly in the operating department. In Woodhead K and Wicker P (eds) *A Textbook of Perioperative Care.* Edinburgh: Elsevier, Churchill Livingstone, pp. 299–311.

Hudsmith J, Wheeler D and Gupta A (2004) *Core Topics in Perioperative Care.* Cambridge: Cambridge University Press.

Joseph Rowntree Foundation (2011) Older people with high support needs: how we can empower them to enjoy a better life. http://www.jrf.org.uk/sites/files/jrf/supporting-older-people-summary.pdf (accessed 26 June 2011).

NCEPOD (National Confidential Enquiry into Patient Outcome and Death) (2010a) Improving the Quality of Medical and Surgical Care. www.ncepod.org.uk (accessed 13 June 2011).

NCEPOD (2010b) Surgery in the Elderly: an age old problem. www.ncepod.org.uk/2010eese.htm.

NICE (National Institute for Health and Clinical Excellence) (2008) *Inadvertent Perioperative Hypothermia. The Management of inadvertent hypothermia in adults* (accessed 18 June 2011).

Office for National Statistics (2011) *Ageing: Fastest increase in the 'oldest old'.* www.ons.gov.uk/ons/rel/mortality-ageing/focus-on-older-people/population-ageing-in-the-united-kingdom-and-europe/rpt-age-uk-eu.html (accessed June 2012).

Phillips N (2007) *Berry & Kohn's Operating Room Technique.* St Louis, MO: Mosby, Elsevier.

Robinson N and Hall G (2007) *How to Survive in Anaesthesia: A guide for trainees.* Oxford: BMJ Books Blackwell Publications.

Tabernacle B, Barnes M and Jinks A (2009) *Oxford Handbook of Nursing Older People.* Oxford: Oxford University Press.

Victor C (2006) What is old age? In Redfern S and Ross F (eds) *Nursing Older People.* Oxford: Elsevier Health Sciences, pp. 7–23.

CHAPTER 29

Bariatric Surgery

Saheba Iaciofano

Thou seest I have more flesh than another man, and therefore more frailty.
(King Henry the Fourth, *Part 1 Act III Scene III – William Shakespeare*)
(National Audit Office 2001)

This chapter provides an adult interventional care pathway for the population of patients who are obese as defined by body mass index (BMI) of at least 30 – calculated as weight (kg)/height (m)^2 (WHO 2011). It is intended to provide physiological management for patients who have thicker layers of adipose tissue covering their organs and skeletal systems, with combined factors of multi-system disease affecting some or all organs. The extra padding in itself poses an anaesthetic challenge, to which are also added perioperative complications such as interactions and reactions of pharmaco-kinetics (AAGBI 2007). This group of patients requires careful preoperative planning and management to minimise risk and complications during surgery.

Background

The World Health Organization (WHO 2003) has declared an epidemic in the increasing number of people globally who are defined as medically obese and this has necessitated that this category of patients is recognised as being a clinical speciality of its own. The National Institute for Health and Clinical Excellence (NICE 2006) also supports this. The National Obesity Observatory defines bariatric surgery as a generic term for weight-loss surgery (National Obesity Observatory 2010). It has also found that bariatric surgery is more effective in achieving weight loss than non-surgical manage-ment, with added likelihood of maintaining weight loss in the longer term.

Bariatric Surgery Criteria

Various research findings and studies show a need for a multi-faceted care pathway to be the gold standard for best practice (NICE 2007). This commences with a multi-disciplinary team made up of nutritionalist, psychiatrist, physician and surgeon, medically

Manual of Perioperative Care: An Essential Guide, First Edition. Edited by Kate Woodhead and Lesley Fudge.
© 2012 John Wiley & Sons, Ltd. Published 2012 by John Wiley & Sons, Ltd.

Table 29.1　BMI is used to define obesity and suitability for surgery.

BMI (kg/m²)	
<25	Normal
25–30	Overweight
30–35	Obese
>35	Morbidly obese

Surgery selection criteria:
- BMI >40 kg/m² or >35 kg/m² with co-morbid conditions
- Failure of non-surgical weight-loss efforts
- Absence of contraindications (medical; e.g. hypothyroidism, Cushing's syndrome or patients who have been on large doses of steroids leading to weight gain and concerns about their psychological state)
- A well-informed, compliant and motivated patient

Adapted and modified from NICE (2007).

assessing all patients considering bariatric surgery to ensure eligibility and thorough preparation of the patient. Obesity is defined in terms of BMI as shown in Table 29.1.

Surgical Treatment for Obesity

To facilitate weight loss surgically, many different types of bariatric procedure methods have been developed and established (National Institutes of Health 2009) which fall into three main categories:

- restrictive procedures that lead to physical reduction, fixed or adjustable in the size of the upper gastrointestinal tract
- malabsorptive procedures that bypass a proportion of the intestine with less physical restriction of food intake
- a combination of the restrictive and malabsorptive, which combines restriction of the upper food pathway with intestinal bypass.

There are four major surgical treatments (Burke *et al.* 2005) that are used after patient selection, assessment, and evaluation to identify and optimally treat medical co-morbidities that may affect perioperative risks and long-term outcomes:

- laparoscopic adjustable gastric banding
- laparoscopic sleeve gastrectomy
- laparoscopic gastric bypass
- laparoscopic duodenal switch.

Patients who are considered to carry too high a risk for surgery can have a less invasive procedure such as placement of an intra-gastric balloon in order to facilitate short-term weight loss, which in turn will mean less dependency on medication and an improvement in the overall wellbeing of the patient, achieving the NICE guidance for bariatric surgery for long-term weight loss.

> **BOX 29.1**
>
> **ASA risk classification**
>
> 1. Healthy patient
> 2. Mild systemic disease, no functional limitation
> 3. Severe systemic disease, definite functional limitation
> 4. Severe systemic disease that is a constant threat to life
> 5. Moribund patient unlikely to survive 24 hours with or without operation
> 6. Emergency status: in addition to indicating underlying ASA status (I–V), any patient undergoing an emergency procedure is indicated by the suffix 'E'
>
> Adapted and modified from NHS (2010).

Anaesthetic Classification

The classification system adopted by the American Society of Anesthesiologists (ASA) for assessing preoperative physical status used to achieve optimal general anaesthetic outcomes is shown in Box 29.1.

As many bariatric patients fall under risk levels 3 and 4, careful selection according to NICE (2006) guidance will ensure risk stratification enabling pre-optimisation prior to surgery. ASA risk classification is also influenced by a person's weight.

Risks Associated with Obesity

Respiratory system

Obstructive sleep apnoea
Redundant fat deposit in the pharynx results in decreased patency and can cause intermittent obstruction of the air passage. Preoperative history with evidence of characteristic increasing snoring with subsequent apnoea and daytime somnolence may be due to obstructive sleep apnoea. All patients undergoing obesity surgery should be suspected of this condition as it can go unrecognised and untreated (Adams and Murphy 2000). To confirm obstructive sleep apnoea, formal sleep studies (polysomnogaphy) can be performed.

Preoperative evaluation must include airway assessment as there is a higher incidence of difficult airway management in these patients due to restricted jaw mobility and mouth opening, short neck and limitation of cervical spine and atlanto-occipital flexion and extension brought about by the fatty deposits (Adams and Murphy 2000).

Cardiovascular system

Obesity may affect the heart through its influence on known risk factors such as: hypertension, ischaemic heart disease (IHD), cardiomyopathies, cardiac failure, arrhythmias and dyslipidaemias (high cholesterol). Venous insufficiency and peripheral vascular disease due to increased atherosclerotic processes may also be present (AAGBI 2007).

Obesity also increases the risk of diabetes by diminishing glucose tolerance as the abnormalities in lipid and glucose metabolism appear to be related to fat distribution and total body weight (Adams and Murphy 2000).

Section 4

Anthropometric evaluation covering blood pressure, waist circumference, weight and height are essential (AAGBI 2007). Laboratory tests include fasting lipid profile, fasting insulin and glucose, haemoglobin A1C, liver profile and thyroid-stimulating hormone evaluation (AAGBI 2007).

Signs of increased jugular venous pressure, added heart sounds, pulmonary crackles, hepatomegaly and peripheral oedema may be difficult to detect due to the large adipose layer of tissue hence, pre-assessment is critical in establishing IHD by performing electrocardiogram and echocardiogram (AAGBI 2007).

Gastro-oesophageal reflux disease

This group of patients may get gastro-oesophageal reflux due to the acid escaping into the oesophagus through a weak or overloaded valve at the top of the stomach. Also, hiatus hernia is more common in this group (National Institutes of Health 2009). These patients have increased intra-abdominal pressure, which displaces the lower oesophageal sphincter and increases the gastro-oesophageal gradient. There is also an association with obesity and vagal nerve function abnormalities causing higher output of bile and pancreatic enzymes, which makes the refluxed stomach acids more toxic to the oesophageal lining (Adams and Murphy 2000).

History of heartburn and difficulty in sleeping flat due to regurgitation may provide some indication of reflux. Non-invasive or conservative treatment is to reduce acid in the stomach using proton pump inhibitors (PPI) which work on stopping the proteolytic enzyme pepsin necessary for hydrochloric acid secretion. Surgical treatment for obesity has proved to be a better intervention for gastro-oesophageal reflux disease (Adams and Murphy 2000).

Communication

Professional and welcoming attitudes will help in maintaining a calm patient. Besides the physical, psychological effects and social burdens of obesity being debilitating, it can lead to a very vulnerable stage and careless comments or remarks can be very hurtful. Having surgery performed in a specialist unit where the medical and nursing staff are sympathetic and understanding to the needs of the obese patient is important (Walsh *et al.* 2008). If invasive monitoring is to be used, informed consent in addition to the surgical procedure must be taken from the patient (Department of Health 2009).

Anaesthetic Management

Because of the engorged extradural veins and extra fat constricting the potential space, less local anaesthetic is needed for epidurals. Between 75 and 80% of the normal dose may well be sufficient (Adams and Murphy 2000).

Venous access, as a routine part of any anaesthetic technique, is technically more difficult in the obese patient, especially central venous access, where ultrasound is particularly useful and should be available (Adams and Murphy 2000). Appropriate gauge of intravenous cannulae and required attachments should be available. Occasionally, a central venous line may be required.

Intraoperative monitoring will need to include pulse oximetry and an appropriately sized blood blood pressure cuff. This should measure 20% greater than the diameter of the patient's upper arm. If the cuff is too small, blood pressure will be overestimated. In morbidly obese patients there may also be a need for invasive monitoring (AAGBI 2007).

Other attachments include electrocardiogram (ECG), bispectral index (BIS) monitor, peripheral neuromuscular monitor and temperature probe (Adams and Murphy 2000).

Airway management and patency is a particular challenge during induction and may contribute to difficulty in mask-ventilation and endotracheal intubation. It is therefore important to have an assortment of equipment available including a 'difficult airway trolley' as a standard within the operating suite (AAGBI 2007). In female patients breast size can interfere in the smooth placing of the laryngoscope (Adams and Murphy 2000). The patient's arms should not be placed across their chest at induction. The key difference in anaesthetic technique is that the patient should be placed in a ramped, head-up position for induction and intubation using an adjustable angled laryngoscope and applying cricoid pressure. It is necessary that there is an adequate selection of bougies and laryngoscope blades close to hand (Adams and Murphy 2000).

These patients will require prolonged pre-oxygenation due to the increased body mass and metabolically active adipose tissue, which leads to increased oxygen consumption and carbon dioxide production. The reduced chest wall compliance increases pulmonary blood volume and splinted diaphragm. The combination of reduced compliance and increased respiratory demand results in an increased respiratory effort. If the oxygen reserve is reduced, these patients are prone to rapid hypoxia. Endotracheal tube intubation is particularly useful in improving oxygenation by reducing small airway collapse providing positive end-expiratory pressure (PEEP). The use of laryngeal mask airways is not recommended (Adams and Murphy 2000).

It is important to also ensure visual inspection of the external chest wall to note normal chest expansion or impaired ventilation.

Patients with cardiovascular co-morbidities will warrant avoidance of hypoxaemia, nitrous oxide and other drugs that may further worsen pulmonary vasoconstriction. Inhaled anaesthetics may be beneficial as they cause bronchodilation and decrease hypoxic pulmonary vasoconstriction (Adams and Murphy 2000). Random blood sugar tests on all obese patients will ensure good perioperative glycaemic control to reduce infection and risk of myocardial events. It is necessary that the patient continues to take statins over the perioperative period as they may help to improve coronary plaque stability (Adams and Murphy 2000). PPI will help reduce gastric volume, acidity or both and help in reducing the risk and complications of aspiration and aspiration pneumonia (Walsh *et al.* 2008).

After intubation, an oesophageal calibration tube is inserted to decompress the stomach (Walsh *et al.* 2008).

Drug Pharmacokinetics

Drug pharmacokinetics is altered in obese patients and depends on changes in volume of distribution, protein-binding properties, increased renal clearance and changes in liver clearance (Adams and Murphy 2000).

It is recommended that drugs with a short half-life are used to guarantee spontaneous ventilation once the medication is stopped. It is also essential to monitor the degree of neuromuscular block to ensure that there is no residual effect on completion of surgery. Opioids and sedatives are used sparingly, maintaining anaesthesia with inhaled gases (desflurane) to ensure rapid recovery following surgery (Adams and Murphy 2000).

Anaesthetic Considerations for Laparoscopic Patients

Pneumoperitoneum causes systemic changes during laparoscopy. The gas most often used for this purpose is carbon dioxide. Positions such as Trendelenburg can worsen the systemic changes of pneumoperitoneum. Systemic vascular resistance is increased with increased intra-abdominal pressure. Treatment options include incentive spirometry, continuous PEEP and pulmonary toilet (AAGBI 2007).

Antibiotic prophylaxis is important because of increased risk of postoperative wound infection due to generally longer operative times causing tissue trauma from excessive traction and exposure. Also adipose tissue has less ability to resist infection (Walsh *et al.* 2008).

More importantly, efforts should be made to continuously improve the anaesthetic techniques and adapt them to the specific surgery by using ultra-short acting anaesthetic and analgesic agents such as remifentanil for easily controllable continuous infusions (Adams and Murphy 2000).

Theatre Care Pathway – Risk Assessment

Sedative premedication is avoided in patients with obstructive sleep apnoea. Venous thromboembolism prophylaxis is also administered preoperatively (Walsh *et al.* 2008).

On the day of the surgery patients who have not been prescribed any premedication and wish to walk are escorted to the operating theatre; alternatively patients are wheeled into the operating theatre on a special trolley accepting weight >220 kg.

Patients are received into the anaesthetic room by the anaesthetic practitioner where the elements of the patient safety checklist based on the WHO Guidelines for Safe Surgery (WHO 2009) are done by the nurse escort and the anaesthetic practitioner. This process is vital as many surgical complications are avoided by following this protocol. Sequential pneumatic compression devices are applied to the calves of the patient along with graduated compression stockings to prevent deep vein thrombosis (AAGBI 2007).

Surgical Intervention

Positioning

Careful patient positioning and pressure area protection are important in the prevention of muscle damage due to arterial occlusion, deep vein thrombosis and dead muscle tissue due to pressure; this damage releases a protein pigment called myoglobin that has potentially harmful effects if it enters the bloodstream, leading to kidney complications. It is important to have the use of specialist equipment such as a hover mattress or Patslide for manual handling (Walsh *et al.* 2008). Given such problems one risk-assessed option to consider is to induce anaesthesia in theatre to avoid such transferring.

Specially designed electrical tables are essential for safe management of patient care and should have the capability of holding up to 455 kg with extra width to accommodate the extra girth. Patients who are obese are at risk of slipping off the operating table during table position changes. It is therefore important that they are well strapped to the operating table and continually observed. The use of vacuum beanbags is recommended; these come in various sizes and shapes and assist in supporting around the patient (Walsh *et al.* 2008).

It is important to protect the patient from tissue damage from pressure and neural injuries, which are more common in this group, especially in the super obese and the diabetic. Brachial plexus and sciatic nerve palsies are caused by extreme abduction of the arms. Sciatic nerve palsy may be caused by prolonged ischaemic pressure from tilting the table sideways. Ulnar neuropathy has been associated with increased BMI (Adams and Murphy 2000).

Surgical requirements

Surgery is technically more difficult in the obese patient due to reduced surgical access, difficult visualisation of underlying structures and excess bleeding. This leads to longer operating times, with poor blood supply to the fatty tissues increasing the chance of both wound infection and wound dehiscence (Walsh *et al.* 2008).

Specifically designed bariatric instruments are preferred and form part of the surgical requirement. There are a variety of single-use instruments available to assist the surgeon in the laparoscopic approach. The laparoscope, scissors, forceps and various ranges of cutting/coagulating equipment are available in longer lengths. The key is to ensure that the equipment is checked for its functionality prior to surgery so there is no need to prolong time on the operating table. These patients may need to be catheterised to empty the bladder (Walsh *et al.* 2008).

It is also important that there is a skilled nominated team who will ensure optimal outcome by paying attention to detail and being intuitive to the surgeon and patient needs perioperatively. Preparation and consideration to the risk of surgical complications such as conversion to open procedure, bleeding and organ perforation form part of the theatre teams' risk assessment and responsibility. There is also evidence that teamwork in surgery links to improved outcomes, with high-functioning teams achieving significantly reduced rates of adverse events.

Post-surgery management

Increased attention and an adequate monitoring during arousal from anaesthesia is an integral part of the perioperative management process. Postoperative pain relief is provided with local anaesthetic wound infiltration of port sites. Patient-controlled analgesia is also used on some patients. The main reason for delayed extubation and postoperative mechanical ventilation is residual curarisation. This occurs because it is routine to keep patients fully relaxed throughout surgery for successful and safe performance of the laparoscopic surgery. Airway obstruction is a likely risk with this group of patients and a skilled recovery team should ensure that the patient is recovered in a sitting position if at all possible, give oxygen and apply continuous positive airway pressure if required (Adams and Murphy 2000). Documentation of care prior to discharge back to the ward/ITU is important, as is an established team in the recovery unit.

Conclusion

Outcome is measured by the success of the procedure and no occurrence of preventable harm. No leakage or return to theatre and adequate pain management that addresses the patient's perception is also a measure. Patient satisfaction does not only depend on the surgical outcome but the whole experience and to ensure that the intended outcome has been achieved it is essential to ensure that the patient is properly prepared to understand that this can only be achieved in partnership.

Section 4

References

AAGBI (Association of Anaesthetists of Great Britain and Ireland) (2007) *Perioperative Management of the Morbidly Obese Patient.* http://www.aagbi.org/sites/default/files/Obesity07.pdf (accessed March 2012).

Adams JP and Murphy PG (2000) Obesity in anaesthesia and intensive care – the General Infirmary of Leeds. *British Journal of Anaesthesia* 85(1): 91–108.

Walsh A, Albano H and Jones DB (2008) A perioperative team approach to treating patients undergoing laparoscopic bariatric surgery. *AORN Journal* 88(1): 59–64.

Burke A, Glass RM and Torpy JM (2005) Bariatric surgery. *JAMA* 294(15): 1986.

Department of Health (2009) *Reference Guide to Consent for Examination or Treatment.* http://www.dh.gov.uk/en/Publicationsandstatistics/Publications/PublicationsPolicyAndGuidance/DH_103643 (accessed March 2012).

National Audit Office (2001) *Tackling Obesity in England: The prevalence and costs of obesity in England.* http://www.nao.org.uk/publications/0001/tackling_obesity_in_england.aspx (accessed March 2012).

National Institutes of Health (NIH) (2009) *Bariatric Surgery for Severe Obesity – NIH Publication No. 08.* http://win.niddk.nih.gov/publications/gastric.htm (accessed March 2012).

National Obesity Observatory (NOO) (2010) *Bariatric Surgery for Obesity.* http://www.noo.org.uk/uploads/doc/vid_8774_NOO%20Bariatric%20Surgery%20for%20Obesity%20FINAL%20MG%20011210.pdf (accessed March 2012).

NHS (2010) *Connecting for Health – ASA physical status classification system code.* https://svn.connectingforhealth.nhs.uk/svn/public/nhscontentmodels/TAGS/Lorenzo_3.5/pub/ContentRelease-2.0.0/archetypes/gen/html/en/openEHR-EHR-OBSERVATION.ASA_patient_status.v1.html (accessed 24 April 2012).

NICE (National Institute for Health and Clinical Excellence) (2006) *Obesity: Full Guidance Final Version (CG43).* http://www.nice.org.uk/nicemedia/pdf/CG43FullGuideline3v.pdf (accessed March 2012).

NICE (2007) *Bariatric Surgical Service for the Treatment of People with Severe Obesity – Commissioning Guide.* http://www.nice.org.uk/media/87F/65/BariatricSurgeryFINALPlusNewToolUpdates.pdf (accessed March 2012).

WHO (World Health Organization) (2003) *World Health Organisation Global Strategy on Diet, Physical Activity and Health – Controlling the Global Obesity Epidemic.* http://www.who.int/nutrition/topics/obesity/en/ (accessed March 2012).

WHO (2009) *Patient Safety – Safe Surgery Saves Lives. The second global patient safety challenge.* http://www.who.int/patientsafety/safesurgery/en/ (accessed March 2012).

WHO (2011) *Obesity and Overweight; Media centre – Fact Sheet No. 311.* http://www.who.int/mediacentre/factsheets/fs311/en/ (accessed March 2012).

CHAPTER 30

Perioperative Care of the Pregnant Woman

Adrienne Montgomery

Urgent and semi-urgent surgery during pregnancy, while not contraindicated, puts mother and fetus at risk. It is recommended that any surgery be delayed until the second trimester or if possible, after delivery (Hart 2005). In order to determine best practice in caring for the pregnant woman who presents for non-obstetric surgery, an understanding of the anatomical and physiological changes that occur is necessary.

Anatomical and Physiological Changes

Anatomical and physiological changes occur in pregnant women to compensate for the needs of fetal development. (It may be useful to review the normal physiology of these systems to fully understand the changes identified in this section.)

Haematological changes

Total blood volume – the combination of plasma and red cell volumes – increases during pregnancy an average of 30–50% (Table 30.1). This increase is noted as early as the sixth week of pregnancy and relates to an increased cardiac output. By weeks 32–34 most of the blood volume increase has occurred with only minimal increase in the later stages. The haematological changes result in hypervolaemia, haemodilution and fall in haemoglobin (physiological anaemia). The rise in plasma volume compensates the increasing circulation demands. For example, increasing blood flow to the skin allows the heat produced by an increase of 20% in the basal metabolic rate to be lost. Hypervolaemia also has a role in maintaining blood pressure and placental perfusion. The red cell content of blood increases naturally by approximately 18% (up to 30% where iron supplements are given), thus enabling adequate oxygen requirements to be met. The haemostatic components of blood change in pregnancy to assist in the prevention of haemorrhage at delivery. However, as these occur early in the pregnancy there is a risk of thromboembolic episode. The total white cell count also rises (Stables and Rankin 2005).

Manual of Perioperative Care: An Essential Guide, First Edition. Edited by Kate Woodhead and Lesley Fudge.
© 2012 John Wiley & Sons, Ltd. Published 2012 by John Wiley & Sons, Ltd.

Table 30.1 Haematological changes.

Total blood volume	↑ >30–50%
Plasma volume	↑ 50%
Red cell volume	↑ 20–30%
Haemoglobin	↓ ±2 g/dL

Table 30.2 Cardiovascular changes.

Cardiac output	↑ 30–40%
Heart rate	↑ 10–15 beats per minute
Stroke volume	↑
Systemic vascular resistance	↓
Diastolic blood pressure	↓ ±15 mmHg
Supine hypotensive syndrome	present
Steinbrook (2002).	

Cardiovascular changes

Dramatic changes occur in the cardiovascular system during pregnancy to meet the needs of the mother and fetus (Table 30.2). The most important of these are the increase in blood volume and cardiac output and the decrease in peripheral resistance. Other changes relate to the position and size of the heart, heart rate, stroke volume and distribution of blood flow. As pregnancy progresses, the mother's heart is moved up and rotated forward so that the apex appears at the 4th intercostal space and the heart volume increases by approximately 12%. The increase in size is related to the increased venous return. These changes may alter some heart sounds, which may be heard as murmurs. Significantly, there is a rapid increase in cardiac output in the first trimester of pregnancy, which is achieved by an increase in heart rate and stroke volume. It is generally agreed that the cardiac output peaks by the end of the second trimester and then levels out. Cardiac output is influenced by the enlarging uterus and related to maternal position. The inferior vena cava is compressed in the supine position, decreasing venous return which in turn decrease cardiac output by 20–30%. While the vena cava is less compressed in the sitting position, the lateral recumbent position is the position of choice for procedures.

Total blood volume (increased plasma and red cell volume) increases from the first trimester through to term. The increase in blood flow is distributed to the uterus, kidneys, skin, liver and breasts. During pregnancy there is little change in the systolic pressure, but a marked fall occurs in the diastolic pressure, lowest at mid-pregnancy, with the return to non-pregnant levels at term. Age and parity (number of pregnancies) can also affect blood pressure. The increased arterial pressure changes lead to an increase in pulse pressure. Venous pressure increases in the femoral veins. This is caused by the weight of the uterus on the iliac veins and inferior vena cava. The rate of blood flow in the legs reduces, leading to risk of varicosities and deep vein thrombosis. The control of cardiovascular changes is part hormonal and part mechanical (Stables and Rankin 2005).

Respiratory changes

During pregnancy, major changes occur in the respiratory system to meet the need for oxygen by the mother and the fetus (Table 30.3). The chest shape changes as a result

Table 30.3   Respiratory changes.

Minute ventilation	↑ 50%
Tidal volume	↑ 40%
Respiratory rate	↑ 15%
PCO_2	↓
FRC	↓ 20%
O_2 consumption	↑ 15–20%

of the relaxation of the muscles and cartilage of the thorax. This allows the accommodation of the diaphragm which rises up to 4 cm and the main work of respiration carried out by the diaphragmatic movement. The changes begin in the first trimester of pregnancy. There are increases in tidal volume, respiratory rate and minute ventilation with decreases in PCO_2 residual volume and functional residual capacity. The increase in oxygen utilisation, by approximately 16%, and the decrease in oxygen reserves give the risk of hypoxia during hypoventilation or apnoea (Stables and Rankin 2005).

Gastrointestinal changes

The anatomical and physiological changes in pregnancy support the nutritional demands of the mother and the fetus. Progesterone affects the cardiac sphincter between the oesophagus and stomach, leading to gastric reflux. Gastric acid secretions are decreased, along with gastric muscle tone and mobility. This results in delayed emptying of the stomach contents and prolonged digestion time for solid foods. Reduced tone and mobility are also found in the biliary tract (Hart 2005, Stables and Rankin 2005).

Musculoskeletal changes

The hormonal effect on the sacroiliac joints and symphysis pubis results in increased mobility of the joints. As pregnancy progresses the pelvis tilts forward, changing the posture and gait and shifting the centre of gravity (Stables and Rankin, 2005).

Common Surgeries

The most common surgeries performed during pregnancy are appendicectomy, cholecystectomy, intestinal obstruction and trauma. The laparoscopic route is the most desired should this be available or appropriate.

Appendicectomy is the most common surgery during pregnancy. Abdominal pain of various origins, such as round ligament pain, urinary tract infection or contractions is common during pregnancy. Appendicitis is, therefore, difficult to diagnose as the symptoms may be masked or present with an altered pattern of pain because the peritoneum is lifted away from the appendix as the abdomen distends with uterine enlargement. Where the appendix is retrocaecal the pain may present as back or flank pain and be confused with early labour or pyelonephritis. It is common, therefore, for peritonitis to be present and thus greater risk to the fetus, with mortality up to 40% if the appendix has perforated (Gambala *et al.* 2008). Early intervention is required if the complications or maternal sepsis, preterm labour and delivery and postoperative complications are to be prevented. Laparoscopic surgery is the approach of choice in the first and second trimester of pregnancy, but as more risk is involved in the third trimester open surgery may be performed (Kuczkowski 2007).

The reduced tone and motility of the biliary tree, associated with the increased progesterone levels, results in bile stasis and therefore increased risk of stone formation. Surgery, usually laparoscopic, is performed during pregnancy if complications such as choledocholithiasis, pancreatitis, cholecystitis or biliary colic present (Kuczkowski 2007).

Trauma in pregnancy is most commonly the result of motor vehicle accidents, although up to 20% may be the result of physical abuse. Maternal mortality is most often from head injury and multiple organ injuries. For example, the risk of liver or splenic rupture is increased because of the displaced viscera, especially in later stages of pregnancy. It is important to note that when intra- or extraperitoneal haemorrhage occurs there is need for a greater volume of blood loss for symptoms to show. Complications of pregnancy also contribute to maternal mortality and morbidity. These include uterine rupture, bladder trauma/rupture and amniotic fluid embolus. In the first trimester of pregnancy the fetus is protected by the bony pelvis and thus fetal mortality is higher in the second and third trimester of pregnancy. The causes of fetal death include skull fractures, intracranial haemorrhage, placental abruption (where the placenta separates from the uterine wall), uterine rupture and maternal hypovolaemia. Where hypovolaemic shock occurs the blood flow is directed away from the uterus and the fetus becomes hypoxic. In the event of blunt abdominal trauma injury may be masked or mimicked with altered patterns of referred pain resulting from the displacement and compression of the abdominal organs (Schick and Windle 2010).

Surgical Risks

Laparoscopy

Laparoscopic procedures have the advantage of exposing the fetus to less toxicity from anaesthetic agents, return to normal respiratory and gastrointestinal function, reduced uterine irritability, less maternal postoperative pain and quicker recovery and mobilisation. Even so, there are risks involved for both mother and fetus as a result of the physiological changes in pregnancy, in particular the decline in respiratory compliance over the course of a pregnancy. The mother is susceptible to hypoxia, hypercarbia and hypotension related to the anaesthetic and the induced pneumoperitoneum. These factors increase the risk of hypoxia in the fetus. To reduce the risks associated with pneumoperitoneum, the carbon dioxide insufflations should be kept as low as possible at no more than 12–15 mmHg. Risks are also associated with the insertion of the Veress needle and trocars depending on the position of the uterus. The left upper quadrant of the abdomen at the mid-clavicular line is recommended as a site of choice once the uterus has reached the level of the umbilicus (Kuczkowski 2007, Schick and Windle 2010).

Anaesthesia

The choice as to whether general or regional anaesthesia is used in based on factors including the safety and urgency of the operative procedure. The availability of newer anaesthetic agents and anaesthetic techniques gives better maternal and fetal outcomes. The maternal risks associated with general anaesthesia are related to intubation and extubation, uterine activity and uterine blood flow. Gastric regurgitation and aspiration should be anticipated on induction of anaesthesia and at extubation. If 25 mL of gastric acid with a pH of less than 7.5 is inhaled, Mendelson's syndrome or acid aspiration syndrome is likely. The administration of antacids or H$_2$ blockers is mandatory pre-anaesthesia (Kuczkowski 2004). Anaesthetic gases, in particular halogenated gases, have the complication of altering uterine tone. This alteration may be either an increase or a decrease and has the effect of reducing uterine perfusion and inducing irritability. Blood flow may also be reduced at induction with the use of barbiturate agents. The risk to the fetus as a result of general anaesthesia is hypoxia due to reduced uteroplacental perfusion and altered uterine tone (Steinbrook 2002).

Regional anaesthesia is the anaesthesia of choice in pregnancy. The advantages are less risk of gastric aspiration, less nausea and vomiting postoperatively and faster recovery. The risks are associated with the increased circulating blood volume. The epidural and subarachnoid spaces decrease in size and diameter during pregnancy, increasing the possibility of intravascular injection of anaesthetic agents. Both spinal and epidural anaesthesia induce hypotension which may lead to reduced uteroplacental blood flow and place the fetus at risk of hypoxia (D'Alessio and Ramanathan 1998). Fetal bradycardia has also been noted as a side effect of spinal and regional anaesthesia (Kuczkowski 2004).

Positioning

The prevention of aortocaval compression is necessary in the second and third trimester of pregnancy. At all times the patient should be tilted to the left lateral position to maintain the natural displacement of the uterus (Steinbrook 2002). Care is also need when positioning the patient in the lithotomy position, taking into consideration the physiological changes to the musculoskeletal and cardiovascular systems. Positioning and repositioning should be a slow transition to reduce the risk of sudden fluctuations in blood pressure, particularly when placing into or out of the Trendelenburg position.

Deep vein thrombosis

During pregnancy the blood is hypercoagulable, placing the patient at risk of developing deep vein thrombosis. Therefore, compression devices, such as anti-embolism stockings, should be employed for all surgery (Schick and Windle 2010).

The fetus

Hypoxia and pre-term labour are the risks for the fetus during surgery. Fetal monitoring is not a requirement of every surgical procedure. It is of more importance to optimise the physiological state of the mother to prevent complications to the fetus. Should monitoring be considered necessary, a midwife and/or obstetrician should be present at surgery (Burlingame 2009).

Conclusions

Perioperative care is assessed, planned and implemented for any patient. But when the patient for surgery is pregnant, good preparation is essential and risk assessment should be conducted to ensure a safe perioperative journey for mother and fetus in which the anaesthetic and surgery time is kept to a minimum (Box 30.1).

Section 4

BOX 30.1

Assessment and planning for the pregnant patient

- Stage of pregnancy
- Blood pressure
- Adequate oxygenation
- Prevention of gastric regurgitation
- Preventing DVT
- Positioning requirements
- CO_2 setting for insufflations
- Fetal monitoring
- Uterine activity
- Vaginal discharge
- Pain management

References

Burlingame B (2009) Pregnant patients undergoing surgery. *AORN Journal* 89(2): 405–406.

D'Alessio JG and Ramanathan J (1998) Effects of maternal anesthesia in the neonate. *Seminars in Perinatology* 22(5): 350–362.

Gambala C, Levine D and Kilpatrick S (2008) Appendicitis in pregnancy: A guessing game? *Contemporary OB/GYN* May: 34–47.

Hart MA (2005) Help! My orthopaedic patient is pregnant. *Orthopaedic Nursing* 24(2): 108–116.

Kuczkowski KM (2004) Nonobstetric surgery during pregnancy: what are the risks of anesthesia? *Obstetrical and Gynecological Survey* 59(1): 52–56.

Kuczkowski KM (2007) Laparoscopic procedures during pregnancy and the risks of anaesthesia: what does and obstetrician need to know. *Archives of Gynecology and Obstetrics* 276: 201–209.

Schick L and Windle PE (2010) *PeriAnesthesia Nursing Core Curriculum*, 2nd edn. St Louis, MO: Saunders Elsevier.

Stables D and Rankin J (eds) (2005) *Physiology in Childbearing*, 2nd edn. Edinburgh: Elsevier.

Steinbrook RA (2002) Anaesthesia, minimally invasive surgery and pregnancy. *Best Practice and Research Clinical Anaesthesiology* 16(1): 131–143.

Further Reading

Porteous J (2008) Oh, by the way, the patient is pregnant. *Canadian Operating Room Nursing Journal* 26(2): 35–42.

Section 5

Different Approaches to Surgery

CHAPTER 31

Key Principles of Laparoscopic Surgery

Joanne Johnson

The need for staff educated and trained specifically in minimal access surgery techniques and skills is well recognised and documented.

This chapter aims to provide an insight into the key principles of laparoscopic surgery to provide specific knowledge in relation to patient care and safety by understanding the technical aspects of the equipment and instrumentation required.

The development of laparoscopic surgery is inextricably linked with advances in the field of medical imaging, instrument development and with the skills of the surgeon and the theatre team.

In 1806, when Philip Bozzini built an instrument which allowed him to look into the human body, lit by a candle, this was the start of the development of endoscopy, although he was years ahead of his time. Still relevant today in laparoscopic surgery is the use of carbon dioxide for insufflation discovered by Richard Zollikofer in 1920 and the rigid rod lens system developed by Harold Hopkins in 1953, which revolutionised videoscopic surgery (Mishra 2011).

These developments have allowed patients to have surgery without the need for large abdominal wounds, which decreases postoperative pain and potentially disfiguring scars. The ability to offer a laparoscopic approach to a patient allows a shortened post-operative recovery in hospital and convalescent time at home. In conjunction with this the development of endoscopic stapling devices has advanced colorectal and bariatric laparoscopic surgery.

Preparing the Environment

Experience has shown that until the team is familiar with the extra equipment and checks required for laparoscopic surgery, additional staff may be required. For theatre practitioners there appears to be much more to do at the beginning and end of a session and less during each procedure There is always the possibility that conversion to open surgery may be necessary, and therefore any additional instruments should be readily available and a full-scale swab and instrument check initiated at the commencement of the laparoscopic procedure.

Manual of Perioperative Care: An Essential Guide, First Edition. Edited by Kate Woodhead and Lesley Fudge.
© 2012 by John Wiley & Sons, Ltd. Published 2012 by John Wiley & Sons, Ltd.

Although each team will determine its own set-up depending on personal preference and theatre size, some general principles can be identified. The use of specially designed stacking systems for equipment is strongly recommended as connections can be maintained between sessions, equipment is positioned at the appropriate height, access is eased and cabling from the unit to the power source is reduced. To maximise function of the stack and for all the team to get the best views of the screen, careful positioning of the equipment is essential.

All equipment must be functioning and positioned correctly prior to commencement.

The insufflator should be checked to ensure there is adequate CO_2 in the cylinder, that it is correctly connected, has been turned on and that the insufflator performs a self-calibration test.

The monitors are positioned on either side of the patient such that the surgeon, assistant and scrub practitioner have a clear, unobstructed view. The surgeon will also need to see the insufflator display panel. Instrument trolleys and stacks, suction equipment, leads, cables and tubing need to be arranged to facilitate access by the theatre team, and to ensure that they do not become tangled or damaged during draping of the patient.

Attention to the placement of technical equipment and room preparation needs to be considered in conjunction with the usual preoperative preparation of the patient.

In minimal access surgery, the positioning of the patient is dependent upon the operation being undertaken. General principles identified include the use of an X-ray translucent table, and a secure patient position.

Medical Imaging

There are five main components to the imaging system:

- video camera and control unit
- scope
- light source, fibreoptic cable
- video monitors
- video recorder/printer.

Video camera and control unit

The video camera and control unit consist of a small lightweight camera head, cable and camera control unit with the following features:

- *Lens*
- *Video imaging chips*: These are one or three charged coupled devices (CCDs) covered in silicone cells (pixels) that are light-sensitive. They emit electronic signals via the camera cable to the camera control unit (CCU) that transforms information into a video signal, which is transmitted to the monitors. Colour, detail and image sharpness (resolution) are governed by the number of imaging chips. A three-chip camera provides greater resolution and a more accurate and natural colour, but is more expensive. Single-chip cameras, however, do now have improved resolution due to advanced electronics in CCDs and also in CCUs due to improved signal processing.
- *Auto shutter*: This controls the amount of light the camera detects at the surgical site. Shutter speed is changed automatically to reduce flare caused by metal reflective instruments passing through the field of view.
- *Focus*: This moves the lens elements in the camera relative to the CCD to sharpen the image (it can be manually controlled using a focus ring on the camera body).

- *Light gain switch*: This helps the camera compensate for low light situations by boosting the video signal amplitude. Unfortunately, the gain switch also boosts unwanted video signal 'noise'.
- *White balance*: This creates a fixed point of reference for all the other colours viewed by the camera which compensates for the type and condition of light source being used.
- *Orienting feature*: This enables operators to keep the image in the correct plane on the monitor.

Scopes

Video endoscopes are designed to transmit the image to a monitor. Within the scope is a negative or objective lens which creates the image at the operative site. A delicate system of rod-shaped glass lenses which are positioned end to end (Hopkins rod lens system) transmit the image along the length of the scope to the ocular lens which magnifies the image. Wrapped around these delicate lenses are thousands of light-carrying fibres, transmitting light to the operative site.

Scopes have different diameters, 5 and 10 mm, and also different angles of view – 0, 30 and 45 degrees.

Warming the scope to body temperature before insertion will minimise fogging of the distal lens. Anti-fog chemicals can also be used or scope-warming devices. The objective lens needs to be cleaned during the procedure if it becomes soiled. Never use abrasives; warm saline and proprietary solutions may be used.

Continuous vision of the operative field is essential, it is particularly important to keep all instruments within sight to avoid accidental damage to tissue. This is particularly pertinent to port insertion and electrosurgery activation.

Light source and fibreoptic cable

The ideal light source emits a light with consistent intensity and balanced colour temperature. Other features include:

- auto and manual control of light output
- infrared filter (heat dissipation)
- standby mode to prolong lamp life
- hours meter for lamp life measurement.

There are two principal lamps used in laparoscopic light source units: metal halide and xenon. The light source and cable produce an intense light beam. The light should be on its lowest setting or switched off unless the laparoscope is in use (standby mode).

Careful handling of the hot end of the light cable reduces the chance of burns to staff or the patient. Retinal damage can be caused by looking directly at the light beam.

Video monitors

Signals are processed by the CCU and displayed via video cables on the monitor. Monitors should be high resolution, medical grade to maintain the quality of the video image and be fully compatible with the imaging devices in use. Most systems now have high definition (HD) monitors.

Note: It is important to be familiar with the sequence of the colour bars on a correctly connected RGB system; it is white, yellow, cyan, green, magenta, red and blue.

Section 5

Video recording/documentation equipment

The procedure may be recorded by attachment of the appropriate cables to the CCU.

Video/Imaging Systems

Recent developments which have improved image and the integration of systems include the following (Leeds Institute for Minimally Invasive Therapy 2002):

- digital camera systems, giving improved image quality and the ability to enhance images while maintaining high quality
- interfaces with other digital equipment and larger images (panoramic view)
- 'intelligent' light sources
- scope recognition
- voice operation (control of light and camera properties without compromising sterile fields)
- digital video recorders (DVR)
- flat screen display devices using plasma technology
- digital printers that can be interfaced with computers
- laparoscopic ultrasound (LYNX) that can be mixed with camera image and displayed as a PIP (picture in picture).

Laparoscopic Instrumentation

Instruments may be described as either 'access' or 'operating' instruments, according to their use.

Most instruments are available as single patient use (spu) or reusable multiple patient use (mpu) (MHRA 2001). The majority of mpu instruments are 'take-apart', to help with the process of cleaning and decontamination. Prior to use, all instruments need to be checked to ensure correct assembly and that each one is functioning as designed. It is also essential to check that insulation is intact, to prevent inadvertent burns to the patient or surgeon.

Access

There are three main methods to gain access to the abdomen: open or closed techniques and under vision.

Veress needle

A Veress needle is used to introduce carbon dioxide gas into the abdomen prior to port insertion. It consists of a blunt inner tube with a spring-loaded outer sheath with bevelled sharp needle and a luer lock at the proximal end for attaching insufflation tubing. The standard diameter of the needle is 2 mm and they are available in different lengths for obese patients and as a spu or mpu.

Instruments

Laparoscopic instruments need to do much the same as open instruments but have to be designed for tissue handling at depth, and through the ports.

There is a wide range of forceps and graspers, some with generic uses and others designed for a specific purpose. Instruments can be either single action, where only one side of the instrument jaw moves, or double action, where both sides move. A choice of handle for most grasping forceps is available – pistol grip or in-line – with the option of a ratchet mechanism which locks the handle, exerting a constant pressure on the tissue being held. The handle may well be a mpu and the instrument spu; this type of instrument is termed a reposable instrument. Any instrument that is to be used with diathermy needs to be insulated. The ergonomics of the instrument need to be designed for ease of use and operator comfort.

Scissors should be checked for blade alignment and that they are sharp if mpu. Needle holders need to be able to grasp and firmly hold a metal needle. They are designed with jaws made of tungsten carbide to prevent the needle rotating.

Care and Handling

The costs associated with the purchase of laparoscopic instrumentation are high and most purchasers have a limited budget. Therefore it is essential that the users are aware of the manufacturer's recommendations for cleaning and sterilisation.

The complexity of laparoscopic instrumentation and the way it is used can make it very difficult to clean thoroughly. All theatre personnel involved in laparoscopic surgery should be aware of the instruments in use in their department and understand the assembly, disassembly and sterilisation method required.

Perioperative staff should be familiar with all technical equipment, products and instruments used. Laparoscopic instrumentation is constantly changing and improving. Perioperative staff need educational resources and product information with instructions that are concise, clear and easy to follow.

The decontamination of reusable instrumentation for laparoscopic surgery needs well-trained staff. Instrument design should allow easy dismantling and rinsing of internal parts. Correct handling and maintenance processes need to avoid damage to the instruments. Protective transport and effective containment reduces the potential for damage to fragile laparoscopic instruments.

Reusable instruments are an economical option, however disposable parts on reusable tubes and handles offer an alternative to complicated or easily damaged working tips (e.g. scissors blades that easily blunt).

Instrument Handles

With instruments that 'take-apart' there are various handles available. Non-ergonomic positioning of the hand and fingers can lead to pressure areas, nerve irritation and rapid fatigue for the surgeon over a period of time.

Ports

A port is a tubular device (cannula) providing access to the internal surgical site, facilitating instrument access via the lumen. Common features include; a stopcock/tap to allow insufflations, a tubing attachment, a seal or valve preventing loss of pneumoperitoneum. Ports are available in a variety of diameters and lengths. Selection is dependent on the surgery being undertaken and individual body dynamics.

Disposable, reposable and reusable versions are available. A variety of trocars are available to enable safe insertion of the port. Trocar selection is dependent on the chosen method of access and on surgeon preference.

Initiating and Maintaining the Pneumoperitoneum

In order to expand actual or potential body spaces to facilitate surgery, carbon dioxide is used because it is cheap, does not support combustion, does not distort the image and is readily soluble and excreted via the lungs.

When initiating closed pneumoperitoneum, using the Veress needle method, it is important to ensure that the scrub practitioner is familiar with the assembly and safety checks necessary on the Veress needle. The procedure is as follows:

1. assemble the two parts of the needle
2. check the point is sharp and not burred
3. check the safety spring in the accepted manner
4. with a syringe of air check the patency of the needle
5. check the tap for stiffness or any missing screws.

There are four main controls to check:

- the CO_2 cylinder gauge
- the pre-set pressure gauge (should never be more than 15 mmHg)
- the patient/abdominal pressure gauge
- the gas flow indicator.

It is important to read the manufacturer's instructions before using the insufflator, to ensure familiarity with the controls and know how to change the cylinder.

In general, the practitioner should check the insufflator tubing and connectors. Ensure there is no fluid in the tubing. Any reusable tubing containing fluid should be discarded as it cannot be guaranteed to be sterile and this could result in an increased risk of contamination to the patient and to the insufflator if back flow occurs. Most hospitals now use single-use tubing with a filter included as standard. The initial pre-set for using the Veress needle is usually a low flow of 1–1.5 L/min and a pre-set of 12 mmHg. Check that there are no contraindications for this pre-set pressure level. When the surgeon is satisfied with the placement of the Veress needle, the insufflator should be switched on. Ensure gas flow through the tubing, can be heard before connecting the Veress needle. Gas should flow to atmosphere for 3–4 seconds before connecting to the patient. The flow should be kept low at 1–2 L/min initially until the surgeon is satisfied that the peritoneal cavity and not the subcutaneous tissue is being insufflated.

If an open insertion technique is being performed (Hassan cannula method) it is possible to insufflate at 16 L/min, but there is an increased risk of anaesthetic complications. It is safer practice to keep the insufflator on low flow (i.e. 7–10 mmHg) until adequate pressure is achieved.

Once the pre-set pressure is achieved and the surgeon is ready to place the primary port, the insufflator should be stopped until gas flow is required. Once the primary port is placed it is good practice to insert the camera to perform a quick laparoscopy to observe for any tissue or vascular damage before attaching the insufflator tubing and turning the gas back on. This reduces the risk of a CO_2 embolus should there be a vascular injury.

It is important for the anaesthetist to observe the patient closely during creation of the pneumoperitoneum, in order for any signs of complications to be quickly diagnosed. While the insufflator is connected to the patient the pressure displays should be monitored and any sudden alterations investigated.

At the end of the operation the insufflator should be disconnected from the patient before switching off to reduce the risk of insufflator contamination. As much gas as possible should be removed from the peritoneum. It is good practice to use suction rather than expelling gas into the atmosphere as some studies suggest the plume and spray generated during surgery can have detrimental effects on the staff. Viruses may remain attached to smoke condensates, which can be inhaled.

The most common effect of the pneumoperitoneum postoperatively is referred shoulder tip pain, which affects about 25% of patients undergoing laparoscopic surgery. It usually resolves in 24–48 hours. The exact cause is unclear but it is possibly caused by retained CO_2 causing diaphragmatic irritation and can cause considerable discomfort following surgery.

The difference between the temperature of standard raw gas of (21 °C) and core temperature (37 °C), and no water vapour versus intra-abdominal steady state saturation, results in alterations that upset normal abdominal homeostasis. The results of this are alterations that influence development of hypothermia, affect recovery room length of stay and postoperative pain. A study has shown that where carbon dioxide gas is heated and hydrated the incidence and severity of postoperative pain and hypothermia are reduced (Mouton *et al.* 2001).

Conclusion

The last 20 years of laparoscopic surgery have advanced greatly due partly to the innovation and development of equipment and instrumentation, often driven by surgeons, as in the past with Bozzini and Hopkins. This chapter has looked at the technical skills and knowledge required to undertake laparoscopic surgery which must be understood to ensure patient safety. That the correct equipment and instrumentation is available at all times is vital to the successful outcome of surgery. It is important that theatre practitioners understand how the equipment works and can use it effectively.

This area of surgery continues to advance and single incision laparoscopic surgery, where access to the abdominal cavity is gained through a single port rather than multiple port sites, is the next development.

References

Leeds Institute for Minimally Invasive Therapy (2002) Course Manual of Practical Skills for Theatre Teams in Laparoscopic Surgery. Unpublished.

MHRA (Medicines and Healthcare products Regulatory Agency) (2001) *Managing Medical Devices*. DB2006(05). http://www.mhra.gov.uk/Publications/Safetyguidance/DeviceBulletins/CON2025142 (accessed March 2012).

Mouton WG, Naelf M, Bessell JR *et al.* (2001) A randomized controlled trial to determine the effect of humidified carbon dioxide insufflation on post-operative pain following thoracoscopic procedures. *Surgical Endoscopy* 15: 579–581.

Mishra RK (2011) History of minimal access surgery. www.laparoscopichospital.com/history_of_laparoscopy (accessed 23 June 2011).

CHAPTER 32

Key Principles of Endoscopic Surgery

Louise Wall

What does the Endoscopy Department Do?

The endoscopy unit cares for patients undergoing gastroscopy, enteroscopy, flexible sigmoidoscopy, colonoscopy, bronchoscopy and percutaneous endoscopic gastrostomy tube (PEG) placement, among others.

What is an Endoscopy?

Endoscopy is a generic word for the examination of an internal cavity. The type of endoscopy and what is to be viewed is reflected in the procedure name. An oesophago-gastro-duodenoscopy (OGD or gastroscopy) examines the oesophagus, stomach, first and second parts of the duodenum; a bronchoscopy the respiratory tract; a colonoscopy the anus, rectum, sigmoid colon, descending colon, splenic flexure, hepatic flexure, transverse colon, ascending colon, the caecum and the ileo-caecal valve. A sigmoidoscopy is a more limited procedure and concludes at the splenic flexure.

Why is Endoscopy Performed?

The purpose of any endoscopy is to give a diagnosis, to evaluate existing conditions or for therapeutic treatment of conditions of the gastrointestinal tract.

Who Refers Patients and Why?

Patients are referred by their general practitioner or hospital doctor for a variety of symptoms. The most common upper gastrointestinal symptoms are gastro-oesophageal reflux (heartburn), dyspepsia, dysphagia (difficulty swallowing), weight loss, anaemia

Manual of Perioperative Care: An Essential Guide, First Edition. Edited by Kate Woodhead and Lesley Fudge.
© 2012 by John Wiley & Sons, Ltd. Published 2012 by John Wiley & Sons, Ltd.

and surveillance of Barrett's oesophagus or oesophageal varices. Lower gastrointestinal endoscopy is performed for investigation of rectal bleeding, change in bowel habit, abdominal pain, surveillance of Crohn's disease, ulcerative colitis and previous colonic polyps. It is also used to screen for potential bowel cancer.

Patients are triaged according to their presenting symptoms and may be seen routinely, urgently or as an emergency.

Where is Endoscopy Performed and by Whom?

Endoscopic procedures of the upper and lower gastrointestinal tracts are performed in hospital endoscopy units, at diagnostic treatment centres and increasingly in GP surgeries by doctors, GPs with a special interest in endoscopy and by nurse endoscopists.

Day-case, Inpatient and Emergency Procedures

Most endoscopies are performed as day-cases, although some patients may require admission to hospital prior to their procedure if they have other co-morbidities or difficulty taking bowel preparations at home.

Inpatient procedures are performed in the endoscopy unit within normal working hours unless the procedure is deemed to be an emergency.

Emergency procedures may be undertaken out of hours. These may be accommodated within the theatres where anaesthetic and surgical support is available if needed.

The Endoscope

The endoscope has a hand-piece (Figure 32.1) which has buttons for suction, air and water insufflation, and additional programmable buttons which can be used for photography and video capture. It also accommodates the angulation wheels which control the movement of the distal tip of the endoscope and which can be locked in position.

The flexible tube of the endoscope carries the light guide bundle, the air and water channel and one or two accessory channels (Figure 32.2).

The accessory channel (Figure 32.3) may also be known as a forcep or biopsy channel and enables the endoscopist to pass accessories such as biopsy forceps, polyp snares, injection needles and retrieval baskets through the endoscope for therapeutic procedures.

The suction channel (Figure 32.4) is controlled via a button on the hand-piece and allows suction, using a vacuum, of fluid to give a clear operative view and to deflate the cavity prior to extubation.

The air and water channels (Figures 32.5a,b) are controlled using a button on the endoscope hand-piece. This enables the endoscopist to insufflate the cavity with air, which is passed through the endoscope, helping to give good views of the mucosa. When the same button is depressed, water is fed through the endoscope to its distal tip and across the lens. This cleans the lens of the endoscope.

The jet channel Figure 32.6 is a Luer lock connection, located at the top of the hand-piece, used to flush water via a large syringe through the endoscope to wash the mucosa.

Section 5

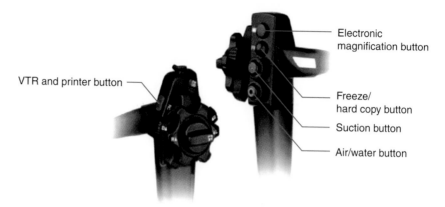

Figure 32.1 Endoscope hand-piece. Reproduced with kind permission from Imotech medical, formerly Fujinon.

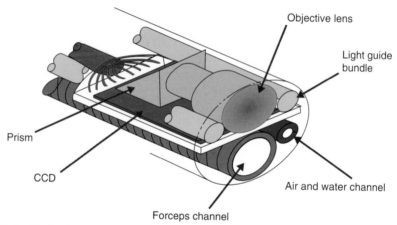

Figure 32.2 The flexible tube of the endoscope. Reproduced with kind permission from Imotech medical, formerly Fujinon.

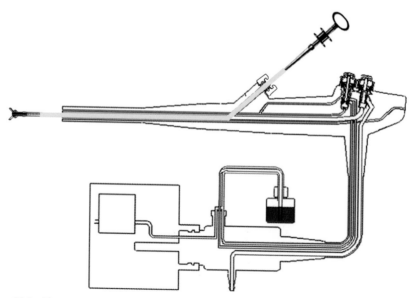

Figure 32.3 The accessory or biopsy channel. Reproduced with kind permission from Imotech medical, formerly Fujinon.

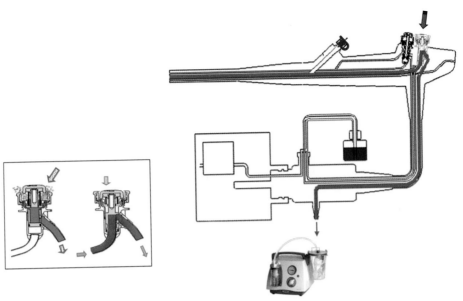

Figure 32.4 The suction channel. Reproduced with kind permission from Imotech medical, formerly Fujinon.

(a)

(b)

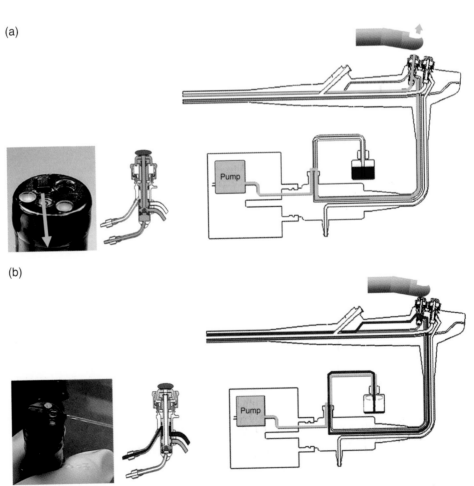

Figure 32.5 The air (a) and water (b) channels. Reproduced with kind permission from Imotech medical, formerly Fujinon.

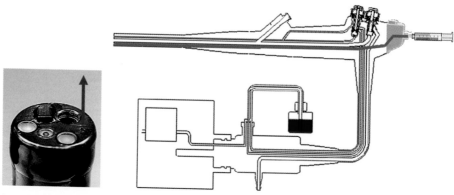

Figure 32.6   The jet channel. Reproduced with kind permission from Imotech medical, formerly Fujinon.

Preparation of the Endoscopy Room

Preparation involves the accumulation of the necessary equipment and checks to ensure it is fully functional, clean and safe to use. The equipment required for an endoscopy will vary according to the type of endoscopy requested and the clinical indication.

The endoscope will need to be processed in an automatic endoscope reprocessor (AER) and used within 3 hours. Processed endoscopes can be stored in an endoscope storage cabinet for a maximum of 72 hours prior to use.

Setting up the Procedure Room

The endoscope is connected directly to a light source (Figure 32.7) and processor (Figure 32.8) which carries the image from the endoscope to a screen. The screen enables the whole team to view the upper or lower gastrointestinal tract.

The endoscope processor and light source are stored on a purpose-built trolley that also acts as a working space for the endoscopy assistant on which can be placed a container of water to test the correct functioning of the endoscope, swabs, mouth guard for gastroscopy, lubricant, specimen containers and a syringe for flushing the endoscope and cleaning the endoscope lens.

Supplementary Equipment

A supply of single-use sterile equipment should be readily available and placed either in the procedure room or in an adjacent area such as:

- biopsy forceps for taking tissue samples
- snares for removing and cauterising (diathermy) polyps
- hot biopsy forceps to cauterise small polyps
- dilation balloons for expanding strictures
- clipping apparatus for control of bleeding points
- injection needles for injecting sclerosing agents, tattooing lesions and lifting polyps to enable a better clearance margin and to reduce the possibility of perforating the colon
- plus a diathermy machine.

Light source XL-4450 functions

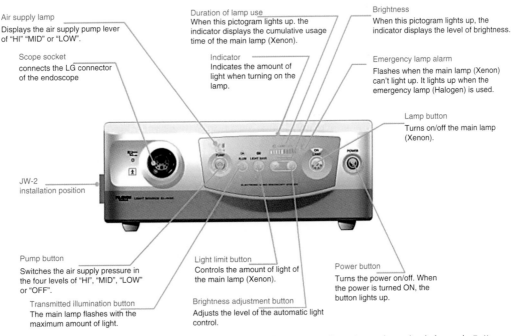

Air supply lamp
Displays the air supply pump lever of "HI" "MID" or "LOW".

Scope socket
connects the LG connector of the endoscope

JW-2
installation position

Duration of lamp use
When this pictogram lights up. the indicator displays the cumulative usage time of the main lamp (Xenon).

Indicator
Indicates the amount of light when turning on the lamp.

Brightness
When this pictogram lights up, the indicator displays the level of brightness.

Emergency lamp alarm
Flashes when the main lamp (Xenon) can't light up. It lights up when the emergency lamp (Halogen) is used.

Lamp button
Turns on/off the main lamp (Xenon).

Pump button
Switches the air supply pressure in the four levels of "HI", "MID", "LOW" or "OFF".

Transmitted illumination button
The main lamp flashes with the maximum amount of light.

Light limit button
Controls the amount of light of the main lamp (Xenon).

Brightness adjustment button
Adjusts the level of the automatic light control.

Power button
Turns the power on/off. When the power is turned ON, the button lights up.

Figure 32.7 Example of light source functions. Reproduced with kind permission from Imotech medical, formerly Fujinon.

Processor VP-4450HD functions

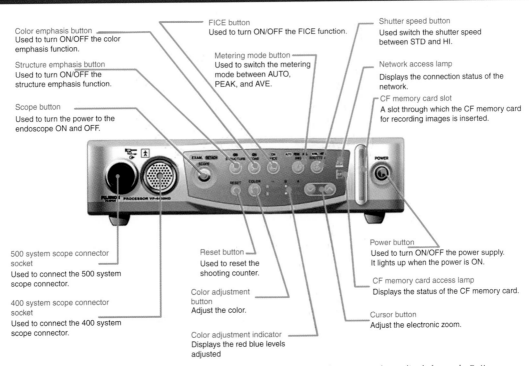

Color emphasis button
Used to turn ON/OFF the color emphasis function.

Structure emphasis button
Used to turn ON/OFF the structure emphasis function.

Scope button
Used to turn the power to the endoscope ON and OFF.

FICE button
Used to turn ON/OFF the FICE function.

Metering mode button
Used to switch the metering mode between AUTO, PEAK, and AVE.

Shutter speed button
Used switch the shutter speed between STD and HI.

Network access lamp
Displays the connection status of the network.

CF memory card slot
A slot through which the CF memory card for recording images is inserted.

500 system scope connector socket
Used to connect the 500 system scope connector.

400 system scope connector socket
Used to connect the 400 system scope connector.

Reset button
Used to reset the shooting counter.

Color adjustment button
Adjust the color.

Color adjustment indicator
Displays the red blue levels adjusted

Power button
Used to turn ON/OFF the power supply. It lights up when the power is ON.

CF memory card access lamp
Displays the status of the CF memory card.

Cursor button
Adjust the electronic zoom.

Figure 32.8 Example of processor functions. Reproduced with kind permission from Imotech medical, formerly Fujinon.

Sengstaken tubes must be available for emergency procedures, where control of oesophageal variceal bleeds may not be possible endoscopically.

Suction

Suction apparatus is required to remove the patient's secretions orally and also via the endoscope, for this reason two independent suction sources need to be available as well as in an emergency setting, where a patient is bleeding profusely, a second patient suction unit is needed as one may not manage the blood flow and maintain a clear patent airway.

Oxygen

Oxygen administration via nasal prongs, nasal catheter or face mask is required either through wall-mounted access points or via a cylinder, as oxygen saturation levels may drop during the endoscopy and recovery period, whether the patient is sedated or unsedated, especially if an opioid has also been administered.

Monitoring

Patient monitoring equipment must be available to measure the pulse, blood pressure, oxygen saturation levels and respiratory rate, which need to be recorded on the care plan along with consciousness levels and pain scores.

The procedure may be performed under sedation, using a topical local anaesthetic spray to numb the patient's throat if not having sedation, or, in an emergency setting, under a general anaesthetic.

Medication

The medications available to the endoscopist will include a sedative such as midazolam, lignocaine throat spray, opioid analgesia for colonoscopy or painful procedures and reversal agents for the sedation and opioid mediations such as flumazenil and naloxone. Nitrous oxide and oxygen (Entonox) is useful for painful procedures, especially in patients who are not well enough to be prescribed sedation or opioid medications. It is also an excellent alternative to sedation and/or opioid medications for day-case patients as the effects are dissipated within 30 minutes of cessation of administration, enabling patients to drive their vehicle from the hospital and return to normal activities without a prolonged recovery period.

Sclerosing agents, such as adrenaline, may be injected into bleeding points within the gastrointestinal tract such as gastric and duodenal ulcers to control bleeding.

Buscopan may be required to relax smooth muscle and reduce spasm within the gut, thus aiding clearer views of the cavity.

Resuscitation

All clinical areas must have resuscitation drugs and equipment. The resuscitation equipment should be latex free and, where appropriate, single use.

In addition to the basic monitoring equipment there must be provision of equipment for the airway and circulation, resuscitation drugs, a defibrillator and stethoscopes. A 12-lead ECG and a blood gas analyser should be available.

Clinical areas should have immediate access to stethoscopes, a device for measuring blood pressure, a pulse oximeter, a 12-lead ECG recorder and facilities for blood gas analysis (Resuscitation Council 2004).

Intravenous fluids may be required, especially for patients who have been nil-by-mouth for long periods or who have taken bowel cleansing preparation as they may become dehydrated. Emergency patients may require colloids (e.g. Gelofusine) or blood transfusion if bleeding.

Photography

The ability to take photographs is helpful but not essential. Photographs enable the endoscopist to record pathology seen during the endoscopy. The patient's future management may not be by the operating endoscopist. A photograph therefore gives the patient's own physician a more detailed picture of the disease process. It may also be necessary for the endoscopy to be repeated, for example to check the healing of an ulcer, and as this may be performed by another endoscopist, a photograph will give the second endoscopist a clear picture of the size and depth of the ulcer thus allowing a more appropriate comparison.

A record of who performed the procedure, what was done and the medication administered is vitally important for follow-up and future patient management. A computer with appropriate reporting software is preferable but not always available away from the dedicated endoscopy unit.

Care of Patient

Pre-procedure

Ensuring that the equipment, personnel and environment are properly prepared also makes sure that the patient episode runs smoothly and is as safe as possible. During their admission the patient must be asked about their past and current medical history, including why the procedure has been requested. Their current drug regime and whether they have any allergies or sensitivities should also be noted and addressed.

Patients who have had spinal or neurological surgery, received growth hormone treatment or who have been exposed to Creutzfeldt–Jakob disease (CJD) will require consultation with the medical and infection control teams, as this could lead to contamination of any endoscopes or equipment used on that patient, including the decontamination apparatus.

Flexible endoscopes cannot be completely decontaminated using current methods and this could lead to cross-infection of other patients. As these endoscopes may be used on future numerous uninfected patients, widespread cross-infection could occur. Any endoscopes or equipment exposed to possible CJD contamination must be quarantined and possibly destroyed. This is not only an inconvenience to the department as the number of available endoscopes is reduced, it also has a major cost implication if the endoscope is destroyed.

Therefore, if a patient is deemed to carry a risk of CJD contamination an alternative investigation should be considered.

Anticoagulation therapy

If the patient is taking anticoagulation therapy their international normalized ratio (INR) will be need to be checked to ensure that the therapeutic procedure can proceed without an increased risk of bleeding. However, the risk of haemorrhage may outweigh the risks of thrombosis if the anticoagulation therapy is stopped (Veitch *et al.* 2008).

Depending on the planned treatment and the indication for the procedure, some patients will need to stop their medication prior to admission. These patients may be prescribed heparin prior to their procedure.

Bowel preparation

Patients undergoing colonoscopy or flexible sigmoidoscopy will need to have a cleansed bowel pre-procedure. Care must be taken when deciding which type of preparation to prescribe. Sodium phosphate bowel preparations are contraindicated in renal, cardiac and elderly patients due to the electrolyte imbalances they cause and the risk of complications (Mun Woo *et al.* 2006).

Elderly patients may not be able to manage bowel preparations due to decreased mobility and poor anal sphincter tone and may need to be admitted to hospital overnight.

Full bowel preparation involves taking a low fibre diet for several days prior to the procedure and taking an oral preparation on the day prior to the procedure. This is indicated for patients undergoing colonoscopy, and for flexible sigmoidoscopy patients where the removal of colonic polyps or endoscopic mucosal resection is expected.

Sigmoidoscopy patients may have an enema to cleanse just the left side of their bowel. This will depend on the extent and indication of the procedure and may be self-administered at home or in the hospital setting.

Consent

The procedure will be explained to the patient by the endoscopist or an appropriately trained assistant, giving clear information of what the procedure entails, how it is to be performed, the possible risks and complications, any alternative investigations available and responding to any questions the patient may have.

The choice of whether gastroscopy is performed using throat spray or sedation is usually the patient's, unless there is a contraindication within their medical history or if they have no adult supervision at home for 24 hours. Emergency procedures may be performed under general anaesthetic depending on the patient's current condition. If intravenous sedation is to be administered secure intravenous access will be required throughout the endoscopy and recovery period.

The patient will be asked to sign a consent form if they agree to the procedure and understand the possible risks, complications and any alternative investigations or procedures (Shepherd and Hewett 2008).

Communication

Pre-procedural checks will determine the patient's identity, fasting time (unless an emergency procedure), allergies, prostheses, loose teeth or dentures. The information gleaned from the patient pre-procedurally is of no benefit if this is not passed on to the team caring for the patient during the endoscopy. It is therefore vital to any team that communication is effective and timely.

Patient positioning

The patient is positioned in the left lateral position on a tipping patient trolley or operating table

During colonoscopy or flexible sigmoidoscopy patients may be asked to turn onto their back or to a right lateral position to assist the endoscopist to pass a difficult bend in the colon or to obtain clearer views.

Assistants

Head-end assistant

The assistant caring for the patient, rather than assisting the endoscopist, is called the 'head-end assistant' and is responsible for the patient's wellbeing throughout the procedure. This will involve taking and recording the pulse, oxygen saturation levels, blood pressure, respiratory rate, pain and consciousness levels pre-procedurally as a baseline, and during the endoscopy. The head-end assistant is also responsible for positioning the patient and supporting them throughout the procedure. They must act as the patient's advocate, a vital role. The head-end assistant will administer oxygen as prescribed by the endoscopist, care for the patient's airway by suctioning any secretions from the mouth during gastroscopy and will alert the endoscopist to any change in the patient's condition during the endoscopy.

Endoscopist's assistant

The endoscopist's assistant is responsible for setting up the equipment and medication necessary for the procedure, the provision of any supplementary equipment and the care of the endoscope during and post-procedurally. This will include the initial decontamination of the endoscope, detailed elsewhere.

Recovery and Discharge

Following the administration of local anaesthetic throat spray, the patient, if feeling well enough, may walk from the endoscopy room to an area designated for the discharge of patients. The patient will be able to eat and drink normally once the effects of the throat spray have worn off, and should be advised initially to take sips of cold water to assess their ability to swallow.

Patients who have received sedation will be transferred to the recovery area by trolley or bed and will need to remain in this area until their basic observations are stable within normal limits, that they are awake, alert, aware of their surroundings and comfortable. If a reversal agent for sedation has been administered the patient must remain in the recovery area for at least 90 minutes as the half-life of the reversal agent, flumazenil, is shorter than the half-life of midazolam, which may cause the patient to become re-sedated as the effects of the flumazenil dissipate.

Patients who have received sedation will require the supervision of a responsible adult for 24 hours post administration of the sedative agent.

When ready for discharge, the patient, now in the discharge area, is given details of the findings of the endoscopy, their post-procedural advice and instructions for their aftercare and transport needs arranged.

Maintenance, Cleaning and Decontamination of Endoscopes

Routine maintenance of the endoscope involves checking the integrity of the coating on the exterior of the endoscope, ensuring the joints are firmly connected, that the channels are patent and that the hand-piece buttons are working efficiently. The buttons have an 'O' ring, which needs to be lubricated to ensure they fit the hand-piece snugly and work efficiently. The distal tip lens will need application of a lens cleaner to ensure clear views and to help reduce the build up of debris.

Section 5

Decontamination of the endoscope commences as soon as it is removed from the patient. The outside of the endoscope should be wiped from the hand-piece to the distal tip using an enzymatic cleaner to remove superficial debris, the distal tip of the endoscope placed in a bowl of enzymatic cleaner, the air/water channel actioned to push debris away from the endoscope and prevent suction of debris into the suction channel. The enzymatic fluid should then be suctioned through the endoscope to clear superficial debris and help prevent the channel blocking.

The endoscope should then be placed in a dirty instrument tray, covered and removed to the cleaning and decontamination area.

Leak testing of the endoscope must occur each time it is cleaned, using a tester specific to the endoscope manufacturer. Testing for leaks in the endoscope prior to immersion in water will prevent damage and contamination of the endoscope through water ingress into the endoscope's patient tube. Any equipment found to have a leak must not be immersed in water or placed in an AER. It should be decontaminated using specially designed wipes and returned to the manufacturer for repair.

The endoscope is placed in a dedicated sink, which is filled with the recommended amount and temperature of water and an enzymatic solution added. The outer surfaces of the endoscope are washed, paying special attention to the angulation wheels. The biopsy channel bung is removed and discarded. The air/water and suction buttons are removed and cleaned. The endoscope biopsy and suction channels and are cleaned internally using a single-use brush until the cleaning brush is visibly clean. Any bridges are manipulated fully, ensuring all debris is removed. The endoscope is then placed in a separate sink dedicated to the rinsing of the endoscope and then placed in the AER and connected according to the manufacturer's instructions (Thompson *et al.* 2009).

The cleaning and decontamination of endoscopes must be performed to the local hospital policy and manufacturers instructions.

Complications

As with all procedures and investigations there are risks associated with endoscopy. The risk of infection has been greatly reduced since the introduction of AERs and endoscope drying cabinets. Manual cleaning is the most important part of the cleaning process. The best equipment in the world will not prevent cross-contamination if the operator fails in their part of the process.

It is vital that all supplementary equipment such as biopsy forceps and snares are single use only and that they are used in accordance with the manufacturer's instructions.

The use of good aseptic technique in percutaneous endoscopic gastrostomy tube placement will help to reduce wound contamination and infection. The mouth and stomach are not sterile cavities and therefore any device that travels through these areas is contaminated. As a result, the risk of contamination can only be contained, not eliminated.

The risk of bleeding is increased if the patient is taking anticoagulation therapy, if they have oesophageal or gastric varices or if they have a gastric or duodenal ulcer. This can usually be controlled by injecting a sclerosing agent, applying endoclips or inserting a Sengstaken tube for varices.

In gastroscopy, pain or discomfort is usually limited to the initial intubation or excessive insufflation with air and does not generally require analgesia.

Colonoscopy or flexible sigmoidoscopy is a more painful procedure than gastroscopy due to the stretching of the colon and insufflation of air, and as a result, colonoscopy patients are usually given a sedative and opioid medications. Flexible sigmoidoscopy patients do not generally require analgesia although the administration of sedation, opioids or Entonox is available if necessary.

The risk of gut perforation is gastroscopy is low, and is more likely to occur where dilatation is required or where large tumours are situated. It is more likely to occur in colonoscopy or sigmoidoscopy where the bowel is stretched, there is diverticular disease, tumours or when removing colonic polyps.

The risk of respiratory depression, respiratory arrest or cardiac arrest is greatly increased when sedative and opioid medications are administered to a patient. To avoid these risks, opioid medications should be given first and the effects observed before a sedative is administered. All medications should be titrated and the dose administered according to the patient's age, existing condition and existing co-morbidity.

References

Mun Woo Y, Crail S, Curry G and Geddes CC (2006) A life threatening complication after ingestion of sodium phosphate bowel preparation. *British Medical Journal* 333: 589–590.

Resuscitation Council (UK) (2004) *Recommended Minimum Equipment for In-Hospital Adult Resuscitation.* www.resus.org.uk/pages/eqipIHAR.htm (accessed 14 December 2011).

Shepherd H and Hewett D (2008) *Guidance for Obtaining a Valid Consent for Elective Endoscopic Procedures.* British Society of Gastroenterologists. http://www.bsg.org.uk/images/stories/docs/clinical/guidelines/endoscopy/consent08.pdf (accessed March 2012).

Thompson L, Allison M, Bradley T, Sjogren G, Green D and Hardman P (2009) *Decontamination Standards for Flexible Endoscopes.* Leicester: National Endoscopy Programme.

Veitch AM, Baglin TP, Gershlick AH, Harnden SM, Tighe R and Cairns S (2008) Guidelines for the management of anticoagulant and antiplatelet therapy in patients undergoing endoscopic procedures. *Gut* 57: 1322–1329.

Further Readings

Cotton PB and Williams CB (2003) *Practical Gastrointestinal Endoscopy: The fundamentals.* Oxford: Blackwell Publishing.

Lam E and Lombard M (1999) *Mosby's Crash Course in Gastroenterology.* St Louis, MO: Mosby.

Resuscitation Council (UK) (2008) *Advanced Life Support.* London: Resuscitation Council (UK).

SGNA (1998) *Gastroenterology Nursing: A core curriculum.* St Louis, MO: Mosby.

Index

Page numbers in bold indicate the main section for a particular term.

Manual of Perioperative Care: An Essential Guide, First Edition. Edited by Kate Woodhead and Lesley Fudge.
© 2012 by John Wiley & Sons, Ltd. Published 2012 by John Wiley & Sons, Ltd.